MEDICAL
INTELLIGENCE
UNIT

THE LIPID HYPOTHESIS OF ATHEROGENESIS

William E. Stehbens, MB, BS, MD, D Phil, FRCPA, FRCPath

The Malaghan Institute of Medical Research
and the Department of Pathology
Wellington School of Medicine
Wellington, New Zealand

R.G. LANDES COMPANY
AUSTIN

MEDICAL INTELLIGENCE UNIT

THE LIPID HYPOTHESIS OF ATHEROGENESIS

R.G. LANDES COMPANY
Austin

CRC Press is the exclusive worldwide distributor of publications of the Medical Intelligence Unit.
CRC Press, 2000 Corporate Blvd., NW, Boca Raton, FL 33431. Phone: 407/994-0555.

Submitted: June 1993
Published: August 1993

Production Manager: Terry Nelson
Copy Editor: Constance Kerkaporta

Please address all inquiries to the Publisher:
R.G. Landes Company, 909 Pine Street, Georgetown, TX 78626
or
P.O. Box 4858, Austin, TX 78765
Phone: 512/ 863-7762; FAX: 512/ 863-0081

ISBN 1-879702-79-7
CATALOG # LN0279

Library of Congress Cataloging-in-Publication Data
Stehbens, William E.
The Lipid hypothesis of atherogenesis / William E. Stehbens
p. cm. — (Medical Intelligence Unit)
Includes bibliographical references and index.
ISBN 1-879702-65-7 (hard): $89.95
1. Atherosclerosis—Pathogenesis. 2. Atherosclerosis—Pathophysiology. 3. Atherosclerosis—Etiology.
4. Lipids—Metabolism—Disorders—Complications.
I. Title II. Series.
[DNLM: 1. Atherosclerosis—etiology. 2. Lipids—metabolism. 3. Risk factors. WG 550 S817L 1993]
RC692.S72 1993
616.1'36—dc20

DNLM/DLC
for Library of Concress

93-26891
CIP

CONTENTS

PREFACE

In technologically advanced countries, atherosclerosis is responsible for a great deal of mental and physical incapacitation, and more seriously, is the primary cause of death in approximately half the population. Currently there are many theories of the etiology of the disease but the lipid hypothesis which came into being early in the century is still at the center of controversy as contention regarding its validity has grown. Some proponents believe it is proven beyond all reasonable doubt. However an increasing number of genuine skeptics are concerned not only with the validity of the lipid hypothesis but also about blanket recommendations for national changes in diet and the administration of powerful drugs of as yet uncertain long term toxicity to a large segment of the community when the evidence for beneficial effect is far from convincing. This book is therefore topical and attempts to provide a rational and scientific basis for discussion and evaluation of the lipid hypothesis.

To assist understanding of the genesis of the lipid hypothesis, its emergence and continuance as a theory is briefly reviewed. Because knowledge of the pathology of the disease is crucial to comprehension and discussion of the cause and pathogenesis, a chapter has been devoted to a brief review of the pathology of atherosclerosis, its pathogenesis and complications from a somewhat heterodox standpoint. This is followed by review of the pathology of relevant lipid metabolic disorders and the experimental evidence for and against the lipid hypothesis.

Since the epidemiological evidence in favor of the lipid theory of atherosclerosis and its prevention is said to be unassailable, most of the text comprises a comprehensive discussion of the nature of the epidemiological evidence and its significance with particular emphasis on the methodology, the need to adhere to fundamental scientific precepts, the relevant vital statistics, the role of risk factors and the difficulties inherent in prevention and regression of atherosclerosis. These aspects must form the basis for the epidemiological study of this chronic progressive disease that is ubiquitous in humans and widespread throughout the animal kingdom.

Such criticisms that are expressed and the new pathological data in evaluation of the lipid hypothesis that is presented in the book will be new to most readers. The book is designed to provide the scientific foundation for the evaluation of current evidence in detail for those involved in atherosclerosis research and for scientists of independent thought. With the passage of time these critical minds will be the final arbiters of what has variously been called the lipid hypothesis, the cholesterol controversy and the cholesterol conspiracy.

—WE Stehbens MD, D Phil, FRCPA, FRCPath

GLOSSARY OF MAJOR ABREVIATIONS

apo	Apolipoprotein
CHD	Coronary heart disease
CVD	Cerebrovascular disease
FDB	Familial defective apoliproprotein B-100
FH	Familial hypercholesterolemia
HDL	High density lipoprotein
ICD	International classification of diseases
IDL	Intermediate density lipoprotein
LDL	Low density lipoprotein
Lp(a)	Lipoprotein (a)
LPL	Lipoprotein lipase
LRC	Lipid Research Clinics
LRCCPPT	Lipid Research Clinics Coronary Primary Prevention Trial
NHBLI	National Heart, Lung and Blood Institute of The National Institutes of Health
NIH	National Institutes of Health
PVD	Peripheral vascular disease
UK	United Kingdom
USA	United States of America
VLDL	Very low density lipoproteins
WHO	World Health Organization

Definition of Cause:
   The cause is the sole prerequisite without which the disease does not occur.

ACKNOWLEDGMENTS

I wish to convey sincere thanks to Mrs. J. Todd and Miss G. Dennis for assistance with the typing of the manuscript, to Mr. B.J. Martin and Mr. G.T. Jones for their assistance with the printing of the photographs and to Mr. D. Harwinkels for preparing the graphs. I am grateful to Mr. T.W. Fitzgerald and Mrs. C. Marshall for their support and particularly to Mr. G. Malaghan and the Trust Board of the Malaghan Institute of Medical Research for their interest and support during the preparation of the manuscript. I also wish to extend my thanks for the assistance provided by Dr. D.W. Liepsch and the Fachbereich 5 of the Fachhochschule München and the Alexander von Humboldt Stiftung during final completion of the manuscript. I acknowledge with gratitude my wife's continued encouragement, assistance and interest throughout the preparation of the monograph.

CHAPTER 1

THE GENESIS OF THE LIPID HYPOTHESIS AND TERMINOLOGY

The lipid hypothesis, currently the most popular and preeminent theory of the etiology of atherosclerosis, has become the most controversial medical subject of recent times. This long-standing controversy has been developing since early in the century, being exacerbated in more recent years by the increase in new knowledge of atherosclerosis and the disappointing results of clinical trials attempting to prevent the development of coronary heart disease (CHD).

We all suffer from atherosclerosis and as most of us will be physically impaired or die from its ill effects, the etiology and management of this disease are of vital importance especially in countries with aging populations. All of us should be aware of the ramifications of the nature, quality and interpretation of the data underlying the recommended changes in our diet and lifestyle.

The scientific status of the lipid hypothesis, and its validity or otherwise, have to be established before implementation of the drastic population based changes in diet advocated by its proponents.

Atherosclerosis is a chronic degenerative disease of blood vessels extending back into human antiquity. It is ubiquitous in man with no proven exception and is regarded as the inevitable fate of all human arteries. It is known to be widespread in lower animals involving mammals (carnivores, omnivores and herbivores) and birds although it varies in severity from species to species and individual to individual. It affects humans in severe degree but advanced disease also occurs in long-living species such as parrots, chimpanzees and gorillas. In advanced technological countries it is considered to be responsible for most deaths from cardiovascular and cerebrovascular disease accounting for almost 50% of all mortality, and responsible for much morbidity and incapacitation.

Vital statistics in the United States of America (USA) indicate that cardiac deaths rose from 8% in 1910 to 30.3% of all deaths by 1945 and further increases were expected.[1] In the United Kingdom (UK) deaths from diseases of the heart and blood vessels[2] were said to have risen from 16.7% to 36.3% between 1910 and 1959. From a previously low level coronary heart disease (CHD) became within 60 years the commonest cause of death in western societies.[3] The increase was regarded as an epidemic[4,5] and this disclosure has been said to be epidemiology's first contribution to the study of atherosclerosis.[6] However this ignores the increase in incidence due to the growth in population, the greater longevity and the dissemination of knowledge of cardiac ischemia, together with changes in diagnostic fashion and alterations in disease terminology according to the International Classification of Diseases (ICD). Nevertheless in aging populations its social and economic importance continues to grow because most deaths of atherosclerotic origin occur after 65 years of age. It is therefore not surprising that much time, effort, and finance have been invested in research into this disease, its cause, pathogenesis, clinical management and attempts at prevention.

THE LIPID HYPOTHESIS

The lipid hypothesis of atherosclerosis theorizes that a diet high in cholesterol and/or animal saturated fat elevates serum cholesterol and low density lipoprotein (LDL) levels, which in turn induce premature severe atherosclerosis and a high incidence of CHD. The dietary fat and elevated blood cholesterol are said to be aided and abetted at times by several other factors. Atherosclerosis is thus considered to be a disease primarily concerned with lipid metabolism in the blood vessel wall. Based on the concept that lipid in the vessel wall came from the blood, it was reasoned that the accumulation of cholesterol and lipid in the wall was due to (i) an augmented influx into the vessel wall from the lumen, (ii) an inability to dispose adequately of or metabolize lipid accumulating in the wall or (iii) some impediment to the efflux of lipid percolating through the interstices of the wall (often thought to be the internal elastic lamina). The basis of this approach reveals that the lipid hypothesis is in reality not a theory of atherogenesis but a theory to explain the influx and accumulation of lipid in the vessel wall, it being assumed that once initiated the gamut of mural changes of atherogenesis will naturally follow together with the complications. A scientific theory of etiology of any disease should explain the initiation, pathogenesis and development of its complications (including intimal tears, ulcerations and aneurysms). In this sense the lipid hypothesis is unsatisfactory and without a unifying thread. It remains but a partial theory and unproven although it has dominated thinking and research in atherogenesis for several decades.

TERMINOLOGY

There is considerable confusion in the literature over the terminology of degenerative diseases of blood vessels and therefore an explanation of terminology is required.

Atheroma is derived from the Greek word "athere" for mush, to indicate the pultaceous, grumous or caseous material of high lipid content in advanced intimal plaques. The disease is now usually referred to as atherosclerosis with the intention of emphasizing the large fibrous tissue component of the lesion. Whilst atheroma is often used synonymously with atherosclerosis, especially in English literature, it has latterly become reserved for the late pultaceous lesion in American terminology, sometimes called an atheromatous abscess or merely "an atheroma". Atherogenesis is a term referring to the initiation and early development (genesis) of atherosclerosis. Arteriosclerosis, meaning literally sclerosis or hardening of the arteries, is sometimes used synonymously with atherosclerosis or generically to include atherosclerosis, diffuse hyperplastic sclerosis and Mönckeberg's sclerosis. It can also be used to indicate the sclerotic changes in the small distributing arteries otherwise known as diffuse hyperplastic sclerosis which is so often forgotten or neglected.

Confusion over terminology stems from the lack of agreement regarding the definition of atherosclerosis and the nature of the earliest demonstrable lesion. It was once thought that the presence of lipid in the intima denoted atherosclerosis and was distinct from the sclerotic changes in arteries that increase with age, but the finding of lipid in the aorta within the first three years of life is inconsistent with such a concept. The confusion over nomenclature is further complicated by the accumulation of lipid not only in large and medium-sized arteries, and in veins (phlebosclerosis or venous atherosclerosis), but also in small peripheral distributing arteries (diffuse hyperplastic sclerosis), arterioles (arteriolosclerosis), cardiac valve cusps (aortic and mitral in particular) and even in the endocardium[7] and intimal thickenings in the thoracic duct (lymphangiosclerosis).[8] Whilst attention is drawn to these observations which must also be explained, concern here will be restricted to atherosclerosis in arteries of large and medium caliber and in veins.

It has long been considered that the presence of lipid in the blood vessel wall was pathognomonic of atherosclerosis, but it can be due to other diseases. Its presence in the vessel wall being the initial lesion is an assumption requiring justification and is not necessarily valid. Even early in the century it was acknowledged that lipid initially appeared deep in the intima. This is an implicit acknowledgment that the intima is thickened and this intimal proliferation was thought to be a "normal" or inherent constituent of the vessel wall. Thus the intimal proliferation preceded lipid accumulation. In recent years with the emphasis on the intimal injury hypothesis[9] smooth muscle proliferation in the intima has been widely though belatedly accepted as an earlier or prelipid phase of the disease.

It is not possible to provide a definition of atherosclerosis that will satisfy all pathologists and investigators in this field. When the cause is established beyond all reasonable doubt, the definition will become self-evident. To some, atherosclerosis is a metabolic disease of lipids, to others it is an inflammatory disorder but the appearance of macrophages and lymphocytes does not make it primarily an inflammation. These cells participate in many human diseases including neoplasms, degenerations and infarcts, their appearance merely representing a biological tissue response that is not understood. Though the definitions of atherosclerosis vary, in general the disorder is described rather than defined. The pathology of the disorder will be described and defined in the next chapter.

CHD (ischemic heart disease or atherosclerotic heart disease) is essentially a generic term for disorders in which the myocardium is deprived of adequate blood supply under normal or augmented physiological conditions. It is not a specific disease, though this is inferred by the widespread usage of the term. Because clinical diagnoses are based on probabilities and many ischemic attacks are silent, the diagnosis is imprecise and gives no indication of the causative disease underlying the development in any individual. In this respect it is like stroke, cerebrovascular disease (CVD) or peripheral vascular disease (PVD), each of which represents a nonspecific group diagnosis not pathognomonic of atherosclerosis. As such CHD is caused by many diseases and is nonspecific in pathological, clinical and etiological terms. Unfortunately it has been incorrectly defined by a panel of experts of the National Institutes of Health (NIH) as coronary atherosclerosis[10] and in loose and imprecise writings on atherosclerosis CHD is used synonymously and interchangeably with atherosclerosis.

Cause in medicine is also often used loosely and misused. Improper and imprecise usage of cause has been considered to be one of the major reasons for the present cholesterol controversy.[11,12] Cause is used in this text as the sole prerequisite without which the disease cannot occur and it follows that the cause must be present in each and every individual and lower animal suffering from the specific disease.

GENESIS OF THE LIPID HYPOTHESIS

Pathologists have long been intrigued by the grumous caseous material of high lipid content within the arterial wall in advanced atherosclerosis, often in association with calcification. Consequently early this century research focused on attempts to produce lipid accumulation and calcification in arteries of experimental animals. However when lipid accumulation was found in the arteries of rabbits fed a diet high in cholesterol or egg yolk,[13] most research was then directed at the cholesterol-fed hypercholesterolemic rabbit in the belief that the vascular lesions were atherosclerotic. This concept was no doubt reinforced by the observation that when the otherwise smooth aortic intima exhibited even such small elevations, lipid was found deep in the intima. Thus it was deduced that the accumulation of lipid was the earliest demonstrable lesion and that with further progression extensive caseous lipid deposits were to be found in irregular elevated fibrous plaques and that ulceration was often found in such lesions in regions of caseation.

The intimal proliferation, consisting of fibromusculoelastic tissue and occurring diffusely in the aortas and as localized lesions at sites of branching in distributing arteries even in infancy, was considered to be an integral part of the vessel because it was ubiquitous and occurred without irregularity of the intimal surface and could therefore be considered "normal".

There was controversy as to whether the lipid accumulation in the cholesterol over-fed rabbit was truly atherosclerotic and Anitschkow[14] in 1933 acknowledged there were differences from the human disease viz the primarily xanthomatous nature of the dietary-induced lesions in rabbits, the paucity of hyaline sclerosis and the absence of complications, but he believed these were not significant. The cholesterol-fed rabbit continued to be accepted as the experimental model of atherosclerosis even by some pathologists. Similar changes to the foam cell or xanthomatous intimal lesion in the rabbit would have been observed in man in familial hypercholesterolemia (FH) and type 2 hyperlipoproteinemia and in other subjects from time to time such as in untreated diabetics on a therapeutic high fat diet associated with extreme hypercholesterolemia and in those with obstructive jaundice. The xanthomatous changes thus observed were probably considered to be variants or the extreme of a spectrum of appearances observed in atherosclerosis of varying severity.

Warnings that the vascular lesions of FH resembled those of cholesterol-fed rabbits and differed from conventional atherosclerosis[15] were ignored. The lipid fervor was developing momentum and unusually severe atherosclerosis was alleged to occur in association with hypercholesterolemia of FH (hereditary xanthomatosis), diabetes mellitus, myxedema and the nephrotic syndrome. Such reports remained anecdotal and detailed pathological assessment of numbers of such patients did not eventuate.

GENESIS OF CORONARY HEART DISEASE (CHD)

Concomitant with the development of the lipid hypothesis on pathological and experimental grounds, knowledge and recognition of myocardial ischemia as a complication of atherosclerosis increased, indirectly giving further momentum to the lipid hypothesis.

After Heberden described angina pectoris in 1772 and Jenner in 1786 attributed the syndrome to coronary artery occlusion,[16] evolu-

tion of further knowledge was slow. Steven[17] in 1887 gave a good account of the features of ischemic necrosis and myomalacia cordis described in 1881 by Ziegler who also related it to coronary artery occlusion.[17] Parkes Weber[18] described an organizing occlusive thrombus in the right coronary artery in a patient who died during a recurrent attack of angina pectoris. At the turn of the century there was still little recognition of CHD, pathological services were poorly developed and the classification of diseases of the heart were (i) valvular heart disease (ii) pericarditis (iii) hypertrophy of the heart (iv) angina pectoris and (v) other diseases of the heart with over 97% being included in the first and fifth.[2]

Review of sporadic papers from the UK early this century revealed that in 1900 rupture of the heart was attributable to acute myocarditis because of acute inflammation in the myocardium and fatty degeneration when there was much fat in the necrotic myocardial fibers.[19] Other papers indicated that left ventricular rupture or angina pectoris was attributed to either pericarditis, fatty myocarditis or fibroid myocarditis (probably healed infarcts) and even to smallpox, enteric fever or septic pneumonia.[20-22] Sir James McKenzie[23] in 1905 attributed angina pectoris to impaired contractility due to excessive strain and in the same year acute myocarditis was associated with several infectious diseases and often progressed to chronic myocarditis on the left side and was frequently transmural in extent.[24] Again in the same year Barr[25] suggested that loss of aortic elasticity resulted in poor coronary blood flow and fatty or fibroid myocarditis. Such views reveal a total lack of understanding of the basic pathology of myocardial ischemia which contributed to the infrequent clinical and autopsy diagnosis despite the fact that the basic pathology of myocardial infarction was already well described in the literature.[17]

At the turn of the century German pathologists had a better idea of the nature of coronary occlusion and myocardial infarction[26] but there was still much confusion in the UK and the US. However in 1910 Osler[27] in his Lumleian Lectures on angina pectoris commented on the remarkable infrequency of the condition and also revealed knowledge and understanding of coronary occlusion and its affect on the heart. Increased clinical awareness of CHD both in the USA and the UK followed a series of papers by Herrick[28-30] between 1912 and 1919. These served to increase awareness of the syndrome of coronary artery occlusion and myocardial ischemia and it is of interest that Bedford,[31] one of England's pioneer cardiologists, indicated it was not even in the medical curriculum in the early 1920s. From 1926 to 1930 deaths attributable to the syndrome increased and in the ICD revision of 1930 for the first time a new classification "diseases of the coronary arteries and angina pectoris" was introduced, there being no equivalent prior to this time. From then into the 1950s reported CHD mortality rose steadily. The crude death rate per million increased fourfold from 1940 to 1960 in the UK. Such increases in national mortality rates led to the belief that there had been an epidemic of CHD, even though the role for "other myocardial degeneration" decreased by two-thirds,[32] indicating that the increased mortality rate was at least in part attributable to a change in the classification of diseases consequent upon increased awareness of the existence of CHD.

Similar increases in CHD occurred in Western countries including the USA, but the radical changes introduced in procedures and classification of causes of death with the 1949 ICD revision invalidates direct comparison of CHD death rates before and after 1949.[33] The difficulty in evaluating the effect on death rates by the broader concept of CHD, better diagnostic facilities and increasing usage of CHD as a cause of death by coroners and medical examiners was appreciated by Lew.[33] He concluded that about 30% of the increase from 1940 to 1955 in the crude CHD death rate was due to aging, 40% to changes in procedures and classifications adopted in 1919 and the remaining 30% to acceptance of a broader concept of CHD, better diagnosis and increasing usage of the term CHD in death certification. Less than 15% was thought to be due to a real increase and the geographic differences in the USA were due to variation in quantity and quality of medical services and greater awareness of CHD among graduates.

Campbell[2,34] indicated that deaths from all causes diminished in England and Wales from 1876 to 1959 in accordance with increased longevity, reduction in mortality from infectious diseases and increased deaths from CHD since the 1920s. Taking into account the increased longevity and the age of death from CHD, he calculated that the expected death rates from diseases of the heart was similar to the actual rates from 1880 to 1959 without having to invoke an epidemic and that on similar grounds this was probably also true for cerebrovascular disease (CVD).

From 1910 to 1932 in the Presbyterian Hospital, New York, there was an increase in the percentage of total autopsies showing lesions of coronary arteries,[32] and an abrupt rise from 1920 to 1931 in clinical diagnoses indicating the greater awareness of the CHD syndrome from 1920. Robb-Smith[32] in a retrospective study reported an almost identical rate of autopsies showing "coronary narrowing" or "severe coronary narrowing" from 1930 to 1960, whereas the number of deaths attributed to CHD had increased 16-fold. There are however serious limitations in this type of retrospective pathological study that also apply to clinical studies and vital statistics.

Robb-Smith[32] analyzed the age specific death rate at ages 45-74 and 75 and over in England and Wales from 1900 to 1960 and concluded that, as in the US, there was no satisfactory evidence to indicate an increase in the severity of atherosclerosis, ischemic heart disease or the age specific incidence of coronary thrombosis or myocardial infarction. The differences in sex incidence of ischemic heart disease were attributed to the lesser severity of atherosclerosis in females in a specific age group and the difference in longevity of the female population reflected similar phenomena. Differences in mortality rates for populations were attributable to different age structures, diagnostic habits and race. Overall no reason for suspecting an epidemic of CHD was found. From as early as 1938 many clinicians and demographers expressed skepticism about the authenticity of CHD death rates,[35-37] classing CHD as a statistical waste-paper basket[38] or merely a convenient or fashionable diagnosis often made solely on clinical history or even guesswork in general practice.[39] The alterations in ICD classifications have altered vital statis-

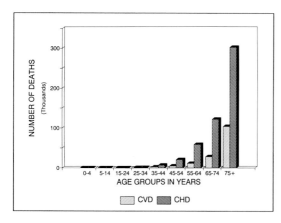

Fig. 1.1. Graph demonstrating the number of deaths from cerebrovascular disease (CVD) and coronary heart disease (CHD) in the U.S.A. for 1988. (From the World Health Statistics Annual 1990.[41])

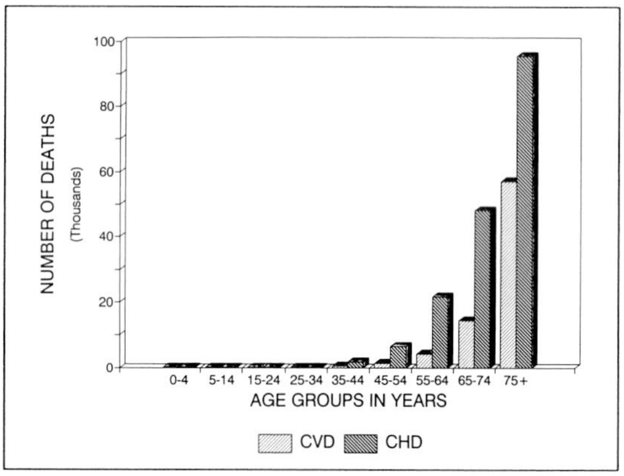

Fig. 1.2. Graph demonstrating the number of deaths from CVD and CHD in the U.K. for 1989. (From the World Health Statistics Annual 1990.[41])

tics substantially with some revisions of more consequence than others. It is difficult to estimate the effect these revisions have on mortality rates from decade to decade and the limitations of vital statistics as indicative of the specific mortality rates for scientific purposes are not generally appreciated. Feinstein[40] concluded that they produce fallacious science.

Overall there appears to be confusion over the prevalence of deaths from CHD and the adjusted age and sex specific mortality rates. Figures 1.1 and 1.2 demonstrate that in both the USA and the UK most deaths from CVD and CHD occur after the age of 55 years. It is readily seen how the total number of deaths from CHD would have increased substantially with an increase in longevity alone. Nevertheless, the increase is attributable to (i) aging of the population (increased longevity), (ii) expanding populations, (iii) true differences in the causes of death due to medical advances particularly with the advent of antibiotics, (iv) changes in diagnostic fashions or customs and (v) the errors in CHD vital statistics. The age and sex specific mortality rates would also be affected by these factors. This being the case, there is no reliable evidence to indicate that there has been an increase or a decrease[42,43] and no justification for the repeated allegation of a CHD epidemic which has supposedly been ravaging technologically advanced countries.[44]

Epidemiologists conceded that some of the

rise may have been fictitious but continued to emphasize a profound real increase in mortality.[4,45,46] The use of only selected age groups by some epidemiologists[5,47] does not validate an increase and the errors inherent in vital statistics remain.

The alleged epidemic of CHD provided the very reason for the search for environmental and life-style factors supposedly responsible. If the epidemic is truly spurious and there is no scientific evidence to the contrary, much time, money and effort have been expended in vain. This concern over the high CHD mortality nevertheless increased research in atherogenesis and stimulated much epidemiological activity related to CHD. Inevitably considerable attention was focused on blood cholesterol levels and dietary fats because of preoccupation with the lipid hypothesis. Consequently much new scientific information on lipids was forthcoming.

THE SPREAD OR PROMULGATION OF THE LIPID HYPOTHESIS

From primarily demographic studies in the first half of the century, a change occurred in the 1950s. Whereas in the past epidemiology was concerned with epidemics and spread of infectious diseases, the high CHD mortality and repeated allegations of an epidemic attracted many from different disciplines to the epidemiological study of CHD in the hope of quick, investigative reward. Perhaps the greatest stimulus was a paper published by Ancel Keys[48] in 1953 in which he reported a striking relationship between the national death rate in six countries for men in two restricted age groups from atherosclerotic and degenerative heart disease and the proportion of fat-calories available in the respective national diets. Yerushalmy and Hilleboe[49] admonished Keys by indicating that (i) the biased selection of only six countries from the 22 for which the information was available greatly exaggerated the importance of any association, (ii) comparison of the data from all of the 22 countries reduced any apparent association and a better correlation existed with animal protein, (iii) comparison of mortality rates for CVD for six selected countries with fat-calories available in the diet revealed an inverse relationship thus contradicting Key's initial report,[48] (iv) in countries with approximately the same proportion of dietary fat, the CHD mortality ranged from 220 to 739 deaths per 100,000 and for an approximate reduction of 10%, countries could range from 100 to almost 700 deaths per 100,000 and Japan with the lowest death rate from CHD had the highest death rate from CVD, (v) the dietary heart disease association was nonspecific and no stronger for fat than other dietary constituents and therefore lacked validity, (vi) fat calories and animal protein calories were negatively associated with noncardiac disease, and (vii) the tenuous association was too weak to provide adequate support for an hypothesis implicating fat as an etiological factor for CHD. Yerushalmy and Hilleboe[50] also indicated that the international statistics on diet and CHD mortality were not sufficiently accurate to contribute materially to knowledge of this relationship. It is also worthy of note that the very restricted age groups used were not representative of the majority of subjects dying from CHD. It was also stressed that statistical associations do not indicate a causal relationship and there was need to demonstrate both specificity and validity, the absence of which detracts from any possible significance in the relationship.[50] A more plausible explanation in their eyes was that environmental factors such as dietary fat and protein are an index of a country's development industrially, nutritionally, medically and technologically.[49] This polite but very telling refutation of Key's

thesis apparently passed unnoticed or was ignored for Key's publication appears to have stimulated a major upsurge in lipid epidemiology which was further encouraged by the Framingham study.

The logical approach to atherogenesis is long, meticulous study, analysis and dissection of the disease and its pathogenesis to determine its cause and underlying mechanisms, aspects which almost invariably precede control and prevention of disease. The epidemiological approach on the other hand attempted to circumvent such a time-consuming project in the hope that taking the short-cut epidemiological approach might reveal some crucial factor, modification of which would dramatically reduce the incidence of CHD and thereby bring fame and fortune to the discoverer. However, few research projects are as simple as originally conceived and the epidemiological approach did not turn out to be the easy short-cut envisaged. Review of this approach and the difficulties encountered will be considered in later chapters. Nevertheless the high CHD mortality in aging populations attracted research funds and the epidemiological approach dominated the field of atherogenesis. The lipid hypothesis has proved to be profitable for many in the food and pharmaceutical industries, whilst dairy and pastoral industries, previously the mainstay of some economies and the basis of good human nutrition have suffered accordingly.

Success has been claimed for this approach as there has been a decline in national mortality rates for CHD in some countries since the late 1960s. Furthermore, within the last few years assertions have been made that the lipid hypothesis is proven.[51,52] These epidemiological studies supported the prevailing view that a high dietary intake of saturated fats and cholesterol results in an elevation of blood cholesterol or LDL levels which are held to be primarily responsible for an enhanced tendency to severe atherosclerosis and CHD. Not only are pathologists attempting to relate risk factors to the pathology of atherosclerosis but the traditional method of determining upper discrimination values for blood cholesterol has been widely abandoned. In effect, cholesterol is claimed to be noxious at all blood levels at which CHD develops.

Intense publicity has brought cholesterol into the working vocabulary of school children and has made the dire consequences of an elevated blood cholesterol level a commonplace in the news media, food advertising and topics for television commercials. Nevertheless there still remains a minority of genuine skeptics who are critical of some conclusions reached by protagonists of the lipid hypothesis, their methods and their writings. National Heart Foundations or Associations concur with the consensus view of many experts world wide and are adamant about the validity of the role of dietary cholesterol and saturated fats in being responsible for many unnecessary premature deaths in western countries. A committee of the World Health Organization[53] has called upon governments to legislate to prevent interference with the implementation of national dietary policies it considers will reduce the financial burden of the high mortality and morbidity of CHD.

This controversy has led to confusion and cholesterol phobia among the general public, personal attacks on dissidents in the lay press and also confusion amongst medical practitioners many of whom acknowledge their inability to assess the arguments for and against. It is therefore appropriate that the essentials of the controversy be presented so that independent scientists and medical practitioners can assess the nature of the argument and the scientific basis of the lipid hypothesis in atherogenesis in as simple and logical a manner as possible.

REFERENCES

1. Moriyama IM. Statistical studies of heart diseases. I. Heart disease and allied causes of death in relation to age changes in the population. Pub Health Rep 1948; 63:537-45.
2. Campbell M. Death rate from diseases of the heart: 1876 to 1959. Br Med J 1963; 2:528-35.
3. Levy RI, Moskowitz J. Cardiovascular research: decades of progress, a decade of promise. Science 1982; 217:121-9.
4. Morris JN. Recent history of coronary disease. Lancet 1951; 1:69-73.
5. Anderson TW, LeRiche WH. Ischaemic heart disease and sudden death. 1901-61. Br J Prev Soc Med 1970; 24:1-9.
6. Strasser T. Atherosclerosis and coronary heart disease: the contribution of epidemiology. WHO Chronicle 1972; 26(1):7-11.
7. Roberts WC, Bujo LM. The frequency and significance of coronary arterial thrombi and other observations in fatal acute myocardial infarction. Am J Med 1972; 52:425-43.
8. Rabinovitz AJ, Saphir O. The thoracic duct. Significance of age-related changes and of lipid in the wall. Circulation 1965; 31:899-905.
9. Ross R. The pathogenesis of atherosclerosis-an update. N Engl J Med 1986; 314:488-500.
10. National Heart, Lung and Blood Institute. Arteriosclerosis. The Report of the 1977 Working Group to Review the 1971 Report by the National Heart and Lung Institute Task Force on Arteriosclerosis. Publication No(NIH)78-1526. Washington:DHEW, 1977.
11. Stehbens WE. Basic precepts and the lipid hypothesis of atherosclerosis. Med Hypoth 1990; 31:105-13.
12. Stehbens WE. Causality in medical science with reference to coronary heart disease and atherosclerosis. Perspect Biol Med 1992; 36:97-119.
13. Anitschkow N. Chalatow S. On experimental cholesterin steatosis and its significance in the origin of some pathological processes. Centrabl für Allg Pathol und Pathol Anat 1913; 24:1-9 Transl by Pelias MZ. Arteriosclerosis 1983; 3:178-82.
14. Anitschkow NN. A history of experimentation on arterial atherosclerosis in animals. In: Blumenthal HT, ed. Cowdry's Arteriosclerosis. 2nd ed. Springfield: CC Thomas, 1967:21-44.
15. Thannhauser SJ. Lipidoses: Diseases of the Cellular Lipid Metabolism. New York: Oxford Univ Press, 1940:81-5.
16. Proudfit WL. Origin of concept of ischaemic heart disease. Br Heart J 1983; 50:209-12.
17. Steven JL. Fibroid degeneration and allied lesions of the heart, and their association with disease of the coronary arteries. Lancet 1887; 2:1153-56, 1205-8, 1255-7.
18. Parkes Weber F. Heart from a fatal case of angina pectoris with thrombosis of the right coronary artery. Trans Pathol Soc London 1896; 47:14-6.
19. Sutcliffe J. A case of rupture of the heart. Br Med J 1900; 1:142.
20. Burgess JJ. Unilateral fatty degeneration of the heart. Br Med J 1902; 1:20.
21. Harris WT. Rupture of the heart from fatty disease of the muscle. Br Med J 1904; 2:1636.

22. James WT. Sudden death from rupture of the heart. Br Med J 1905; 1:132.

23. McKenzie J. An enquiry into the cause of angina pectoris. Br Med J 1905; 2:845-7.

24. Dreschfeld J. A discussion on the diagnosis and treatment of degeneration of the heart apart from valvular disease. Br Med J 1905; 2:1023-7.

25. Barr J. Arteriosclerosis. Br Med J 1905; 1:53-7.

26. East T. The Story of Heart Disease. London: W Dawson & Sons, 1958.

27. Osler W. The Lumleian Lectures on angina pectoris. Lancet 1910; 1:697-702, 839-84, 973-7.

28. Herrick JB. Clinical features of sudden obstruction of the coronary arteries. JAMA 1912; 59:2015-20.

29. Herrick JB. Thrombosis of the coronary arteries. JAMA 1919; 72:387-90.

30. Herrick JB, Nuzum FR. Angina pectoris: Clinical experience with two hundred cases. JAMA 1918; 70:67-70.

31. Bedford DE. Harvey's third circulation. De circulo sanguinis in corde. Br Med J 1968; 4:273-7.

32. Robb-Smith AHT. The enigma of coronary heart disease. London: Lloyd-Luke, 1967.

33. Lew EA. Some implications of mortality statistics relating to coronary artery disease. J Chr Dis 1957; 6:192-209.

34. Campbell M. The main cause of increased death rate from diseases of the heart: 1920 to 1959. Br Med J 1963; 2:712-7.

35. Atkinson HC. The changing emphasis in heart disease. JAMA Georgia: July 1938; 257-60.

36. Page IH, Stare FJ, Corcoran AC et al. Atherosclerosis and the fat content of the diet. Circulation 1957; 16:163-78.

37. Editorial: The convenient coronary. N Engl J Med 1960; 262:149-50.

38. Woolsey TD, Moriyama IM. Statistical studies of heart disease. II. Important factors in heart disease mortality trends. Pub Health Reports 1948; 63:1247-73.

39. Walford PA. Sudden death in coronary thrombosis. J Roy Coll Gen Pract 1971; 21:654-6.

40. Feinstein AR. Clinical epidemiology II The identification rates of disease. Ann Int Med 1968; 69:1037-61.

41. World Health Statistics Annual 1990. Geneva: WHO, 1990.

42. Stehbens WE. An appraisal of the epidemic rise of coronary heart disease and its decline. Lancet 1987; 1:606-11.

43. Stehbens WE. Review of the validity of national coronary heart disease mortality rates. Angiology 1990; 41:85-94.

44. Stamler J. Epidemiology of coronary heart disease. Med Clin North Am 1973; 57:5-46.

45. Morris JN. In: Uses of Epidemiology. 3rd ed. Edinburgh: Churchill Livingstone, 1975.

46. Epstein FH. Epidemiology of coronary heart disease. In: Jones AM. ed. Modern Trends in Cardiology. London: Butterworths, 1960:155-71.

47. Alderson MR. Mortality in heart disease. Br Med J 1963; 2:934.

48. Keys A. Atherosclerosis: a problem in newer public health. J Mt Sinai Hosp 1953; 20:118-39.

49. Yerushalmy J, Hilleboe HE. Fat in the diet and mortality from heart disease. N Y State J Med 1957; 57:2343-53.

50. Yerushalmy J, Palmer CE. On the methodology of investigations of etiologic factors in chronic diseases. J Chr Dis 1959; 10:27-40.

51. Dock W. Why do we pretend the pathogenesis is mysterious? Circulation 1974; 50:647-9.

52. Simons L. The lipid hypothesis is proven. Med J Aust 1984; 140:316-7.

53. WHO Technical Report of Expert Committee Prevention of Coronary Heart Disease Report 732. Geneva: WHO, 1982:2-53.

CHAPTER 2

THE PATHOLOGY OF ATHEROSCLEROSIS AND EXPERIMENTAL ATHEROSCLEROSIS

In considering any etiological theory of a disease, familiarity with its pathology is essential. This chapter therefore reviews the pathological features of spontaneous and experimental atherosclerosis, because, to be viable, the lipid hypothesis must be consistent with current knowledge of the earliest demonstrable lesion, the topography, the natural history of the disease, its progression, the development of complications in end-stage disease and its experimental reproduction.

THE NATURE OF ATHEROSCLEROSIS

Atherosclerosis is a chronic degenerative disease of blood vessels and the inevitable fate of all human arteries. It is ubiquitous in humans, there being no evidence of an exception to this rule although the severity varies from individual to individual. The disease is widely spread in the animal kingdom (carnivores, omnivores and herbivores) with generally lessened severity in lower animals. However it has long been recognized that chimpanzees (Fig. 2.1), gorillas and parrots and other birds can develop moderately severe atherosclerosis despite their almost exclusively vegetarian diet.[1,2]

Though atherosclerosis has been regarded as a focal disease of the intima of large arteries, in reality it involves large and small arteries, veins and even the heart[3] itself. Whilst it commences initially as focal areas of involvement of the intima, it rapidly becomes diffuse, with the focal lesions coalescing and progressively involving all coats of the blood vessel wall.

THE PATHOLOGY OF ATHEROSCLEROSIS

Atherosclerosis may be considered to have two phases. The first is the silent or developmental stage commencing in utero and extending to about the sixth decade (Fig. 2.2). The second is the stage of complications which tend to make their presence felt clinically and cause high morbidity and mortality with increasing age.

The disease is most severe in the aorta in the abdominal segment particularly and the iliofemoral arteries. The coronary arteries are the next most severely affected and cerebral arteries after that. Other arteries such as the splenic and those of the lower limb are also severely affected.

(A) LOCALIZATION OF ATHEROSCLEROSIS

The topographical distribution of the disease can provide clues to etiology and early pathologists recognized that atherosclerosis had a special predilection for certain areas in the vascular system.[2]

1. Atherosclerosis is most severe in the systemic arterial circulation where pressure is higher than in pulmonary arteries and is least severe in veins where the pressure and blood velocity are lowest.

2. In the systemic circulation there is variation in severity from vascular bed to vascular bed even within the same individual. Severe disease in lower limb arteries is common whereas in the upper limbs severe atherosclerosis with ischemia is rare. Variation in collateral circulation cannot explain this disparity in severity of involvement but it requires explanation if the blood lipid levels are of prime importance.

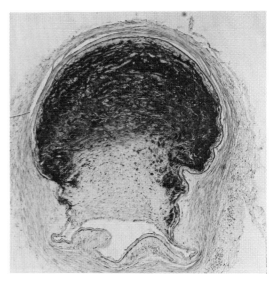

Fig. 2.1. Transverse frozen section of an atherosclerotic middle cerebral artery of a female chimpanzee that died of a ruptured berry aneurysm.[1] The dark material in the eccentrically thickened intima is lipid. Note the very severe involvement of the artery despite the normal intima devoid of thickening of the adjacent and opposite wall (stained with hematoxylin and Oil red O). (From: Stehbens WE. J Pathol Bacteriol 1963; 86:168-8).

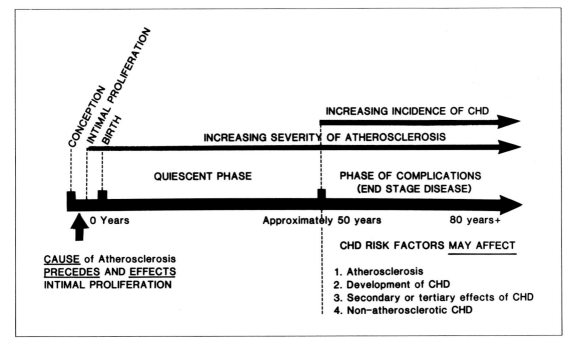

Fig. 2.2. Diagram to demonstrate the two phases of atherosclerosis in humans with reference to age, its inception with intimal proliferation, the quiescent phase, the development of complications and their relationship to causation and risk factors. (From: Stehbens WE. Perspect Biol Med 1992; 36:97-119 with permission of the Univ. of Chicago Press).[4]

3. Within any circulatory bed the severity of atherosclerosis is proportional to the caliber of the vessel.

4. In the limbs the severity is said to be augmented by usage and diminished in a paralyzed limb.[5,6] In right-handed individuals the severity is greater in the right radial artery and vice versa in the left-handed.[7] These anecdotal observations are consistent with recent experimental findings.[8]

5. Hypertension aggravates the severity of the disease in the systemic, pulmonary and venous systems. In aortic coarctation the severity of atherosclerosis is greatly augmented in the blood vessels directly supplied by the proximal aorta and reduced distally where the pulse pressure is dampened.[2]

6. The disease affects all coats of the vessel wall with the intima most severely affected and the adventitia least.

7. The disease is more severe in the distal aorta and iliofemoral arteries than in the proximal aorta due to the high pulse pressure distally.

8. It has a predilection for forks, junctions, curvatures and fusiform dilatations (carotid sinus).

9. It runs an accelerated course in berry aneurysms.[9]

10. A single umbilical artery predisposes the homolateral common iliac artery to premature atherosclerosis in infancy due to the augmented blood flow and associated blood pressure changes.[10]

11. Atherosclerosis develops at an accelerated rate in the afferent artery of chronic femoral arteriovenous fistulas,[11] an observation confirmed experimentally.[8]

12. Veins used for venous bypass grafts develop severe atherosclerosis within 18 months to 10 years whereas when the internal thoracic (internal mammary) artery is used, it proves to be more resilient, having a longer survival time and being less susceptible to atherosclerosis than veins because it is architecturally designed to withstand the arterial hemodynamics inherent in the bypass.

Veins, believed by many physicians to be relatively immune to atherosclerosis because of their minimal involvement, develop premature severe disease when used in arteriovenous shunts[12] or bypass grafts irrespective of blood lipid levels. Architecturally they are not designed to withstand arterial hemodynamics or the stresses of a shunt and the pathological changes so induced must therefore be attributable to the hemodynamic stresses rather than circulating humoral factors. If left intact like other veins elsewhere in those same subjects, they would have shown only minimal involvement for the remaining years of life. These are two fundamental inconsistencies that cannot be explained on the basis of some circulating humoral agent.

In Figure 2.1 from a chimpanzee, severe atherosclerosis is obvious on one side of the vessel wall and yet directly opposite, the intima is not even thickened. Similar phenomena occur in humans as may be seen in longitudinal section in Figures 2.3 and 2.4. It is implausible that such localization could be the consequence of a circulating lipoprotein or noxious agent. Invoking a mass action effect with delayed removal is inconsistent with the lesser or minimal involvement of pulmonary vessels and veins. These observations all suggest that atherosclerosis is closely associated with hemodynamics. Though generally regarded as a localizing factor, the topographical lesion distribution as outlined above and its iatrogenic production suggest it is of more basic etiological significance.

MORPHOLOGY

Initially the aorta has a smooth intimal surface in neonates and infants but within two decades four changes become manifest to a varying degree.

(i) In every fetus intimal proliferation develops about the ostia of branch sites, on the lesser curvature of the aortic arch and about the orifice of the ductus arteriosus.[10] This fibromusculoelastic thickening replaces the previously thick internal elastic lamina (Fig. 2.5) and at birth or by three years of age exhibits some lipid histologically. There is often elevation of the proximal aspect of the ostia of the branches and masking of the U-shaped flow divider ultimately resulting in narrowing and deformation of the branch orifice. This is due to progressive intimal proliferation about the ostia and the distal extensions merge with those of the proliferation about the next segmental branch.

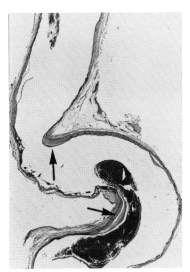 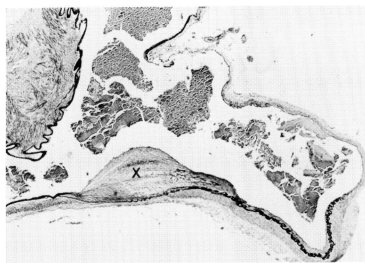

Fig. 2.3. (above, left) Low magnification of longitudinal section through the carotid siphon demonstrating atherosclerotic thickening at sites where flow separation is likely to occur (arrows) and thinning at sites where flow is likely to impinge on the vessel wall (Flow is from below upwards) (Verhoeff's elastic stain and eosin). (From: Stehbens WE. Pathology of the Cerebral Blood Vessels, St Louis: CV Mosby, 1972).[9]

Fig. 2.4. (above, right) Low magnification of a longitudinal section through a cerebral arterial fork, with extensive mural thinning and loss of elastica where the blood would impinge. Note the large lateral pad (x) with extension distally along the adjacent wall of the daughter branch with absence of underlying media. Note the absence of intimal thickening in the stem immediately proximal to the lateral pad. Flow is from the left (Verhoeff's elastic stain and eosin). (From: Stehbens WE. Histopathology of cerebral aneurysms. Arch Neurol 1963; 8:272-85. American Medical Association).[13]

(ii) Transversely oriented elevations and depressions produce areas of transverse wrinkling (Fig. 2.6), sometimes on the posterior wall but frequently elsewhere and they can often be seen in the common iliac arteries. These are flow-induced and resemble the wavy patterns observed on wind-swept sands or river beds. The elevations exhibit alternating mounds of musculoelastic proliferation denser than the loose almost edematous tissue beneath the intervening troughs (Fig. 2.7 and 2.8). Lipid may appear in foam cells beneath the troughs[10] or can be closely related to a thin secondary subendothelial elastic lamina over the mounds (Fig. 2.9) or deeper in the intima (Fig. 2.10). No doubt due to the flow-induced stresses in the troughs, a new discrete layer of intimal proliferation develops in the troughs and eventually extends over the entire surface flattening and masking the wrinkling (Fig. 2.8). In more advanced and fibrous intimal thickening lipid is usually diffuse and extracellular often with

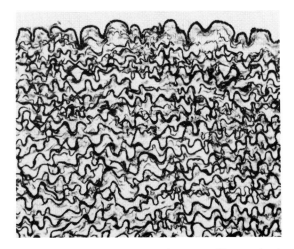

Fig. 2.5. Transverse histological section of human fetal aorta stained to demonstrate the thick internal elastic lamina (at the top) and successive medial elastic laminae below (Verhoeff's elastic stain and eosin).

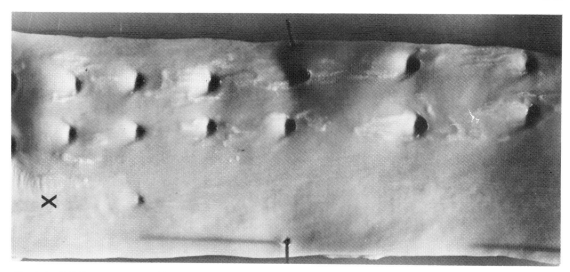

Fig. 2.6. Child's aorta opened longitudinally with flow from left to right. Note the raised dots and fatty streaks predominantly related to the posterior wall between the orifices of the segmental branches. Transversely orientated ridges and hollows are present at x.

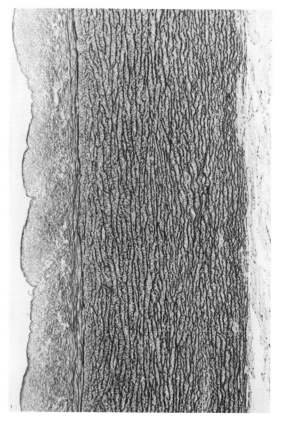

Fig. 2.7. Longitudinal section of human aorta through zone of wrinkling showing musculoelastic intimal thickening with loose intimal tissue related to floor of troughs. Flow from above down (Verhoeff's elastic stain and eosin).

relatively little intracellular lipid (Fig. 2.11).

(iii) Yellow, mostly slightly elevated, fatty streaks and dots appear in varying patterns along the posterior wall of the descending aorta, especially in the abdominal segment and between and closely related to the ostia of the segmental branches (Fig. 2.6). There are small quantities of lipid either in the interstitial tissue of the intimal proliferation between the ostia and near the poles of the nuclei of smooth muscle cells (probably lysosomal) (Fig. 2.12). Large macrophages heavily laden with multiple lipid vacuoles are believed to be derived from monocytes and appear secondarily. Small aggregates of these macrophages occur but the streaks never consist of a mass of foamy macrophages as in the cholesterol-fed rabbit or in homozygous FH. Lipid progressively increases as the intima thickens and can be seen in the media as well as in nonelevated regions of the intima (Fig. 2.12). Lipid is also found in the ostia of branches. With progressive thickening and fibrosis particularly about the ostia, atherosclerotic plaques eventually appear and involve areas where fatty streaks previously existed. Lipid accumulation becomes more pronounced and dense accumulations (Fig. 2.13) are observed particularly where the intima is hyaline, relatively acellular and often with few lipid-laden macrophages (lipophages). It is probable that the lipophages,

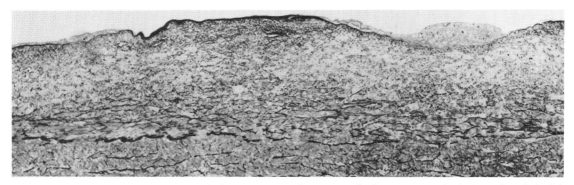

Fig. 2.8. Higher magnification of ridges which contain more dense musculoelastic tissue and a distinct subendothelial elastic lamina. The intima beneath the troughs is relatively loose and on the floor of both troughs there is loose intimal proliferation appearing to be superimposed on the preexisting intima. This loose layer of intimal tissue often extends over the ridges and troughs tending to smooth out the surface irregularities (Verhoeff's elastic tissue stain and eosin).

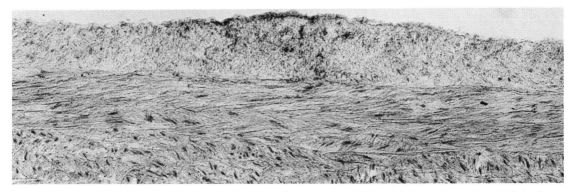

Fig. 2.9. Frozen section demonstrating lipid in the ridge of an area of wrinkling of the aortic intima, particularly about the subendothelial elastic tissue over the summit of the ridge (Hematoxylin and Fett rot).

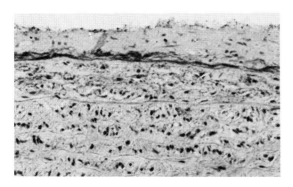

Fig. 2.10. (left) Frozen section of aortic intimal thickening showing a dark zone of fat along elastic laminae in the middle of the thickened intima (Hematoxylin and Oil red O).

Fig. 2.11. (below) Denser more fibrous intimal thickening in the human aorta exhibiting diffuse mostly extracellular fat (Hematoxylin and Fett rot).

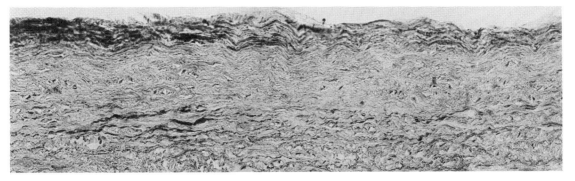

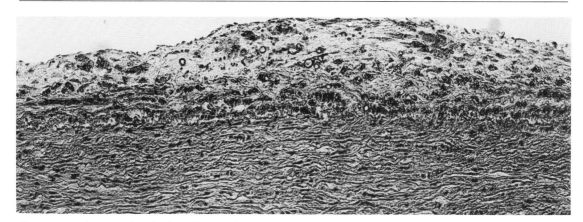

Fig. 2.12. Dark material in thickened intima from a zone of fatty streaking. Note the localized deposits represent cellular lipid, some being macrophages. Some smooth muscle cells also contain lipid believed to be lysosomal from phagocytosis of intercellular matrix vesicles. Diffuse lipid is extracellular. There is also lipid in the underlying media. Note that these lipid deposits are not essentially foam cell or xanthomatous lesions (Hematoxylin and Fett rot).

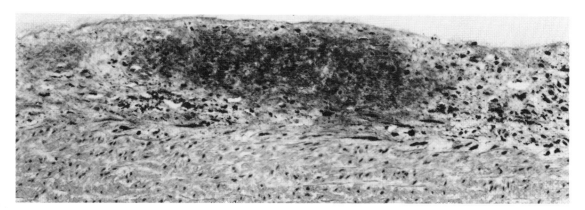

Fig. 2.13. More advanced lipid accumulation in aortic intimal proliferation. Some lipid appears to be intracellular but a large zone of dense lipid is mostly extracellular. Note that the lipid is not the most salient feature and to suggest that it is lipid that accumulates in the intima to produce narrowing of the lumen is misrepresentation (Hematoxylin and Fett rot).

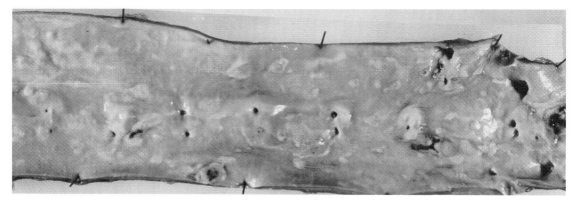

Fig. 2.14. Thoracic aorta exhibiting moderate atherosclerosis. Some irregular thickenings are related to the ostia of segmental branches which are generally narrowed and distorted. There are a few small tears and ulcers. Flow is from left to right.

like the smooth muscle cells, undergo granulo-vesicular disintegration. Ultimately the entire aortic surface is affected in varying degrees of severity and in association with progressive ectasia.

Even within the first decade, slight irregularities (nodules or flat elevations) of the aortic intimal surface can be observed. Though few initially, they increase in frequency and are sometimes within the ostia. They may be precursors of fatty streaks since they are not yellow and are apparently enveloped or masked by progressive intimal proliferation.

(iv) In the common and internal iliac arteries transversely orientated tears in the internal elastic lamina develop in late fetal life. After birth they develop in large arteries such as the internal carotid artery and splenic arteries and more distally in the external iliac and femoral arteries. Calcification in the margins of these elastic tears extends into the elastic lamina but not into the space or gap formed by retraction of the edges of the tear. Interconnecting tears form and the gaps are prone to lipid deposition. This is pronounced in the common iliac artery when there is but one umbilical artery. Overt atherosclerosis has been observed in the common iliac artery in infancy on the side of a single umbilical artery.[10] It is not known whether the tears occur in the aorta during fetal life. However, they appear to be similar to those initiating cerebral arterial dissecting aneurysms[9] and to the tears at the apex or crotch of cerebral arteries and they can be produced experimentally within a few days following alteration of the blood flow pattern.[14-17] The evidence is that such tears are due to mechanical failure of the tissue, there being no evidence of elastolytic activity.[18] The periodicity is relatively regular and reminiscent of the transverse wrinkling but there is no evidence that the tears precede the wrinkling although the hemodynamic conditions may be similar in both situations.

The above phenomena appear to be flow-related and intimately associated with hemodynamic stress. The aortic intima progressively thickens, becomes increasingly fibrotic and both lipid and mineral content continue to increase with irregularity of the intimal surface and a variable degree of medial thinning. The fibrous tissue proliferation is thickest about the ostia of

the aorta and obviously incorporates both the wrinkling and the fatty streaks with narrowing and distortion of the ostia (Fig. 2.14).

Atherosclerosis in smaller arteries commences as fibromusculoelastic intimal proliferation with medial thinning and loss or disruption of elastic tissue and progresses insidiously to overt atherosclerosis.[13] As seen in Figures 2.3 and 2.4 the lesions have specific localization and are not essentially foam cell or xanthomatous lesions. In advanced lesions the intima is primarily sclerotic but also heavily infiltrated with lipid (Fig. 2.15).

COMPLICATIONS

Atherosclerosis manifests itself clinically as a result of (i) thromboembolic occlusion of an artery resulting in ischemia of vital tissues such as the heart and brain, (ii) rupture of an aneurysm leading to fatal hemorrhage or less com-

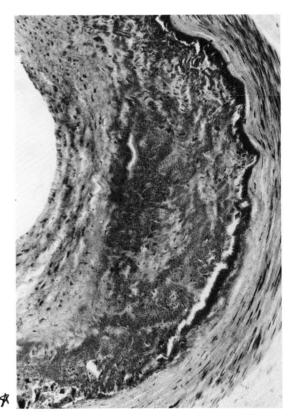

Fig. 2.15. Frozen section of a cerebral artery exhibiting extensive fat infiltration deep in the sclerotic intima. Note the fat is mostly extracellular and some dense lipid is related to the internal elastic lamina (Hematoxylin and Fett rot).

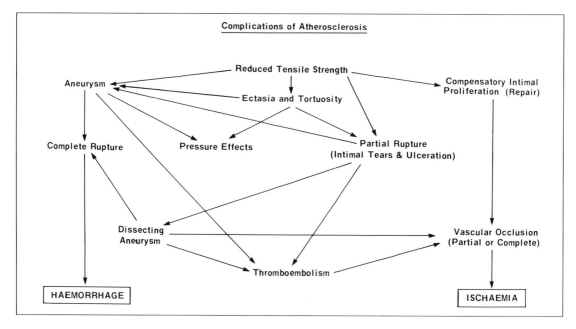

Complications of Atherosclerosis

Fig. 2.16. Diagram indicating the inter-relationship of complications of atherosclerosis which can all be basically attributed to reduced tensile strength. (Modified from Stehbens WE. Hemodynamics of the Blood Vessel Wall. Courtesy of Charles C. Thomas, Publisher, Springfield, IL:1979.)

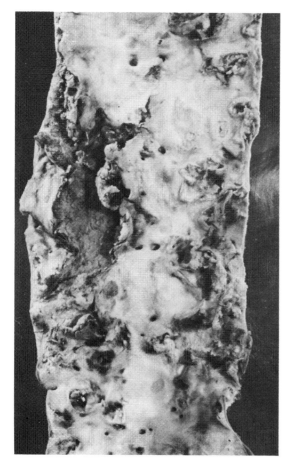

monly (iii) ectasia and tortuosity with displacement leading to pressure effects on nerves etc (Fig. 2.16).

About the sixth decade intimal tears develop when there is considerable irregularity of the surface. The tears are associated with thrombus deposition and some extravasation of blood and fibrin about the tear. These phenomena become more prevalent and eventually large patches of aortic intima slough off (Fig. 2.17) with mural thrombosis and atheroembolism. Continued shedding of thromboemboli leads to occlusion of vessels distally with secondary ischemia of tissues and progressively there is disruption of distal circulatory beds since some permanent occlusions result. Mural thrombus rarely occludes the aorta because of its large diameter, although this can occur in the iliofemoral arteries (Fig. 2.18). When there is an ulcer or intimal tear of an atherosclerotic

Fig. 2.17. An extreme degree of aortic ulceration with undermining of the edges of the tears, secondary thrombosis on the exposed subintimal surface and obliteration of the orifices of segmental branches. (Reproduced with permission from Stehbens WE. Speculations in Science and Technology. 1988; 11:89-99.)[19]

plaque in a coronary or cerebral artery, thrombotic occlusion is likely to result producing myocardial ischemia or infarction of the myocardium causing a heart attack and in the brain, causing a stroke.

The important question to ask is why should the aorta tear or ulcerate when the pressure required to burst the aorta or any other artery is many more times the highest systolic pressure ever sustained during life? No artery should tear or ulcerate spontaneously under normal physiological conditions. By analogy a severe injury may result in a bone fracture but if someone's femur fractures spontaneously whilst walking the dog, an underlying weakness responsible for the pathological fracture should be sought. Similarly most humans from the sixth decade onwards harbor intimal tears or ulcers subclinically without their being subjected to any trauma. Weakening of the aortic wall has been recognized as a phenomenon that occurs with age, and the intimal tears are analogous to the spontaneous stress fractures of the bones and tendons of joggers, sports persons and marathon runners. The intimal tissue of torn or fractured coronary arterial intima is of lower tensile strength than the neighboring wall.[20] These intimal tears or ulcers can be regarded as pathological fractures or tears due to an acquired underlying weakness of the tissue just as is the case with pathological fractures of bone. The thromboembolic phenomena that follow these intimal tears or ulcerations are secondary phenomena but the primary underlying abnormality is the intimal weakness or, in the engineering sense, the acquired loss of tensile strength of the connective tissues.[2]

Some intimal tears initiate dissecting aneurysms but rarely direct rupture, and occasionally a small saccular aneurysm may develop from the base of an ulcer following yielding of the attenuated medial remnants and adventitia. Alternatively a fusiform aneurysm (Figure 2.19) may develop as the result of yielding of a larger area of the severely atherosclerotic wall and as with distension of an inner tube, the gradual,

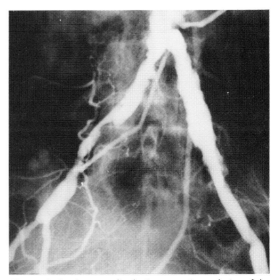

Fig. 2.18. Angiogram displaying gross irregularity of the lumen of the lower abdominal aorta and ilio-femoral arteries with stenoses and thrombotic lesions narrowing the arteries and some small branches. (By courtesy of Mr. P. Meech.)

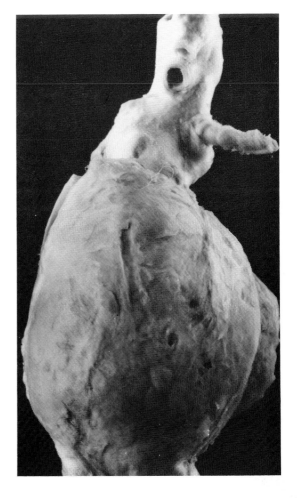

Fig. 2.19. A large fusiform aneurysm of the abdominal aorta due to atherosclerosis. The sac had caused considerable pressure erosion of the vertebral column.

localized bulging of the wall must be due to an acquired weakness of the arterial wall with the conditions that caused the weakness and yielding of the wall in the first place being responsible for the progressive enlargement and eventual rupture of the aneurysm with hemorrhage.[2] Ectasia, aneurysms and dissecting aneurysms occurring beyond an arterial stenosis or a valvular stenosis are now recognized as nonspecific manifestations of the hemodynamic stresses in a poststenotic zone, the result of mechanical failure due to an engineering fatigue-like phenomenon.[2,21,22] These observations indicate that hemodynamic stresses can be more intimately and fundamentally associated with atherogenesis than merely acting in the guise of a localizing factor.

Aneurysms are frequently preceded by ectasia, lengthening of the artery due to medial thinning, weakening, and loss of elasticity. These changes cause tortuosity and the displaced, sclerotic and sometimes calcified wall can cause pressure symptoms.

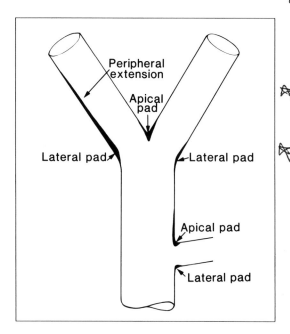

Fig. 2.20. Diagram to illustrate the localization of intimal thickenings or pads at forks in fetal and infant cerebral arteries. The lateral pad on the left main branch has been thickened and extended to show how it grows in later life. The apical pad on the small side branch (right) extends peripherally and is thicker in the main stem but it is less extensive within the branch.

This line of argument contends that the essential clinical manifestations of atherosclerosis can be explained by an acquired weakness or loss of tensile strength of the vessel wall (Fig. 2.16).

INTIMAL PROLIFERATION AT ARTERIAL FORKS

The intimal proliferation at branching sites does not occur as a diffuse involvement about arterial forks. In fetal cerebral arteries intimal proliferation develops over the flow divider preceded by pale staining, thinning and lacy appearance or fragmentation of the internal elastic lamina.[23] Thickening also occurs at lateral angles just beyond where the side wall of the stem curves into the outer or lateral wall of the daughter branch, i.e., where boundary layer separation and eddy currents would be expected. These intimal pads or cushions progressively coalesce and the lateral thickenings extend peripherally along the adjoining wall of the daughter branch (Fig. 2.20) producing, when cut in cross section, an eccentrically located lesion. These thickenings are ubiquitous in humans[2] and the lower animals so far examined. They are consistent in their localization and vary in size according to the angle at which the branch arises from the parent stem, again suggesting that hemodynamic factors are important in their localization, if not in their etiology. Serial sections of a large number of cerebral arterial forks from fetus to old age indicate that the intimal proliferations progress to overt atherosclerosis without any distinctive line of demarcation.[9,13]

Investigation of several extracranial forks from rabbits reveals similar intimal proliferation over the flow divider but at some forks lateral angle thickening is absent or minimal and, according to the configuration of the fork[2,24] so the proliferation varies, but commonly the thickening extends peripherally from either the flow divider or the lateral angle thickening (cushion or pad) (Fig. 2.20).

The localization of intimal proliferation about the forks of human arteries is essentially similar to that in the cerebral arteries and lipid is preferentially deposited in these thickenings.[24,25] Even in the earliest thickenings Levene[26] found the underlying media was substantially thinned if the vessels were perfusion-fixed and the internal elastic lamina was usually disrupted. The most plausible explanation for these intimal thickenings is that they constitute reparative thickening to compensate for the medial and elastic loss.[2,9]

In experimental animals these intimal proliferations at forks and curvatures[27] were found to be sites of predilection for lipid deposition whether spontaneous or dietary induced.[24-27] Consequently it has become increasingly recognized that this intimal proliferation in the fetus and neonate is an integral part or an important precursor of atherosclerosis. Ross[29] emphasized that intimal proliferation is the key event in the development of atherosclerosis and its advanced lesions, the intimal injury hypothesis being a belated acceptance that intimal proliferation precedes lipid deposition. The localization of these intimal thickenings is important to our understanding of atherogenesis. Hemodynamics can explain the consistent localization[2] if not the pathogenesis. In different experimental models of surgically fashioned arterial forks and curvatures intimal proliferation developed at sites analogous to those occurring naturally in human fetal and infant arteries.[17,27,30,31]

ULTRASTRUCTURE OF INTIMAL PROLIFERATION AND ATHEROSCLEROSIS

This intimal fibromusculoelastic proliferation at branching sites has been considered an integral part of the arterial wall but even in the neonate there are signs of degeneration. There is disruption of the internal elastic lamina[23] and also cell debris derived primarily from smooth muscle cells, thickening and reduplication of basement membrane and separation of basement membrane from the muscle cells.[32] Similar changes are also seen in intimal thickenings at rabbit arterial forks.[33] These changes progress with thickening and extension of the intimal proliferation, together with thinning of the media. As atherosclerosis progresses there is further thickening and lamination

of the endothelial basement membrane (Fig. 2.21), development of bizarre shaped smooth muscle cells often with thin elongated cytoplasmic extensions, evidence of muscle degeneration and cell death. Small membrane-bound vesicles of varying size are shed from the muscle cells in enormous numbers and at times whole cells disintegrate into a myriad of vesicles (granulovesicular degeneration).[32] These matrix vesicles as they are now called are believed to be due to plasma membrane fragility[34] since plasma membrane fragments are found mixed with matrix vesicles and other cellular debris (Fig. 2.22).

Basement membrane material about the smooth muscle cells is irregularly thickened, multilaminated, sometimes reticulated and often unassociated with cells (Fig. 2.21). The hyaline appearance corresponds to the abundant dystrophic basement membrane material. Collagen fibrils are frequently short, bent, haphazardly arranged and exhibit the abnormal shapes (Fig. 2.22) characteristically seen in hereditary connective tissue disorders associated with vascular fragility.[35,36] Collagen is less abundant than expected by virtue of the sclerotic texture of the tissue at autopsy which must be accounted

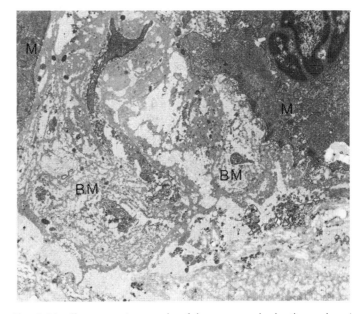

Fig. 2.21. Electron micrograph of human cerebral atherosclerosis showing abnormally shaped smooth muscle cells in the intima (M), irregular (grey) thick laminated basement membrane material (BM) with cell debris and disorganized intercellular matrix and collagen (C). No elastic tissue is present.(x 15,000)

for to a large extent by the abundant basement membrane material.

Endothelial cells exhibit partial separation from one another and areas of separation from the basement membrane material.[31] This is frequent with the smooth muscle cells. These abnormal changes are consistent with loss of cohesion of the mural connective tissues and are associated with progressive loss of the intimal elastic tissue.

Cell debris, consisting of small electron dense granules and membrane-bound vesicles, has been observed in the blood vessel wall for many years. Stehbens[2,31-33] refers to it as vesiculogranular debris and has demonstrated[31] that there is a progressive accumulation of this debris in cerebral blood vessel walls, apparently due to inadequate phagocytosis.[2] It is more pronounced in the intima and occurs particu-

larly where smooth muscle cells are absent. Similar material has been identified in a variety of tissues including cartilage, bone and dentine,[2] where the vesicles are referred to as matrix vesicles and thought to represent the initial locus of calcification in these tissues. Whether or not the matrix vesicles in blood vessels are identical to those in the skeletal system is uncertain, but at present those in cartilage and bone appear to be produced for the purpose of calcification. The presence of these vesicles in blood vessels has been virtually overlooked despite their occurrence in enormous numbers.

Matrix vesicles have been reviewed elsewhere.[2] Their location correlates well with the already documented augmented mitotic activity and smooth muscle cell turnover at arterial forks and branchings.[2] Matrix vesicles have been observed in the aorta of aging rats,[37] in the small pulmonary arteries following experimental hypertension[38] and in the media of hypertensive rats.[39] They accumulate in the human blood vessel wall with age[32] and occur in other vascular lesions such as berry aneurysms[40] and arteriovenous aneurysms of man.[12] I consider the occurrence of matrix vesicles or cellular debris to be effects of hemodynamic stress and not specifically an age phenomenon.[2,41] This concept is supported by their ready production in large numbers in experimental aneurysms[42] and in the anastomosed vein of arteriovenous fistulas.[43]

Some vesicles have electron dense contents considered to be calcium phosphate. Calcification in atherosclerosis is thought to be associated with mineralization of matrix vesicles[2] and an x-ray microanalysis of mineralized matrix vesicles in experimental saccular aneurysms has revealed the presence of calcium phosphate and at times a small quantity of magnesium.[44] It has been shown that the early appearance of extracellular lipid in cerebral arteries is associated with the transformation of these membrane-bound vesicles to relatively electron-translucent, closely-packed, round membra-

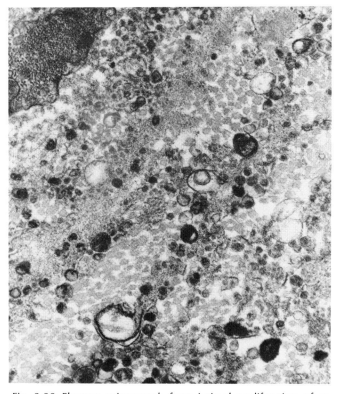

Fig. 2.22 Electron micrograph from intimal proliferation of an experimental aneurysm produced in a rabbit. Portion of a smooth muscle cell is at the top left with little basement membrane distinguishable. There are abundant matrix vesicles elsewhere, segments of cell membranes and abnormal shaped collagen fibrils in cross section suggesting plasma membrane and collagen fragility. (x 60,000).

nous profiles larger than the denser vesicles.[41,43] The phenomenon occurs simultaneously with the disappearance of matrix vesicles or cellular debris. The matrix vesicles accumulate progressively in the vessel wall and fail to undergo phagocytosis. Plasma lipoproteins, the low density lipoproteins (LDL) in particular, may become incorporated within the vesicular cytoplasm possibly due to altered plasma membrane permeability to LDL after being separated from the cell of origin. The arterial intima would be an excellent environment for the continued activity of plasma membrane enzymes of the vesicles and this difference in environment from that in cartilage, bone and dentine could account for the preponderance of lipid accumulation in vascular matrix vesicles and of calcification in the skeletal system. Even so chondrocytic vesicles show an enrichment of total lipids, cholesterol, phospholipid and glycolipid but no capacity to synthesize lipid.

Vascular matrix vesicles have been regarded as cell debris, rather than a physiological product of smooth muscle cells and endothelium.[2] Their association with apparent defects in the plasma membrane fragments in the matrix[34] supports the concept of debris. Accumulation of lipid in the vesicles does not require the presence of hyperlipidemia. Such accumulation may be nonspecific though altered by high levels of plasma lipid or minerals but the extent to which this occurs in man is unknown. Pathologists have for years taught medical students that non-phagocytosed cell debris has an affinity for lipid deposition and calcium salts. This appears to be the mechanism for lipid accumulation in tuberculosis and in the vessel wall which can occur in normolipidemic subjects[2,41] and even herbivorous animals with low blood cholesterol levels.

There is no evidence that hyperlipoproteinemia induces the production of matrix vesicles or that dietary-induced hypercholesterolemia in rabbits induces matrix vesicles to enlarge. The contents become electron translucent, but there is no increased production of vesicles suggesting that the underlying mechanism or pathogenesis for lipid accumulation differs from that in true atherosclerosis.[45]

These ultrastructural changes characterize the essential proliferative changes of atherosclerosis which occur with increasing age in humans.

THE ATROPHIC LESION

In the study of human cerebral arterial forks, preaneurysmal changes were observed primarily in middle-aged subjects.[9,13] They consisted of mural atrophy with extreme loss of ectasia and a variable degree of thinning extending to complete attenuation and loss of medial muscle (Fig. 2.4). The adventitia was also thinned. These atrophic lesions occurred primarily adjacent to the apex where the flux of blood impinged on the arterial wall. This change, often affecting a large segment of the wall, could occur on both sides of the apex. These atrophic lesions have been mistaken for congenital defects but the evidence that they are acquired lesions seems conclusive[9] and they can proceed to frank aneurysmal dilatation. Many early aneurysms in human cerebral aneurysms are thin walled consisting of endothelium and a thin layer of fibrous tissue. Superimposed on this, intimal proliferation can develop and progress to atherosclerosis indicating a close relationship between the atrophic and proliferative lesions.

HEMODYNAMICS AND THE BLOOD VESSEL WALL

It was postulated in 1958 that atherosclerosis was the combination of degenerative and reparative changes[46] in the blood vessel wall consequent upon ongoing hemodynamically-induced mechanical fatigue or failure of the blood vessel wall and that lipid accumulation in the wall was but one of the manifestations of the disease and of secondary importance to the effects of hemodynamically induced vibrations of the vessel wall.

To demonstrate the validity of the fatigue hypothesis it was necessary to accelerate the development of lesions in an experimental model in which wall vibrations were of higher frequency or of greater amplitude or both. In the first model, arteriovenous fistulas in sheep, vibratory activity was gross. In 1974 I demonstrated that atherosclerosis morphologically identical to human atherosclerosis can be induced in the anastomosed vein of an experimental arteriovenous fistula in herbivorous sheep[47] which normally have serum cholesterol levels less than 100 mg/dL. Lipid deposition and calcium were present, and also aneurysmal dilatation, intimal tears, mural thrombosis and profound degenerative changes in the blood vessel wall.

In an ultrastructural study[43] the changes in the anastomosed veins of sheep with an experimental arteriovenous fistula were morphologically identical to those of human atherosclerosis as demonstrated in human material.[32,40] The human counterpart of this disease is the anastomosed vein of therapeutic arteriovenous fistulas used for renal dialysis.[12] Again we demonstrated that changes in the anastomosed vein were identical to atherosclerosis, and that they developed prematurely and at an accelerated rate when subjected to the augmented hemodynamic stresses for which they were not architecturally designed.

The second model used was the experimental aneurysm because vibratory activity in aneurysmal sacs is of low amplitude and high

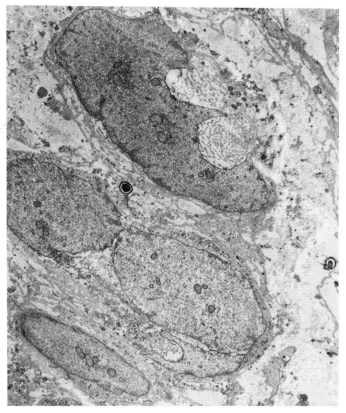

Fig. 2.23. Ultrastructure of intimal proliferation in an experimental aneurysm in a rabbit showing bizarre shaped muscle cells, abundant grey multilaminated, reticulated and redundant basement membrane material with separation from the muscle plasma membrane. Note the dense calcospherite near the center and to the right of the figure. Matrix vesicles are scattered about in the matrix. Compare with Fig. 2.21. (x 15,000).

frequency[48] such as to produce high pitched musical murmurs (inaudible without amplification). Berry aneurysms develop postnatally, mostly in middle age and the sac often contains atherosclerosis macroscopically, whereas the parent vessel may be free.[9] This suggests that atherosclerosis in such sac walls develops at an accelerated rate. Three types of experimental aneurysms were produced in stock fed rabbits by microvascular surgery using venous transplants according to the techniques described by Stehbens.[49] Over one to four years atherosclerosis morphologically identical to human atherosclerosis both histologically[50,51] and ultrastructurally[42] develops in these aneurysms. Increase in size, thrombosis and rupture also occur. In experimental aneurysms, I demonstrated bizarre shaped muscle cells ultrastructurally, abundant matrix vesicles, dystrophic basement membranes with separation of basement membranes from the cellular constituents (Fig. 2.23), abnormal collagen fibers (Fig. 2.22),[35] lipid deposition, calcification and thrombosis. There was evidence of cell fragility with disrupted muscle cell membranes and fragments of cell membrane in the matrix[34] associated with matrix vesicles (Fig. 2.22).

Hemodynamics is usually considered to be a localizing factor and hypercholesterolemia is held responsible for the atherosclerotic process. The above experiments provide evidence against this contention as the animals were on a stock diet and lipid deposition occurred despite the low serum cholesterol levels. However by producing arteriovenous fistulas and aneurysms in rabbits and subsequently placing them on a high cholesterol diet, lipid is preferentially deposited in the anastomosed veins of the fistulas[52] and in the aneurysmal sacs[53] but histologically the picture is that of a foam cell infiltration superimposed on the degenerative changes and it is not typical of spontaneous atherosclerosis.

The third model, analogous to tortuosities, is the U-shaped bend.

In the S-shaped carotid siphon in longitudinal section (Fig. 2.3) there is thinning and calcification of the wall on the greater curvature of the bends and a proliferative atherosclerotic lesion beyond the lesser curvature of the bends. I classified these lesions as "atrophic" and "proliferative" respectively and regard both as lesions of atherosclerosis. The sites correspond to regions of scouring and sedimentation respectively at the bends of a meandering stream. In experimental arteriovenous fistulas the afferent artery becomes enlarged, tortuous and thin-walled and aneurysmal dilatation may occur.[2,47,52] This is associated with gross elastic tissue fragmentation and loss of media. It is regarded as an atrophic lesion in contradistinction to the proliferative lesion in the anastomosed vein. By producing U-shaped loops surgically in rabbits and sheep Stehbens[31] reproduced atrophic and proliferative lesions at the bends at sites analogous to those in the carotid siphon of man. Moreover the atrophic lesions in the rabbit were histologically identical to the "mural thinning" and the funnel-shaped lesions in cerebral arteries of man which Stehbens has shown to be the early changes in the formation of cerebral berry aneurysms.[9,13]

We thus demonstrated that the atrophic lesions of atherosclerosis which constitute the early changes of berry aneurysm formation in the cerebral arteries of man occur (i) in the afferent artery of experimental arteriovenous fistulas[47,52] and (ii) on the greater curvature of experimental U-shaped bends in rabbits.[31] Similar atrophic lesions have been demonstrated by Hazama et al[54] at arterial forks after producing an imbalance of flow with or without hypertension or lathyrism. We have also demonstrated (by scanning electron microscopy) that the earliest demonstrable manifestation of these atrophic lesions is the development of predominantly transverse tears in the internal elastic lamina five days postoperatively in carotid-jugular fistulas[14] and U-shaped bends[15] and at two days in femoral arteriovenous fistulas.[16] These tears are remarkably similar to those described by Meyer et al[10] in the common and internal iliac and carotid arteries of infants and neonates. They seem to be analogous to the disruptions in the internal elastic lamina in the crotch or apex of cerebral arterial forks of infants and

to those which initiate intracranial arterial dissecting aneurysms.

The tears, initially covered with thrombus, rapidly became endothelialized. The tears in the internal elastic lamina in older animals increased in size and extent and ultimately became confluent with one another but left islands of elastic lamina which could have retained little functional capacity. Following chemical de-endothelialization of the afferent arteries of carotid arteriovenous fistulas, scanning electron microscopy of the internal elastic lamina revealed predominantly straight tears with sharp margins.[18] Even in chronic fistulas the tears, despite propagation, retained their sharp margins and there was little evidence of repair with reconstitution of the lamina. The tears commenced by rupture of the elastic trabeculae traversing the fenestrae. Enzymatic digestion of the internal elastic lamina did not resemble the hemodynamically induced tears and no evidence of elastolytic enzyme activity was detected in the arterial wall of fistulas. If enzymatic digestion had been responsible, further erosion of the sharp edges would have been expected but they remained quite sharp even months postoperatively. The abnormally stressed elastic tissue undergoes some structural alteration leading to a reduction in its tensile strength and the acquired fragility results in tears.[18]

The establishment of an arteriovenous fistula is accompanied by profound alterations in local hemodynamics, much depending on the size of the fistula and its proximity to the heart. The proximal artery manifests an initial fall in blood pressure and soon increases in diameter. In chronic fistulas the pressure approaches normal levels and is elevated on rare occasions.[2] It is often associated with an augmented pulse pressure (water hammer effect) and the blood flow may be increased more than 10 times.[2] In chronic fistulas the pressure in the distal artery gradually increases from the initial low level until eventually it approximates that in the proximal segment. The changes in the anastomosed artery therefore cannot be attributed to hypertension being more probably flow related and due to changes in the pulse, pulse pressure and/or velocity. In the distal artery, flow becomes retrograde and is also increased in chronic fistulas although an increase in girth is infrequent. Likewise the frequency of elastic tears is less than proximally although the amount of collateral circulation may be a determining factor.

In femoral fistulas tears of the internal elastic lamina develop within two days[16] but in the long-term they progress to severe mural atrophy with loss of arterial structure, severe ectasia and incipient aneurysm formation.[8] In addition the intimal thickenings at forks and branching sites (even in the aorta) enlarge, extend distally and progress to frank atherosclerosis with lipid accumulation, calcification and fibrin infiltration of the wall. Similar changes involve the femoral artery near the fistula diffusely. These observations support the hemodynamic theory of atherosclerosis particularly since the experiments were performed on herbivorous rabbits on a stock diet.[8]

THE DIETARY-FED HYPERCHOLESTEROLEMIC RABBIT

The presence of lipid in the blood vessel wall has long been considered the hallmark of atherosclerosis and so the production of lipid deposits in rabbit blood vessels by a diet rich in cholesterol or egg yolk which caused hypercholesterolemia lent support to the simplistic concept that the essential feature of atherosclerosis was lipid imbibition into the arterial wall.[55] Cholesterol-rich diets are still the principal though not the only means of inducing both hypercholesterolemia and lipid-containing lesions still considered atherosclerotic by most investigators.

A crucial problem of research into the etiology of atherosclerosis is that of relating ex-perimental lesions in short-lived animals to those which occur in long-lived humans. Caution is always essential in extrapolating from animal experiments to humans even though atherosclerosis is not species specific. The essential feature is that the experimental model must reproduce the disease and its complications with the same pathogenesis and under conditions similar to those prevailing in man. These features seem straightforward enough but even Anitschkow,[56] whose name will forever be connected with the introduction of the lipid hypothesis, admitted there were differences viz (i) no fatty infiltration of the elastic lamella is ever observed (ii) much larger quantities of foam cells occur than in the human disease (iii) neither the hyalinization nor the fibrous sclerosis are prominent (iv) no ulceration with thrombus is ever observed in the dietary-induced disease and (v) the distribution of the disease is different and cerebral arteries are never involved.

There are, in fact, many other differences quite recently reviewed[57,58] which overall can be classified as (i) irreconcilable morphological (Fig. 2.24 and 2.25) and topographical differences between the two disorders, (ii) the notable absence of complications, intimal tears and ulcerations with secondary thromboembolic phenomena and aneurysms in the rabbit, (iii) extravascular lipid storage phenomena and hemolytic anemia that are not a feature of atherosclerosis, (iv) the essential pathogenetic features of the atherosclerosis (bizarre smooth muscle cells, loss of elastic tissue, granulovesicular degeneration and matrix vesicles, dystrophic collagen and basement membrane, separation of

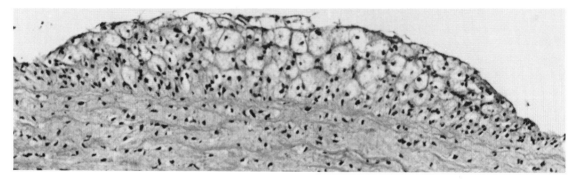

Fig. 2.24. Photomicrograph of lipid lesion in intima of a cholesterol-fed animal, the thickening consisting entirely of lipid-laden macrophages—the so-called foam-cell lesion. Note how dissimilar this rabbit lesion is to the lipid-containing lesions in humans and even the lipid streaks (Fig. 2.12) (Hematoxylin and eosin).

basement membrane from endothelial and smooth muscle cells) are absent, and (v) Stehbens and Ludatscher[45] demonstrated that in cholesterol-fed rabbits, the lipid accumulation in the matrix of intimal thickenings about renal arterial forks was predominantly lipid infiltration with separation of the cellular and noncellular constituents but was without the accumulation of matrix vesicles, bizarre muscle cells and the associated collagen and basement membrane changes that denote atherosclerosis (Fig. 2.25).[45] The basic features of the dietary induced disease are characteristic of a fat storage disease. This disease can be mimicked by storage of methyl cellulose[59] and other high molecular weight polysaccharides.[7]

Some other animal species require thiouracil therapy or thyroidectomy together with a high cholesterol diet to induce extreme hypercholesterolemia but many investigators prefer to use primates or other animals such as pigs or pigeons because they develop overt atherosclerosis spontaneously and therefore by overfeeding cholesterol, they produce lesions which seem more similar to the human disease. In other words they develop a mixed lesion. Characteristically the intima, as Anitschkow stated, always has a high population of foam or xanthoma cells (Fig. 2.24). Cliff[60] calculated that an average man would need to eat 110 eggs daily to consume an intake of cholesterol equivalent to experimental cholesterol feeding of rhesus monkeys. Constantinides and colleagues[61,62] acknowledged that the large quantity of dietary cholesterol was noxious and to prevent the rabbits dying prematurely, they subjected them to only intermittent periods of cholesterol feeding.

Vesselinovitch,[63] reviewing different animal models based on dietary-induced hypercholesterolemia, admitted "it is rare to find an animal that is satisfactory in all respects for the study of atherosclerosis. There are always some features that differ somewhat from those in human disease." Carey[64] conceded that cholesterol feeding of experimental animals fails to reproduce atherosclerosis, admitting that models are chosen for experimental purposes to express one or more aspects of the human disease. To ignore such differences in pathology and pathogenesis is to deny scientific exactitude and Carey appears unaware that results from experiments where the pathogenesis is different have no applicability to atherosclerosis. This "approximation" appears to be the common approach. The lesions are still called atherosclerosis and from them deductions are made regarding atherosclerosis in man such that it is common for the majority of illustrations of atherosclerosis in textbooks to be from dietary-induced animal experiments.

It is also no longer valid to invoke a species or time factor to explain differences since accel-

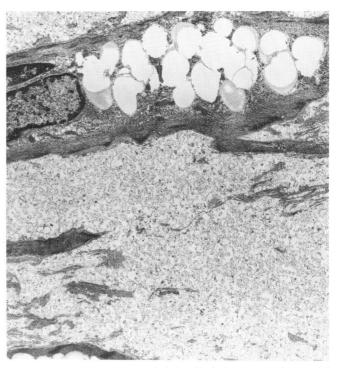

Fig. 2.25. Electron micrograph from the intimal pad of the renal arterial fork from a cholesterol-fed rabbit showing lipid accumulation in the smooth muscle cells (top and bottom of the micrograph). Note abundant intracellular (lysosomal) lipid accumulation without the bizarre muscle cells, the dystrophic basement membrane changes and abnormal collagen seen in spontaneous atherosclerosis (Fig.s 21 and 23). Matrix vesicle production is not increased and the extracellular lipid is merely infiltration with separation of pre-existing tissues. No foam cells are seen. (x 16,000) (From: Stehbens WE, Ludatscher RM. The susceptibility of renal arterial forks in rabbits to dietary-induced lipid deposition. Pathology 1983; 15:475-85).[45]

erated lesions similar to the human disease can be produced experimentally in normocholesterolemic animals as well as iatrogenically in humans when venous bypass grafts are used for CHD and when arteriovenous shunts for renal dialysis are fashioned[12] and the ensuing lesions never resemble a fat storage disease.

The differences between dietary-induced lesions and atherosclerosis are so fundamental that it is unwise to regard the former in any sense as atherosclerotic lesions especially so since they differ in pathogenesis. Neither should it be assumed that they have the same etiology. Any extrapolation from such experimental models to atherosclerosis must be fallacious and similarly it would be invalid to use such evidence in support of deductions made from epidemiological studies.

HYPERCHOLESTEROLEMIA AND ATHEROSCLEROSIS IN HUMANS

Clinical reports early this century contended that premature severe atherosclerosis occurred frequently in a group of diseases associated with hypercholesterolemia viz familial hypercholesterolemia (FH), diabetes mellitus, obstructive jaundice, hypothyroidism and the nephrotic syndrome.[55,65] These anecdotal assertions were used to support the causal role of hypercholesterolemia in atherogenesis. The pathological evidence underlying these associations, therefore, warrants review.

FAMILIAL HYPERCHOLESTEROLEMIA

This is a relatively common inherited metabolic storage disease of lipid characterized by an elevated plasma cholesterol level and xanthomatosis. It is genetically transmitted by an autosomal dominant gene and caused by the presence of a mutant allele at the low density lipoprotein (LDL) receptor locus. The homozygous form occurs about once in a million. There is a virtual absence of LDL receptors or the receptors have an inability to bind and take up LDL. Heterozygotes have a frequency of about 1 in 500 but in some populations (South Africa, Syria) it is closer to 0.5%. The heterozygote take up or binds LDL at approximately half the normal rate.

The homozygotes have a blood cholesterol level between 600 and 1200 mg/dL with the excess cholesterol entirely in the LDL fraction. Heterozygotes have blood cholesterol levels ranging from 270 to 550 mg/dL (with a mean of 340 to 370 mg/dL) and there is relatively little overlap with the general population.[66] The plasma triglyceride level, often slightly elevated in homozygotes, is normal in heterozygotes.

The homozygous form is said to be the purest form of FH and the most cogent illustration of the causal relationship between high serum cholesterol levels and coronary heart disease (CHD)[67] and coronary atherosclerosis.[68] FH has been known as essential or hereditary hypercholesterolemic xanthomatosis. The vascular lesions have repeatedly been reported as dissimilar to atherosclerosis and likened to those of the subcutaneous and tendon xanthomata or the cholesterol-fed rabbit. The aortic lesions have been referred to as xanthomatosis or xanthelasma of the aorta, thus emphasizing the xanthomatous or foam cell nature of the lesions. Even Goldstein and Brown[68] admitted that "atheromas" are composed of foam cells and referred to xanthomatous plaquing of arteries. These descriptions do not characterize atherosclerosis.

Autopsy of a fetus of 20 weeks with homozygous FH[69] revealed multifocal lipid deposition particularly involving stromal cells of the thymus, spleen, skin and both stromal and parenchymal cells of the kidney and only one minute focus of intimal lipid in the aorta and coronary arteries. Foam cells were observed in the epicardium, aortic adventitia, perithymic and perirenal tissue, liver, lymph nodes, bone marrow, skeletal muscle, colonic subserosa and the placenta.

The homozygous form runs a rapid course, most dying of myocardial infarction or congestive heart failure by 30 years of age there being no evidence of variation in susceptibility of the sexes. Though heterozygotes may live into the eighth decade, they also have a predisposition to premature CHD, the mean age of onset in males being 43 years and 53 years in females.[70] At least 50% of males have clinical CHD by the age of 50 years with somewhat fewer females similarly affected by that age (Table 2.1).

The subjects with FH constitute a distinct clinical entity sufficient to question the rationale of grouping them with the rest of the population in studies of CHD. However variations in severity of the xanthomatous lesion is attributable to genotypic variation at the LDL receptor locus[73] and probably inclusion of subjects with familial defective apolipoprotein B-100.

Buja et al[69] contended that the lipid accumulation results primarily from cellular overloading with plasma LDL. Slack[74] noted qualitative differences in FH stating that it may not represent an acceleration of the "normal" atheromatous process and the large "cushions" obliterating the sinuses of Valsalva[75] are not features of atherosclerosis.

The effect of homozygous FH on the heart and blood vessels is quite profound and differs substantially from that of atherosclerosis, these differences being tabulated for convenience (Table 2.2). The topography and morphology of the vascular lesions differ from those of atherosclerosis and the infrequency of thromboembolic phenomena, ulcerations and diffuse sclerotic changes that characterizes atherosclerosis is not accentuated.[85] The infrequency of cerebral and peripheral vascular disease is a further difference from atherosclerosis.

The foam cell (Fig. 2.26 and 2.27) has been regarded as the predominant intimal cell type[79,86] whereas in atherosclerosis it is undoubtedly the smooth muscle cell that predominates. Hueper[87] said, "the foam cell proliferations in the smaller arteries are sometimes so extensive that they may occlude the vascular lumens, while they may narrow considerably the lumens of large arteries". Foam cell infiltration in the disrupted

aortic media (Fig. 2.28) is not a feature of atherosclerosis. In the first 12 communications in the literature[85] giving autopsy details of homozygotes, the vascular lesions were xanthomatous (or characterized by foam cells) and in 2, the authors specifically likened the lesions to those of the cholesterol-fed rabbit. Subsequently this early emphasis was not continued possibly due to longer survival, or modification by developing atherosclerosis or therapy or a combination of the three.

The total absence of any abdominal aortic aneurysms in the literature in homozygotes and great rarity in heterozygotes argue against the vascular lesions being atherosclerotic. In view of the profound effect hemodynamic stress has on the blood vessel wall experimentally[47,48] and the progressive granulovesicular degeneration of smooth muscle cells and other degenerative changes in the aortic intima with age even by the age of 30, pronounced degeneration with secondary fibrosis and even caseation must be expected secondary to a large foam cell lesion or xanthomatous infiltration of the intima or cardiac valve leaflets. The monocytes are not protected by basement membranes, other matrix fibrous proteins and the viscoelastic properties of the normal arterial matrix. If smooth muscle and endothelial cells have an augmented turnover even though they are designed to withstand normal hemodynamic stresses, monocytes when laden with lipid must be at a much greater mechanical disadvantage particularly

Table 2.1. Tabulation of the percentage of male and female heterzygotes with familial hypercholesterolemia and familial defective apolipoprotein B-100 who will develop myocardial ischemia before reaching specific ages

Authors FH	Age	Males	Females
Slack[70]	30 years	5	0
Goldstein & Brown[68]	40 years	20%	3%
Yamamoto et al[71]	50 years	80%	20-30%
Slack[70]	50 years	51%	12%
Goldstein & Brown[68]	50 years	45%	20%
Slack[70]	60 years	85%	58%
Goldstein & Brown[68]	60 years	75%	45%
Authors FDB	**Age**	**Males**	**Females**
Tybjaeg-Hansen & Humphries[72]	50 years	40%	20%

Table 2.2. Differences between homozygous familial hypercholesterolemia and atherosclerosis in humans
(Modified from Stehbens & Martin 1991)[76]

CHARACTERISTICS	HOMOZYGOUS FH	ATHEROSCLEROSIS
Frequency	One in one million	Ubiquitous in *Homo sapiens*
Inheritance	Autosomal dominant gene	No specific genetic inheritance
Age of clinical disability	18 months to 30 years	Rare before the sixth decade
Heart		
Aortic valve	Stenosis 55%, ejection murmur 87%[77] Spongy, yellow, xanthomatous deposits, ultimately becoming fibrotic and calcified Possibly widening of commissures and valvular incompetence	No association
Mitral valve	Raised, yellow xanthomatous infiltration Incompetence 9.5%	Ordinarily not significantly affected, only fibrotic thickening and diffuse interstitial lipid especially of anterior leaflet
Pulmonary valve	Xanthomatous patches	No association
Ischemia, myocardial infarction and sequelae	Usual outcome	Common
Endocardial deposits	Left ventricle, atrium, chordae tendineae[78]	Rare
Cerebrovascular disease	Rare if ever	Common concomitant
Peripheral vascular disease	Nil	Common concomitant
Aorta		
Distribution	Severe proximally	Severe distally
Aneurysm	Nil	Common
Ectasia, tortuosity	Nil	Usual
Morphology	Yellow-orange, discrete, raised sessile lesions (described as xanthelasmatous or xanthomatous)[79]	Pale, not discrete, merges with adjoining fibrotic intima
Xanthomata	May be nodular or even tumor-like mass and can cause supravalvular aortic stenosis or obliterate sinuses of Valsalva. Also involves ostia of coronary arteries	No association
Early lesion	Xanthomatosis	Interstitial lipid deep in intima
Late lesion	Eventually fibrotic but plentiful foam cells. Calcification not pronounced	Sclerotic and atheromatous. Fibrin insudation common. Calcification often extensive
Ulcers, tears, thrombi	Infrequent superficial erosion with mural thrombosis	Usual outcome in endstage disease. Fibrin insudation common. Extensive mural thrombosis frequent
Foam cells	Initially almost exclusively xanthomatous. Later extensive infiltration in intima and moderate infiltration of media and to lesser extent the adventitia	Less frequently in the intima, rarely in adventitia
Stenosis of coronary ostia	Common	Not significant
Cellularity	Advanced lesions quite cellular, monocytes and lipophages	Advanced lesions peculiarly acellular and hyaline, occasional giant cells. Hemosiderin-laden macrophages and some round cells
Smooth muscle cells	Extensive (bipolar) lipid vacuolation in intima and media	Lipid vacuolation (bipolar) in fatty streaks but not prominent feature in advanced disease
Media	Thinned beneath plaques and extensively disrupted in a patchy fashion with crowding of residual elastic laminae	Elastic tissue fragmentation. Thinning common
Adventitia	Thickened and fibrotic beneath plaque, perivascular foam cells	May have hemosidern-laden macrophages
Adventitial round cells	More likely to be macrophages lesions	Often perivascular, common in advanced lesions

CHARACTERISTICS	HOMOZYGOUS FH	ATHEROSCLEROSIS
Vasa Vasorum	Proliferation with perivascular fibrosis and foam cell accumulation, with severe interruption of elastic lemellae within media. Those in adventitia may be surrounded by lipophages and some round cell infiltration	Proliferation with some perivascular fibrosis and interruption of elastic tissue but not pronounced
Degenerative changes	Commonly exhibit endarteritis obliterans (arteriosclerosis) of small arteries associated with plaques, elsewhere unaffected	No significant change
Coronary arteries	Severely affected, patchy involvement. Initially xanthomatous. Advanced lesion cellular, usually some medial thinning and foam cell infiltration. Foam cell accumulations appear to be independent of intimal proliferation at branching sites.	Severe, diffuse involvement. Initially fibro-muscular elastic intimal proliferation commencing about branching sites
	Advanced lesions focal with minimal conventional diffuse changes elsewhere and in small vessels	Advanced lesions diffuse and in presence of severe small vessel disease
Calcification	Infrequent or mild	Often extensive
Ectasia	Only one instance (may be due to post-stenotic effect[80]	Usual
Ulceration, thrombosis	Rare	Common
Smooth muscle cells	Fat vacuoles at poles of nuclei of muscle cells prominent in intimal proliferation and subjacent media.	Seen in early lesion but not prominent in advanced disease. Intimal smooth muscle cells thin, attenuated, malshapen Also lipofuscin
Adventitia	Proliferation of vasa vasorum and can have extensive foam cell infiltration	Proliferation of vasa vasorum. Foam cells rare, only seen when atheromatous debris herniates into adventitia
Interstitial lipid	Mostly in advanced stages	Abundant
Intracellular lipid	Foam cells abundant	Foam cells relatively sparse
Intimal tears, ulceration and thrombosis	Very infrequent	Common
Stenotic intimal lesions	Usual	Common
Xanthomatous lesions in pulmonary arteries	May be extensive in absence of pulmonary hypertension – less severe than in systemic circulation	Infrequent in absence of pulmonary hypertension
Veins	No reported involvement	Very mild, aggravated by venous hypertension
Small vessel disease		
Arteriosclerosis or diffuse hyperplastic sclerosis	Only associated with xanthomatous aortic lesions and in splenic arterioles	Usual and proportional to the severity of atherosclerosis in large vessels
Intimal xanthomatous change	May occlude small vessels	Nil
Vascular lesions — general		
Similarity to tendon xanthomata	Yes	No
Predominant cell type	Macrophage—foam cell	Smooth muscle cell
Cellularity	Pronounced	Pronounced acellularity
Xanthomata	Correlation of severity of extravascular xanthomata and vascular lesions	No association
Similarity to cholesterol-fed rabbit	Yes	No
Similarity to WHHL rabbit	Yes	No
Extravascular Xanthomata		
Cutaneous and tendon	Usual—may interfere with manual dexterity and use of feet	No association
Visceral	Common but variable	No association
Miscellaneous		
Hypercholesterolemia	Gross elevation	Can occur at any level
Migratory polyarthritis	56%—large peripheral joints[81]	No association
Uricemia	Increased in approximately one third[82,83]	No special association
Elevated erythrocyte sedimentation rate	Common[84]	No association
Hypertension	No specific association	Aggravated severity

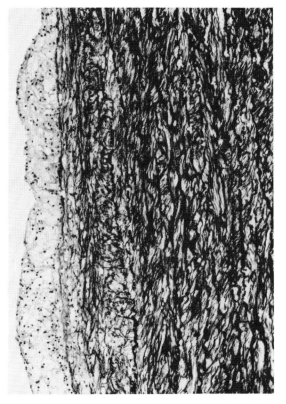

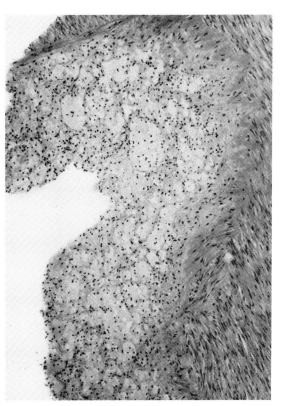

Fig. 2.26. Superficial foam cell lesion with lack of fibrous tissue in the aorta of a young homozygous boy with FH. Note vacuolation of smooth muscle cells in deep intima on left. Compare with Fig. 2.24 (Verhoeff's elastic tissue stain).

Fig. 2.27. Intimal foam cell lesion of coronary artery (homozygous FH) similar to early lesion of cholesterol-fed rabbit (Hematoxylin and eosin). (From: Stehbens WE, Martin M. The vascular pathology of familial hypercholesterolemia. Pathology 1991; 23: 54-61.)[76]

Fig. 2.28. Gross disruption of aortic medial lamellar units by extensive foam cell infiltrations. Gradua-tions exist between such changes and small zones of vacuolated smooth muscle cells. Foam cell infiltration of the adventi-tia external to such lesions is frequent (Verhoeff's elas-tic tissue stain and eosin). (From: Stehbens WE, Mar-tin M. The vascular pathol-ogy of familial hyper-cholesterolemia. Pathol-ogy 1991; 23: 54-61.)[76]

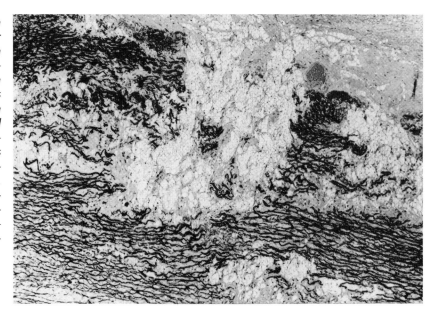

when present in a massive accumulation with little interstitial tissue. Their disintegration would attract more monocytes even without our having to speculate on the chemotactic effect of oxidized LDL particles.

The high incidence of aortic valve stenosis, migratory polyarthritis, elevated erythrocyte sedimentation rate, uricemia and extravascular xanthomatosis is consistent with a lipid metabolic disorder.[76,88] Moreover the frequency of CHD in FH does not make the vascular lesions atherosclerotic (Fig. 2.29) and the pathogenesis of CHD differs fundamentally from that in atherosclerotic CHD which is associated with an intimal tear with secondary thrombotic occlusion. It cannot be alleged that the lesions are fulminant and therefore differ from the usual atherosclerosis. Accelerated atherosclerosis induced surgically in humans and experimental herbivorous animals does not differ from conventional slowly developing lesions and such lesions are not xanthomatous unless subjected to severe hypercholesterolemia.

The homozygous form requires most emphasis but the more numerous heterozygotes are of interest. These subjects also have an unduly high frequency of aortic and mitral valvular disease with greater severity of atherosclerosis proximally than distally in the aorta. The characteristic features of FH seen in homozygotes are not so pronounced in heterozygotes and by virtue of their greater longevity the vascular lesions exhibit a greater contribution by atherosclerosis. Detailed pathological and biochemical study both qualitative and quantitative of the vascular lesions of heterozygous FH and also of other hyperlipoproteinemias by experienced vascular pathologists is wanting. However,

based on present knowledge, the heterozygote must be considered to have mixed lesions. The vascular lesions of FH and atherosclerosis are not identical and differ in kind rather than degree.

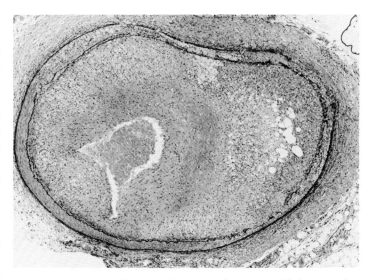

Fig. 2.29. Low magnification of section of a stenosed left circumflex coronary artery exhibiting pronounced cellularity in the intima, and even in the adventitia. The vessel appears to be peppered with foam cell nuclei. The large fat spaces are believed to be secondary to breakdown of lipophages due to hemodynamic stress (Verhoeff's elastic tissue stain and eosin (From: Stehbens WE, Martin M. The vascular pathology of familial hypercholesterolemia. Pathology 1991; 23:54-61.)[76]

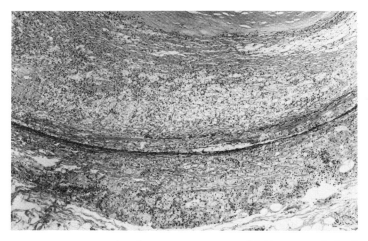

Fig. 2.30. Section of right coronary artery exhibiting gross intimal thickening (above), hyalinization, extensive foam cell infiltration through the full thickness of the wall including the adventitia (below). Note the peppering of most of the wall and the thin media with nuclei of macrophages (Verhoeff's elastic tissue stain and eosin). (From: Stehbens WE, Martin M. The vascular pathology of familial hypercholesterolemia. Pathology 1991; 23:54-61.)[76]

FAMILIAL DEFECTIVE APOLIPOPROTEIN B-100

Plasma levels of LDL are considerably increased in FH in which the LDL receptors are deficient numerically or defective. They may also be increased by the inability of the receptors to interact with the ligand apo B-100 of the LDL particles due to defects in the ligands. This abnormality called familial defective apolipoprotein B-100 (FDB) is a dominantly inherited genetic disorder resulting in elevated serum LDL levels. The blood cholesterol levels of such subjects are above the 95th percentile usually being 320 to 450 mg/dL but occasionally under 300 mg/dL. The LDL receptors are not defective and it is thought they constitute about 3% of subjects labeled as FH.[72,89] Subjects so far examined are all heterozygous and it is thought they have a frequency of 1 in 500 or 1 in 700 of the population.

Clinically these subjects have remarkably similar features (including CHD, xanthomata and arcus senilis) to those of FH. Whereas FH has many different genetic mutations, FDB has but one defect due to substitution of the amino acid glutamine for arginine in codon 3500. Little is known of the pathology of this disease but from the basic molecular defect, it is highly likely that it is not only similar to FH in both homozygous and heterozygous forms, but has in the past been mistaken for FH and is also associated with the premature development of CHD (Table 2.1).

THE WATANABE HERITABLE HYPERLIPIDEMIC RABBIT

In the Watanabe heritable hyperlipidemic (WHHL) rabbits[90] which constitute a spontaneous animal model of FH, Buja et al[91] reported the absence of cell membrane LDL receptors from cultured fibroblasts and hepatic and adrenal gland cells. The WHHL rabbit differs from FH in that the affected animals also have hypertriglyceridemia as well as hypercholesterolemia.[68] Lipid was present in the aorta of newborn WHHL rabbits and more extensive macroscopic lipid deposits were demonstrable by lipid staining of gross specimens from rabbits of four months of age and older. The pathology of the lesions was basically similar to that of cholesterol overfed rabbits. Xanthomata

were observed in skin and tendons although visceral lipid deposition (liver, lymph nodes, spleen) was milder than in cholesterol-fed animals. Despite their remarkable similarities to the lesions of cholesterol-fed rabbits and of homozygous patients with FH, the vascular lesions were referred to as atherosclerotic. Buja et al[91] considered them to be different from the dietary-induced lesions as indeed they may be but the WHHL rabbit vascular lesions are still not atherosclerotic. By two or three years WHHL rabbits develop severe stenosis of the ostium of the left coronary artery and also of its stem and branches resulting in myocardial ischemia and fibrosis. In true atherosclerosis in humans intimal tears and ulceration with thrombosis are the primary features of myocardial infarction which is not the case in either FH or the WHHL rabbit.

Several other inherited lipid disorders with lipid storage characteristics have been found in other animal species or produced experimentally in transgenic mice. Whilst they may be useful models for studying genetic lipid disorders, the vascular lesions are directly due to the lipid dystrophy, and do not support the lipid hypothesis of atherogenesis.

DIABETES MELLITUS

It is accepted that diabetes mellitus exhibits unusually severe atherosclerosis and in the International Atherosclerosis Project, despite geographic variations, the severity in the aorta and the coronary arteries was greater in diabetics than in nondiabetics.[92] Lipid infiltration of renal arterioles is pronounced and diabetic microangiopathy is manifested by thickening and irregular lamination of capillary basement membranes similar to that occurring in atherosclerosis.

Diabetics, with their high incidence of hypertension and obesity, have a particular propensity for CHD and the probability is that diabetes predisposes to atherosclerosis independently of hyperlipemia and hypertension. With its disturbance of lipid, carbohydrate and protein metabolism and a high susceptibility to infections, it is not surprising that the disease has an adverse effect on atherogenesis.

In preinsulin days when diabetics were given a high fat diet therapeutically, profound hypercholesterolemia (above 1300 mg/dL) was associated with a creamy plasma and widespread cutaneous xanthomatosis.[93-96] A familial occurrence of xanthomatosis diabeticorum was noted and xanthomatous vascular lesions with severe stenosis were reported. The intimal thickening of coronary arteries contained abundant foam cells, specifically described as yellowing xanthomatous patches of closely packed foam cells with the aortic and mitral valves similarly affected. This extravascular storage disease was very pronounced in such subjects with foam cells even in the walls of lymphatics. The similarity to the cholesterol-fed rabbit was recognized[94,95] and obviously there were similarities to FH, and yet this diabetic hypercholesterolemic xanthomatosis has been almost forgotten since the advent of insulin therapy. The condition was a lipid storage phenomenon superimposed on atherosclerosis, i.e., a mixed disease rather than the hypercholesterolemia merely accentuating and promoting atherogenesis.[85]

OBSTRUCTIVE JAUNDICE

It is not commonly known that obstructive jaundice may be associated with xanthomatosis. In 1873 Fagge[97] reported widespread cutaneous xanthomatosis (skin, tendons, larynx, trachea, left atrium, aorta, and the pulmonary, carotid, subclavian and innominate arteries) and said, "it would be a matter of indifference whether we should speak of the cutaneous disease as an atheroma of the skin or of the arterial lesion as a xanthelasma of the aorta". He added that in such cases he had never seen aortic ulceration as would be expected in atherosclerosis. Similar cases have been reported still with the widespread xanthomatosis and even giant foam cells as in the cholesterol-fed rabbit.[98,99]

Primary biliary cirrhosis of the liver without extrahepatic obstruction and secondary infective cholangitis is a rare but specific disease. A few of the subjects develop cutaneous xanthomata with the syndrome being called xanthomatous biliary cirrhosis.[99] There is no familial association and no history of familial CHD. Tendon xanthomata are lacking and extreme hypercholesterolemia is rare. In older literature severe generalized cutaneous xanthomatosis was at times seen without severe coronary lesions and vice versa. The critical

serum cholesterol level appeared to be 1800 mg/dL above which xanthomatosis occurred, this level being exceeded only in cases with the most severe hepatic damage.[99] Whilst there are reports of xanthomatous lesions of the heart and blood vessels, there has been no recent scientific comparison of the vascular lesions with atherosclerosis and the possibility exists that these isolated anecdotal cases may have had coexistent FH. If the syndrome (xanthomatous biliary cirrhosis) is authentic, then the evidence indicates that the vascular lesions were not truly atherosclerotic but rather mixed lesions due to superimposed lipid storage.

MYXEDEMA

The "myxedema heart" is at times associated with angina pectoris without severe coronary atherosclerosis.[100] Untreated myxedema may be associated with hypercholesterolemia as severe as in subjects with homozygous FH and xanthomatosis.[87,101,102] However this phenomenon occurred in a bygone era. The evidence is again anecdotal and the severity of atherosclerosis a subjective appraisal which should be addressed with caution since most myxedematous subjects are middle-aged or elderly when severe atherosclerosis is to be expected. Adequate controls are essential. Blumgart et al[103] reviewed 150 hypothyroid patients and concluded that the associated hypercholesterolemia did not appear to augment the severity of atherosclerosis. There was no xanthomatosis and the accompanying hypertension or renal disease may aggravate atherosclerosis rather than the hypercholesterolemia.

Hypothyroidism facilitates lipid deposition in the blood vessels of cholesterol-fed dogs, rats and other animals but there is no scientific evidence indicating augmentation of true human atherosclerosis by the hypercholesterolemia of myxedema. Instances in past literature purporting to support this causal relationship may have had a familial lipid disorder prior to and independent of hypothyroidism.[104]

THE NEPHROTIC SYNDROME

Hypercholesterolemia is recognized in the nephrotic syndrome and the allegation that there is an increased frequency of CHD in this syndrome is perpetuated in the literature without substantiating evidence. Even so Oppenheimer and Fishberg[94,95] considered the xanthomatous vascular lesions in nephrosis, like those of diabetes mellitus and obstructive jaundice, were identical in morphology and distribution to those of cholesterol-fed rabbits. There is no detailed study of the severity of atherosclerosis in nephrotic patients with adequate control material and until this is forthcoming, hypercholesterolemia associated with nephrosis cannot be accepted as accentuating atherosclerosis.

It must be concluded that there is insufficient evidence to support the thesis that (i) hypercholesterolemia associated with diabetes mellitus, chronic obstructive jaundice, myxedema and the nephrotic syndrome causes severe premature atherosclerosis and (ii) in the past when extreme hypercholesterolemia was present for whatever reason, the vascular lesions had characteristics of lipid storage similar to that in FH.[85]

FAMILIAL TYPE III HYPERLIPOPROTEINEMIA

This rare form of hyperlipoproteinemia has several synonyms including familial hypercholesterolemic xanthomatosis with hyperlipemia. There is both hypercholesterolemia and hypertriglyceridemia but the underlying metabolic defect has not been identified. The principal abnormal lipoproteins are ß-very low-density lipoproteins, differing from very low-density lipoprotein (VLDL) in apoprotein content with a higher proportion of cholesterol relative to triglyceride. Most have a deficiency of apolipoprotein E3. The age of detection has varied from 12 to 70 years with the mean age being 40 years in males and 49 years in females.[105,106] Characteristically there is yellow xanthomatous lipid deposition along the creases of the palm and possibly of the elbows, wrists, axillae, groin, knees, toes and breasts. Patients also develop tuberose xanthomata on their elbows, knees and buttocks, subperiosteal xanthomata over the tibial tuberosities and less often xanthomata of the Achilles tendons or extensor tendon of the hands. Xanthelasma palpebrarum and corneal arcus are sometimes present.[107] Hyperuricemia and an abnormal glucose tolerance test are features in almost half of the subjects.

Morganroth et al[106] reported 49 affected patients of whom 37% had ischemic heart disease and 27% peripheral vascular disease (11% having both). Cerebrovascular disease had become clinically manifest in only 10%. In three pooled series, Fredrickson et al[107] found ischemic heart disease in 33% and peripheral vascular disease in 27%. However the true incidence is difficult to estimate because ischemic heart disease was the reason for referral to the clinics and the incidence in a dermatology clinic is less.[105]

In the most detailed autopsy study[108,109] a 57-year-old woman also had diabetes mellitus, cholesterolosis of the gall bladder, numerous ceroid-containing foam cells in the enlarged spleen and bone marrow and subendocardial xanthomatous deposits in the left atrium. Foam cell infiltrations of the coronary arteries were pronounced and several vessels were occluded by foam cells which no doubt contributed to her recurrent myocardial infarction but there was no mural thrombosis. Cholesterol clefts and pultaceous deposits were absent. The mitral valve was affected and the aorta and iliac arteries exhibited complicated plaques but no mention was made of ulcerations and thrombi.

Other reports support the general findings of xanthomatous vascular disease including cardiac valvular involvement, extravascular involvement and extravascular xanthomatous infiltrations.[105,110-112] Intimal foam cells have been seen in vasa vasorum.[110] These observations suggest the disorder is characterized by lipid storage in blood vessels and extravascular tissues. In type III hyperlipoproteinemia there is no doubt that vascular storage occurs but the age distribution of these subjects indicates that combined atherosclerosis will be present. It cannot be assumed that these subjects or those with FH are free from atherosclerosis. As with heterozygous FH, there is a need for a detailed, qualitative and quantitative comparative study of the vascular lesions with atherosclerosis of normolipidemic individuals.

The histology of the obstructing lesions has in some cases been characterized by a plethora of foam cells simulating the cholesterol-fed rabbit.[112] The apparent amenability to therapy is of interest and reminiscent of dietary-induced lesions in rabbits although nothing is known of the histological sequelae following resorption of lipid from the vessel wall in type III.

When rabbits, dogs, swine, rats and monkeys[113-117] are subjected to high cholesterol diets, they develop lipoproteins equivalent to ß-VLDL with an excess of cholesterol in relation to triglyceride, and are rich in apoprotein E, poor in apoprotein C and abundant in apoprotein B.[105] This similarity to type III in man raises further doubts about the applicability of the cholesterol-fed rabbit and type III hyperlipoproteinemia to human atherosclerosis.

TYPE I HYPERLIPOPROTEINEMIA

The rare familial type I syndrome, genetically discrete and consistent in its clinical manifestations,[118] is also termed familial hyperchylomicronemia and familial lipoprotein lipase deficiency. It has been attributed to diminished activity of lipoprotein lipase (LPL) which catalyzes an important step in the extrahepatic removal of triglyceride-rich lipoprotein from the blood. Massive accumulations of chylomicrons develop in the plasma with a corresponding increase of plasma triglyceride concentrations and low levels of low density and high density lipoprotein. The very low density lipoprotein level is normal. Heterozygotes exhibit a 50% decrease of lipoprotein lipase activity with normal or only slightly elevated plasma triglyceride levels.[119]

Recurrent attacks of pancreatitis are a feature,[119,120] as are manifestations of extravascular lipid storage viz papulo-eruptive xanthomatosis, foam cell infiltration of bone marrow, lymph nodes, liver and spleen (with hepatosplenomegaly), and lipemia retinalis.[107,109,121] Despite moderate hypercholesterolemia there is no clinical evidence of premature severe atherosclerosis.[109,119] Autopsy material is minimal and though atherosclerosis develops, it was not unduly severe in the five cases so far studied.[119] Subendocardial lipid deposition has been reported in a 30-year-old male but no macroscopic arterial lesions were found.[109,122,123]

Though type I patients are not thought to have a propensity for CHD, Malmros et al[120] reported angina or myocardial infarction clinically in a few of their patients. Most were well within the age range when these complications of atherosclerosis are to be expected, i.e., over 60 years of age, and there is no evidence of undue severity of atherosclerosis in the young.[124]

TYPE IV HYPERLIPOPROTEINEMIA

Type IV is genetically heterogeneous and not necessarily a familial disorder. It is characterized by an increase in plasma VLDL (hyperprebetalipoproteinemia) of normal composition and mobility and is probably the most common lipid abnormality. The total plasma cholesterol is either normal or increased and triglycerides are markedly elevated. Most patients exhibit moderate obesity, abnormal glucose tolerance or overt diabetes mellitus, hyperuricemia and hypertension.[118] Only rarely are xanthomata, hepatosplenomegaly and lipemia retinalis observed but arcus corneae and xanthelasma are frequent. Though the disorder is believed to be associated with a propensity for premature severe atherosclerosis, the nature of this increased risk is uncertain. To some authors CHD is prevalent, but the risk has not yet been evaluated accurately.[109,122] To others coronary disease is not particularly prominent in type IV families.[125] Cerebral and peripheral vascular disease occur much less frequently. Though no firm data regarding the qualitative or quantitative nature of the arterial lesions in type IV hyperlipoproteinemia exists, in view of the frequency of hypertension, diabetes mellitus and hyperuricemia, it is not surprising that the development of a degenerative disease of blood vessels such as atherosclerosis is enhanced.

TYPE V HYPERLIPOPROTEINEMIA

This lipid abnormality is relatively uncommon and represents a small percentage of patients with CHD.[118] It is characterized by a mixed hyperlipemia with elevated chylomicrons and pre-ß lipoproteins in the fasting state. Plasma cholesterol and triglyceride concentrations are elevated but variable.[126] Nikkilä[119] regards primary type V as a genetic syndrome not a separate disease.

Typically the type V subject is an adult, possibly middle-aged, with a family history of diabetes mellitus and CHD. Most (80%) have an abnormal glucose tolerance test and hyperuricemia. Bouts of abdominal pain or pancreatitis occur in severe cases[107] and about one-third have hepatomegaly. Some have a peripheral neuropathy which is ill understood and hypertension is prevalent.[119] Eruptive xanthomata may occur in up to half of the subjects[119] and hepatomegaly in 57%. Xanthomatous retinopathy and foam cell infiltration of the bone marrow have also been reported.[119]

There is doubt as to whether type V subjects are prone to develop premature severe atherosclerosis.[107,118] The reported frequency of ischemic heart disease clinically has varied between 15 and 24%.[119] However the abnormal glucose tolerance test, the hyperuricemia, hypertension and the possibility of a familial tendency to atherosclerosis and CHD independently of the lipid metabolic defect could account for enhanced atherosclerosis severity if it exists.

FAMILIAL STORAGE DISEASES OF STEROLS OTHER THAN CHOLESTEROL

There are two storage diseases of sterols other than cholesterol.

(I) CEREBROTENDINOUS XANTHOMATOSIS

Cerebro-tendinous xanthomatosis is a rare familial sterol storage disorder believed to be transmitted as an autosomal recessive trait and characterized by xanthomata of tendons, lungs and brain despite a normal or low plasma cholesterol level.[127] Cholestanol and cholesterol accumulate in every tissue secondary to an abnormality in cholesterol metabolism.[128]

Small amounts of cholestanol have been found to accompany cholesterol in virtually every mammalian tissue and it is believed to be synthesized solely from cholesterol. The underlying metabolic mechanism, though unclear, is thought to be due to a defect in bile acid synthesis.[128] The plasma cholesterol level is usually normal and the plasma cholestanol level is characteristically elevated, but both are stored in excess in virtually all tissues.[127,128] There may be some defect in the incorporation of cholesterol into the cell membrane of myelin and the tissues, some of the cholesterol being replaced by cholestanol but there is certainly more cholesterol than cholestanol in the xanthomatous lesions. Cholesterol esters account for up to 49% of the total esterified sterols in abnormal brain tissue and cholestanol accounts for up to 11% of total sterols in tendon xanthomata, 6% of the total plasma sterols being associated principally with the LDL.[127]

Tendon xanthomata occur as early as 15

years superficially resembling those of FH but severe cerebral manifestations dominate the disease, with the patients incapacitated by the fourth or fifth decade generally.[128] Death usually occurs between the fourth and sixth decades. Tuberose and palpebral xanthomata may be present. Histologically they are indistinguishable from those in other hyperlipoproteinemias. Granulomatous lesions containing cholesterol crystals, multinucleated giant cells and large foam cells have been observed in the lung and bones. Lipid and foam cell deposits are common about blood vessels. Several patients with this disease have died following myocardial infarction (aged 60, 46, 48 and 36 years) but in many others evidence of cardiovascular disease was absent or not mentioned. Salen[129] recorded two deaths from myocardial infarction, both in males (aged 36 and 48 years). They were said to have "extensive atheromatous infiltrations" throughout the coronary arteries but no mention of thrombosis was made or of severity or distribution in the aorta. The aorta and atherosclerotic lesions in one patient contained 2% and 2.8% of total sterols as cholestanol, the highest level being in the plaques.[129] Another patient of 46 years died of cardiac arrhythmia six weeks after suffering an acute myocardial infarction but no pathological detail was provided regarding vascular disease.[130]

Though the incidence of CHD is low, the possibility exists that lipid storage in the arteries may be enhanced, at least in some patients, despite normal or low serum cholesterol levels.[128] The absence of aneurysms, ulceration, thrombosis and cerebral involvement is consistent with this. Involvement of the coronary arteries that leads to ischemic changes is particularly the case in fat storage diseases. A similar tendency in cerebrotendinous xanthomatosis is as yet unproven. If deposition of these sterols occurs in this metabolic disorder however, it only indicates the nonspecificity of lipid localization in arteries in such storage diseases.

(II) SITOSTEROLEMIA AND XANTHOMATOSIS

This is a rare familial disorder of which only 16 cases have been recorded.[127,128] The metabolic defect has yet to be determined. The three plant sterols (phytosterols) viz ß-sitosterol, campesterol and stigmasterol are usually found only in plant lipids but small quantities are absorbed naturally by man and excreted in bile and skin secretions. Though normally only small amounts are present in the blood of humans, during infancy larger amounts of sitosterol can be found in the blood. They have been detected in the aortas of infants fed vegetable oil-rich diets.

High blood levels of the three plant sterols, particularly ß-sitosterol, occur in this disorder and have been attributed to enhanced intestinal absorption and possibly diminished excretion[128] but other metabolic defects may occur concurrently. Possibly the augmented levels of the plant sterol interfere with normal lipoprotein sterols, thus favoring tissue deposition secondary to hypercholesterolemia and hyperbetalipoproteinemia.[128,129]

Major clinical manifestations are tendon and subcutaneous xanthomas including xanthelasma and at times arthritis.[131] However, premature severe atherosclerosis has been suggested as a complication.[128] One affected 29-year-old male had normocholesterolemia, hemolysis, hypersplenism, an aortic systolic murmur and premature coronary atherosclerosis requiring triple coronary bypass surgery.[132] A 12-year-old girl afflicted with xanthomatosis had aortic stenosis and angina pectoris[123] reminiscent of the storage phenomena of FH but the coronary arteries were reported as normal.

Bevans and Mosbach[134] fed two rabbits ß-sitosterol for four weeks but found no aortic lesions. This experiment cannot be regarded as conclusive. Evidence of a predisposition to vascular disease in the case of human sitosterolemia is not conclusive either but the finding of severe arterial lesions in at least four subjects (one with aortic stenosis also) and at times an associated arthritis is reminiscent of homozygous FH. The cell membrane fragility in this disease (hemolytic anemic) could theoretically aggravate lipid deposition in the vessel wall by enhancing the production of matrix vesicles.[41] Qualitative and quantitative morphological studies of the vascular changes are needed and also chemical analyses of the lesions. Comments regarding the significance of vascular lesions in cerebrotendinous xanthomatosis are equally applicable to this disorder.

TANGIER DISEASE (FAMILIAL HDL DEFICIENCY)

Tangier disease is a rare disorder, apparently due to an autosomal recessive gene (consanguinous matings in 25% of cases). There is an absence of normal high density lipoprotein (HDL) in plasma and storage of cholesterol esters in histiocytic foam cells in many tissues viz liver, spleen, lymph nodes, thymus, intestinal mucosa, skin and cornea, bone marrow etc. There is a low plasma cholesterol level and normal or elevated triglyceride levels in patients with enlarged yellow-orange tonsils and adenoid tissue.[135,136] The small amount of HDL in the plasma differs quantitatively and qualitatively from normal HDL, particularly regarding apolipoprotein content (low apo A1 levels). Abnormal catabolism of HDL by macrophages has been recognized. Neurological disturbances are prevalent but clinical vascular disease is not a striking feature of homozygotes or heterozygotes with Tangier disease at 40 years or younger. There is evidence of CHD in a few older patients[136,137] and some are hypertensive. The paucity of significant data precludes any generalization regarding premature atherosclerosis in this disease associated with a low blood level of HDL.[135,136] The absence of any firm evidence of an aggravating effect on atherosclerosis does not support the thesis that an elevated blood HDL level independently aggravates or promotes atherosclerosis.

WOLMAN'S DISEASE AND CHOLESTEROL ESTER STORAGE DISEASE

These two diseases are associated with prodigious amount of cholesterol esters and often triglyceride in lysosomes.[138,139] Wolman's disease is the more severe form inherited as an autosomal recessive trait. Only some 25 cases have been reported. It is usually fatal within six months and associated with enlarged calcified adrenal glands. Apart from anemia and acanthosis there is an accumulation of lipid in the liver, heart and muscle and foam cells in the spleen, lymph nodes, tonsils, thymus, bone marrow, adrenals, intestinal wall, kidneys, leptomeninges, thyroid and gonads. Foam cells have been found in the circulating blood and lipid is demonstrable in vascular endothelium, neurones etc. Some lipid deposition has been recorded in the aorta of a few infants[140,141] but frank atherosclerosis has not been alleged. The bulk of the lipid accumulated is cholesterol.[138] Plasma cholesterol and triglycerides are normal in most patients who are considered to have a deficiency in acid cholesterol ester hydrolase activity.[142]

Cholesterol ester storage disease, a rare familial disorder of uncertain inheritance, is also characterized by hepatosplenomegaly and accumulation of cholesterol esters and triglycerides, mainly in lysosomes in liver, spleen, lymph nodes, intestinal mucosa and other tissues. The disease may not be recognized until adulthood. There is hypercholesterolemia and some degree of hypertriglyceridemia. Lipid deposition is abnormal in many cells including hepatocytes, adrenal cortical cells, smooth muscle cells of the lamina propria of the gastrointestinal tract, blood vessels, endothelial cells, the reticuloendothelial cells in liver, spleen, lymphoid tissue and bone marrow and occasionally in neutrophils and lymphocytes and cultured fibroblasts.[138] There may also be cirrhosis and portal hypertension. None of the 24 patients so far reported have had clinical evidence of premature severe atherosclerosis[142] although three patients who have come to autopsy had severe disease. One patient (aged 21) had up to 75% stenosis of coronary arteries as well as cerebral atherosclerosis of less severity and some myocardial necrosis but died of aortic valvular stenosis.[142,143] The other patient, who died at nine years of age, had a few elevated yellow plaques in the ascending aorta.[144] The similarity to FH (aortic stenosis and involvement of the proximal aorta) is noteworthy although no xanthomata occur in this disease. The lipid accumulation in endothelial and smooth muscle cells is similar to the dietary-induced lesions in the rabbit.[138,142] Assman and Fredrickson[142] have suggested that most patients with cholesterol ester storage disease may be under increased risk of developing premature atherosclerosis but the evidence for such a claim is poorly founded. It is possible that atherosclerotic changes occurring spontaneously in these patients may be aggravated by the superadded accumulation of lipid since this is a lipid storage disease and by virtue of the generalized metabolic defect likely to affect all cells.

LIPOPROTEIN LIPASE DEFICIENCY— FAMILIAL COMBINED HYPERLIPIDEMIA

Lipoprotein lipase (LPL) is a key enzyme involved in the metabolism of triglyceride-rich lipoproteins and occasionally severe hypertriglyceridemia occurs due to a deficiency in either apo C11 or LPL. It is thought that mutations in the LPL gene may make a significant contribution to the development of hyperlipidemia and atherosclerosis in the general population.[145] The homozygous form occurs in about one in a million individuals but the blood triglyceride levels are not particularly high. The lipoprotein pattern is of a mildly elevated blood cholesterol with or without elevated triglycerides, a lipid pattern referred to as familial combined hyperlipidemia. The link with atherosclerosis is based on epidemiological not pathological grounds. An aggravating effect on atherosclerosis has yet to be demonstrated and the effect of a mildly elevated blood cholesterol level on atherogenesis is unproven but any genetic metabolic defect might aggravate a chronic degenerative disease to some extent. This however has to be proven by pathological and experimental evidence not on the assumed validity of weak epidemiological correlations using inappropriate methodology.

OTHER HERITABLE METABOLIC DISORDERS

Several nonlipid heritable metabolic disorders affect blood vessels and exhibit tissue storage of a metabolite (often in blood vessels) with widespread cellular and connective tissue dysfunction. A generalized metabolic disorder will affect some viscera more than others depending on the metabolic pathway but some aggravate naturally occurring degenerative diseases involving blood vessels, cardiac valves and joints, e.g., Fabry's disease, homocystinuria, Hurler's syndrome, Scheie's syndrome, Morquio's syndrome and alkaptonuria.[85]

These metabolic storage diseases are associated with sclerotic vascular disease and storage phenomena (often in blood vessels). Mostly these disorders have considerable sclerotic intimal thickening, aortic valve stenosis, arthritic disorders and at times aneurysms, varicosities, vascular occlusions and stenoses of the coronary ostia with ischemic changes. Lysosomal storage of metabolites is common and the term thesaurosclerosis has been suggested and their similarity to "cholesterol storage" noted.[146] Whilst their vascular effects have some similarities to atherosclerosis, they are superimposed on, but not identical to atherosclerosis, and in this respect are analogous to FH.

Lysosomal storage may be detrimental to cell function in the vessel wall but generalized metabolic disorders can cause connective tissue dysfunction with an adverse effect on "wear and tear" degenerative diseases, hence the propensity for involvement of cardiac valve cusps (on the left side), arteries and joints.

Other metabolic diseases such as Menke's kinky hair disease, homocystinuria, progeria, Werner's syndrome and hereditary connective tissue diseases simulate atherosclerosis and produce some of its complications but the metabolic effect, when known, aggravates or is superimposed on atherosclerosis. In any epidemiological or pathological study these disorders should be considered in separate categories as should FH, FDB and type III hyperlipoproteinemia.

COMMENTARY

On present evidence the lipid hypothesis does not explain the pathology of atherosclerosis, its pathogenesis, topography or complications. The most significant inconsistency is the development of accelerated atherosclerosis in venous bypass grafts and arteriovenous shunts for renal dialysis when the veins, if left intact like veins elsewhere in the body, would have remained virtually unaffected for the remaining years of life. This unexplained inconsistency alone necessitates review of the premises on which the lipid hypothesis rests.

Not many years ago there was much emphasis on Fredrickson's types IV and V hyperlipoproteinemia and other lipid dystrophies but there is no evidence that they have a causal relationship to atherosclerosis. This may be the reason interest in their relationship to CHD and atherosclerosis waned.

Emphasis has shifted more to FH and various apolipoproteins and their variants. It is acknowledged that some apolipoproteins may be detrimental but like FH they are abnormalities of lipid or lipoprotein metabolism, and as

such cannot be causal. Their pathological effects must be demonstrated and cannot be assumed by associating their presence, or any excess or deficiency with variation in blood LDL or HDL levels.

There is sufficient evidence to doubt the validity of the common allegation that hypercholesterolemia associated with diabetes mellitus, obstructive jaundice, myxedema and the nephrotic syndrome accelerates the development of premature atherosclerosis. The presence of lipid in the blood vessel wall is not pathognomonic of atherosclerosis being associated with several pathological states or diseases. Scientifically the onus is on the pathologist to determine the underlying disease responsible rather than assuming that atherosclerosis is responsible for most instances.

Atherosclerosis and the vascular lesions of FH are not identical and their etiology, pathogenesis and pathological differences cannot be ignored. Since the homozygous form is the purest form of FH and the strongest clinical evidence that hypercholesterolemia causes CHD and premature severe atherosclerosis, most emphasis has to be placed on comparisons between homozygous FH and atherosclerosis in normolipidemic individuals. The evidence provided suggests that the vascular lesions peculiar to FH and indeed other extreme hypercholesterolemic states from whatever cause are lipid storage phenomena superimposed on ubiquitous atherosclerosis. Other metabolic disorders briefly discussed with or without tissue storage of some metabolite display variable features which have something in common with atherosclerosis. However it would be erroneous to allege that the vascular manifestations of these diseases are all atherosclerotic. Some storage diseases have much in common with FH and such features are nonspecific reactions that differ substantially from atherosclerosis. The ill-effects of tissue storage in the blood vessel wall can have secondary consequences such as fibrosis and calcification but it would still be scientifically misleading to classify the vascular lesions of FH as atherosclerotic. An infection (cholangitis) complicating an obstructive biliary cirrhosis produces a mixture of two diseases. The combination is not biliary cirrhosis pathologically.

Pathologists of independent mind and free from preconceived ideas would have to conclude from the available evidence that the vascular lesions of the cholesterol-fed animal and of FH are not atherosclerotic pathologically.[57,58,76,85] Most investigators seemingly are unaware of the extent of the differences in pathology and differences in the occurrence of complications of spontaneous atherosclerosis and the widespread extravascular storage phenomena of experimental dietary induced lesions and those of FH. Excessive preoccupation with lipid in the lesions has led to the neglect of the fundamental differences which are of kind and not of degree.

The pathological differences between atherosclerosis and the vascular lesions of dietary-induced lipid deposition in experimental animals cannot be ignored. Since pathologically it is necessary at times to resort to electron microscopy, special stains, histochemistry and immunological techniques to reach a correct diagnosis, it is incongruous that such differences indicated above and reviewed in more detail elsewhere[57,58] continue to be ignored. Acknowledging differences between the vascular lesions of cholesterol-fed animals and human atherosclerosis whilst continuing to refer to the dietary-induced lesions as atherosclerosis is scientific misrepresentation and misleads those in other disciplines. This widespread misrepresentation of the pathology of dietary-induced lipid deposition and of FH has been in large part responsible for the dominance of the lipid hypothesis which in atherosclerosis research has excluded alternative and more profitable avenues of investigation.

This review and the conclusions reached do not preclude considerations of an adverse role of lipids in atherogenesis. It has been indicated that hypercholesterolemia in rabbits can retard repair in the vascular wall and excessive lysosomal storage of lipid in endothelial and smooth muscle cells may be detrimental to their other cellular functions or make the cells more susceptible to hemodynamic stress by having several large lipid vacuoles in their cytoplasm. The massive subendothelial accumulation of lipid-laden lipophages and extracellular lipid would not provide the viscoelastic properties of the wall that are necessary to withstand hemodynamic stresses and thus cell degeneration and necrosis could ensue with secondary fibrosis and calcification. The lipid accumulation could also act as a space occupying lesion much as occurs in FH and the cholesterol-fed rabbit and causes myocardial ischemia. The lipid dystrophies may have an aggravating effect on cell metabolism which would be aggravated by any chronic degenerative disease. Each of these possibilities is plausible and realistic but some require substantiation.

THE LIPID HYPOTHESIS

The lack of pathological and experimental support for the lipid hypothesis undermines its validity. Unless these criticisms can be adequately countered by scientific evidence to the contrary, the lipid hypothesis must be revised or discarded. However, as indicated, lipid and cholesterol are important constituents of the vessel wall and participate in the pathogenesis of atherosclerosis as do the other normal mural constituents (collagen, elastin, proteoglycans, glycolipids, minerals, endothelium, smooth muscle cells, monocytes, etc), but it is inappropriate and implausible to invoke a dominant or causal role for any one of these constituents in the etiology of atherosclerosis. All are interrelated participants in this ubiquitous degenerative disease.

References

1. Stehbens WE. Cerebral aneurysms of animals other than man. J Pathol Bacteriol 1963; 86:161-8.

2. Stehbens WE. Hemodynamics and the Blood Vessel Wall. Springfield: C C Thomas, 1979.

3. Roberts WC, Bujo LM. The frequency and significance of coronary arterial thrombi and other observations in fatal acute myocardial infarction. Am J Med 1972; 52:425-43.

4. Stehbens WE. Causality in medical science with particular reference to coronary heart disease and atherosclerosis. Perspect Biol Med 1992; 36:97-119.

5. MacCallum WG. Arteriosclerosis. Physiol Rev 1922; 2:70-91

6. Moschcowitz E. The cause of arteriosclerosis. Am J Med Sc 1929; 178:244-67

7. Hueper WE. The relation between etiology and morphology in degenerative and sclerosing vas-

cular diseases, Biol.Sympos 1945; 11:1-42.

8. Stehbens WE. Experimental induction of atherosclerosis associated with femoral arteriovenous fistulae in rabbits on a stock diet. Atherosclerosis 1992; 95:127-35.

9. Stehbens WE. Pathology of the Cerebral Blood Vessels. St Louis: CV Mosby, 1972.

10. Meyer WW, Walsh SZ, Lind J. Functional morphology of human arteries during fetal and post natal development. In: Schwartz CJ, Werthessen NT, Wolf S. eds. Structure and function of the circulation. Vol 1 New York: Plenum Press, 1980:95-379.

11. Eisenbrey AB. Arteriovenous aneurysm of the superficial femoral vessels. JAMA 1913; 61:2155-7.

12. Stehbens WE, Karmody AM. Venous atherosclerosis associated with arteriovenous fistulas for hemodialysis. Arch Surg 1975; 110:176-80.

13. Stehbens WE. Histopathology of cerebral aneurysms. Arch Neurol 1963; 8:272-85.

14. Greenhill NS, Stehbens WE. Scanning electron-microscopic study of experimentally induced intimal tears in rabbit arteries. Atherosclerosis 1983; 49:119-26.

15. Greenhill NS, Stehbens WE. Haemodynamically induced intimal tears in U-shaped arterial loops as seen by scanning electron microscopy. Br J Exp Pathol 1985; 66:577-84.

16. Greenhill NS, Stehbens WE. Scanning electron mocroscopic investigation of the afferent arteries of experimental femoral arteriovenous fistulae in rabbits. Pathology 1987; 19:22-7.

17. Stehbens WE, Martin BJ, Delahunt B. Light and scanning electron microscopic changes observed in experimental arterial forks of rabbits. Int J Exp Pathol 1991; 73:183-93.

18. Martin BJ, Stehbens WE, Davis PF et al. Scanning electron microscopic study of hemodynamically induced tears in the internal elastic lamina of rabbit arteries. Pathology 1989; 21:207-12.

19. Stehbens WE. Atherosclerosis—Its cause and nature. Speculations Sc Technol 1988; 11:89-99.

20. Lendon CL, Davis MJ, Born GVR et al. Atherosclerotic plaque caps are locally weakened when macrophage density is increased. Atherosclerosis 1991; 87:87-90.

21. Heath D, Edwards JE, Smith LA. The rheologic significance of medial necrosis and dissecting aneurysm of the ascending aorta in association with calcific aortic stenosis. Proc Staff Meet Mayo Clin 1958; 33:228-34.

22. McKusick VA, Logue RB, Bahnson HT. Association of aortic valvular disease and cystic medical necrosis of the ascending aorta. Circulation 1957; 16:188-94.

23. Stehbens WE. Focal intimal proliferation in the cerebral arteries. Am J Pathol 1960; 36:289-301.

24. Stehbens WE. The renal artery in normal and cholesterol-fed rabbits. Am J Pathol 1963; 43:969-85.

25. Jaffé D, Hartroft WS, Manning M et al. Coronary arteries in newborn children. Acta Paediat Scand 1971 (Suppl); 219:3-28.

26. Levene CI. The pathogenesis of atheroma of the coronary arteries. J Pathol Bacteriol 1956; 72:83-6.

27. Imparato AM, Lord JW, Texon M et al. Experimental atherosclerosis produced by alteration of blood vessel configuration. Surg Forum 1961; 12:245-7.

28. Stehbens WE. Intimal proliferation and spontaneous lipid deposition in the cerebral arteries of sheep and steers. J Atheroscl Res 1965; 5:556-68.

29. Ross R. The pathogenesis of atherosclerosis—an update. N Engl J Med 1986; 314:488-99.

30. Nathan I, Imparato AM. Vibration analysis in experimental models of atherosclerosis. Bull N Y Acad Med 1977; 53:849-68.

31. Stehbens WE. Experimental arterial loops and arterial atrophy. Exp Mol Pathol 1986; 44:177-89.

32. Stehbens WE. Cerebral atherosclerosis: Intimal proliferation and atherosclerosis in the cerebral arteries. Arch Pathol 1975; 99:582-91.

33. Stehbens WE, Ludatscher RM. Ultrastructure of the renal arterial bifurcation of rabbits. Exp Mol Pathol 1973; 18:50-67.

34. Rogers KM, Stehbens WE. The morphology of matrix vesicles produced in experimental arterial aneurysms of rabbits. Pathology 1986; 18:64-71.

35. Stehbens WE, Martin BJ. Ultrastructural alterations of collagen fibrils in blood vessel walls. Connect Tissue Res 1993; In press.

36. Martin BJ, Leppien B, Stehbens WE. Changes in collagen fibril morphology in experimental aneurysms and arteriovenous fistulae in sheep. Int J Exp Pathol 1993;In press.

37. Cliff WJ. The aortic tunica intima in ageing rats. Exp Mol Pathol 1970; 13:172-89.

38. Esterly JA, Glagov S, Ferguson DJ. Morphogenesis of intimal obliterative hyperplasia of small arteries in experimental pulmonary hypertension. Am J Pathol 1968; 52:325-47.

39. Aikawa M, Koletsky S. Arteriosclerosis of the mesenteric arteries of rats with renal hypertension. Am J Pathol 1970; 61:293-322.

40. Stehbens WE. Ultrastructure of aneurysms. Arch Neurol 1975; 32:798-807.

41. Stehbens WE. The role of lipid in the pathogenesis of atherosclerosis. Lancet 1975; 1:724-7.

42. Stehbens WE. The ultrastructure of experimental aneurysms in rabbits. Pathology 1985; 17:87-95.

43. Stehbens WE. The ultrastructure of the anastomosed vein of experimental arteriovenous fistulae in sheep. Am J Pathol 1974; 76:377-400.

44. Greenhill NS, Presland MR, Rogers KM et al. X-ray microanalysis of mineralized matrix vesicles of experimental saccular aneurysms. Exp Mol Pathol 1985; 43:220-32.

45. Stehbens WE, Ludatscher RM. The susceptibility of renal arterial forks in rabbits to dietary-induced lipid absorption. Pathology 1983; 15:475-85.

46. Stehbens WE. Intracranial arterial aneurysms and atherosclerosis. Thesis, Univ of Syd. 1958.

47. Stehbens WE. Haemodynamic production of lipid deposition, intimal tears, mural dissection and thrombosis in the blood vessel wall. Proc Roy Soc (London) Ser B, 1974; 185:357-73.

48. Ferguson GG. Turbulence in human intracranial saccular aneurysm. J Neurosurg 1970; 33:485-97.

49. Stehbens WE. Experimental production of aneurysm by microvascular surgery in rabbits. Vasc Surg 1973; 7:165-75.

50. Stehbens WE. Chronic vascular changes in the walls of experimental berry aneurysms of the aortic bifurcation in rabbits. Stroke 1981; 12:643-7.

51. Stehbens WE. Chronic changes in experimental saccular and fusiform aneurysms in rabbits. Arch Pathol 1981; 105:603-9.

52. Stehbens WE. Experimental arteriovenous fistulae in normal and cholesterol-fed rabbits. Pathology 1973; 5:311-24.

53. Stehbens WE. Predilection of experimental arterial aneurysms for dietary-induced lipid deposition. Pathology 1981; 13:735-47.

54. Hazama F, Hashimoto N. An animal model of cerebral aneurysms. Neuropathol Appl Neurobiol 1987; 13:77-90.

55. Page IH, Stamler J. Diet and coronary heart disease. Mod Concepts Cardiovasc Dis 1968; 37:119-23.

56. Anitschkow NN. A history of experimentation on arterial atherosclerosis in animals. In: Blumenthal HT. ed. Cowdry's Arteriosclerosis. Springfield: CC Thomas, 1967:21-44.

57. Stehbens WE. An appraisal of cholesterol-feeding in experimental atherogenesis. Progr Cardiovasc Dis 1986: 29:107-28.

58. Stehbens WE. Vascular complications in experimental atherosclerosis. Progr Cardiovasc Dis 1986; 29:221-37.

59. Stehbens WE, Silver MD. Arterial lesions induced by methyl cellulose. Am J Pathol 1965; 48:483-501.

60. Cliff WJ. Experiments on animals and human populations. In: Cliff WJ, Schoefl GI, eds. Coronaries and Cholesterol. London: Chapman and Hall, 1989:55-74.

61. Constantinides P, Booth J, Carlson G. Production of advanced cholesterol atherosclerosis in the rabbit. Arch Pathol 1960; 70:712-24.

62. Constantinides P, Chakaravarti RH. Rabbit arterial thrombosis production by systemic procedures. Arch Pathol 1961; 72:197-208.

63. Vesselinovitch D. Animal models and the study of atherosclerosis. Arch Pathol 1988; 112: 1011-7.

64. Carey KD. Nonhuman primate models of atherosclerosis. In: Strong WB, ed. Atherosclerosis. New York: Grune & Stratton,1978, 41-83. 65. Katz LN, Stamler J. Experimental Atherosclerosis. Springfield: CC Thomas, 1953.

66. Dawber TR. The Framingham Study. The Epidemiology of Atherosclerotic Disease. Cambridge: Harvard Univ. 1980.

67. Oliver MF. Serum cholesterol—the knave of hearts and the joker. Lancet, 1981; 2:1090-5.

68. Goldstein JL, Brown MS. Familial hypercholesterolemia. In: Stanbury JB, Wyngaarden DS, Fredrickson DS et al. eds. The Metabolic Basis of Inherited Disease. 5th ed. New York: McGraw Hill, 1983:672-712.

69. Buja LM, Kovanen PT, Bilheimer DW. Cellular pathology of homozygous familial hypercholesterolemia. Am J Pathol 1979; 97: 327-58.

70. Slack J. Risks of ischaemic heart-disease in fa-

milial hyperlipoproteinaemic states. Lancet 1969; 2:1380-2.

71. Yamamoto A, Kamiya T, Yamamura T et al. Clinical features of familial hypercholesterolemia. Arteriosclerosis 1989; 9 Suppl 1:1-66; 1-74.

72. Tybjäerg-Hansen A, Humphries SE. Familial defective apolipoprotein B-100: a single mutation that causes hypercholesterolemia and premature coronary artery disease. Atherosclerosis 1992; 96:91-107.

73. Thompson GR, Seed M, Niththyananthan S et al. Genotypic and phenotypic variation in familial hypercholesterolemia. Arteriosclerosis 1989;(Suppl 1) 9:1-75; 1-80.

74. Slack J. Inheritance of familial hypercholesterolemia. Atherosclerosis Rev 1979; 5: 35-66.

75. Allen JM, Thompson GR, Myant NB et al. Cardiovascular complications of homozygous familial hypercholesteraemia. Br Heart J 1980; 44:361-8.

76. Stehbens WE, Martin M. The vascular pathology of familial hypercholesterolemia. Pathology 1991; 23:54-61.

77. Khachadurian AK, Uthman SM. Experiences with the homozygous cases of familial hypercholesterolemia. Nutr Metabol 1973; 15:132-40.

78. Thannhauser SJ, Schmidt G. Lipins and Lipidosis Physiol Rev 1946; 26:275-318.

79. Hess FO. Allgemeine Xanthomatose, Herztod infolge schwerer xanthomatöser Veränderungen des Gefässsystems. Münch Medizin Wochenshr 1934; 13:579-80.

80. Mabuchi H. Tatami R. Haba T et al. Homozygous familial hypercholesterolemia in Japan. Am J Med 1976; 65:290-7.

81. Khachadurian AK. Migratory polyarthritis in familial hypercholesterolemia (type II hyperlipoproteinemia) Arthritis Rheum 1968; 11:385-393.

82. Adlersberg D. Hypercholesterolemia with predisposition to atherosclerosis. Am J Med 1951; 11:600-14.

83. Harris-Jones JN, Jones EG, Wells PG. Xanthomatosis and essential hypercholesterolaemia. Lancet 1957; 1:855-7.

84. Khachadurian AK. A general review of clinical and laboratory features of familial hypercholesterolemia (Type II hyperlipoproteinemia). Protides Biol Fluids 1971; 19:315-8.

85. Stehbens WE, Wierzbicki. The relationship of hypercholesterolemia to atherosclerosis with particular emphasis on familial hypercholesterolemia, diabetes mellitus, obstructive jaundice, myxedema and the nephrotic syndrome. Progr Cardiovasc Dis 1988; 30:289-306.

86. Hess FO. Über allegemeine Xanthomatose. Verhand deutsch Gesselschaft inn Med 1934; 46:355-9.

87. Hueper WC. Arteriosclerosis. Arch Pathol 1944; 38:162-81, 245-85, 350-64: 1945; 39:51-65, 117-31, 187-216.

88. Stehbens WE. The lipid hypothesis and the role of hemodynamics in atherogenesis. Prog Cardiovasc Dis 1990; 33:119-36.

89. Schuster H. Rauh G. Kormann B et al. Familial defective apolipoprotein B-100. Comparison with familial hypercholesterolemia in 18 cases detected in Munich. Arteriosclerosis 1990; 10:577-81.

90. Watanabe Y. Serial inbreeding of rabbits with hereditary hyperlipidemia (WHHL-rabbit). Atherosclerosis 1980; 36:261-8.

91. Buja LM, Kita T, Goldstein JL et al. Cellular pathology of progressive atherosclerosis in the WHHL rabbit, an animal model of familial hypercholesterolemia. Arteriosclerosis 1983; 3: 87-101.

92. Robertson WB, Strong JP. Atherosclerosis in persons with hypertension and diabetes mellitus. Lab Invest 1968; 18:538-51.

93. Smith MG. Hyperplasia of lipoid-holding cells in diabetes with lipemia. Bull Johns Hopk Hosp 1925; 36:205-11.

94. Oppenheimer BS, Fishberg AM. Lipemia and the reticulo-endothelial apparatus. Arch Int Med 1925; 36:667-81.

95. Oppenheimer BS, Fishberg AM. Lipemia and reticulo-endothelial apparatus. JAMA 1925; 84:1775.

96. Thannhauser SJ. Lipidoses: Diseases of the Cellular Lipid Metabolism. New York: Oxford Univ Press, 1940:81-5.

97. Fagge CH. General xanthelasma or vitiligoidea. Pathol Soc Lond Transact. 1873; 24:242-50.

98. Pye-Smith PH. Xanthelasma. Guy's Hosp Rep 1877; 22:97-132.

99. Weidman FD, Boston LN. Generalized xanthoma tuberosum with xanthomatous changes in fresh scar of an intercurrent zoster. Arch Int Med 1937; 59:793-822.

100. Vanhaelst L, Bastenie PA. Heart and coronary artery disease in hypothyroidism. Am Heart J

1968; 76:845-8.

101. Craig LS, Lisser H, Soley MH et al. Report of two cases of myxedema with extreme hypercholesterolemia; one complicated by xanthoma tuberosum. J.Endocrinol 1944; 4:12-6.

102. Bronstein IP. Studies in cretinism and hypothyroidism in childhood. JAMA 1933; 100:1661-3.

103. Blumgart HL, Freedberg AS, Kurland GS. Hypercholesterolemia, myxedema and atherosclerosis. Am J Med 1953; 14:665-73.

104. Thannhauser SJ. Xanthomatoses. J Mt Sinai Hosp 1950; 17:79-97.

105. Brown MS, Goldstein JL, Fredrickson DS. Familial type 3 hyperlipoproteimemia (dysbetalipoproteinemia). In: Stanbury JB, Wyngaarden JB, Fredrickson DS et al. eds. The Metabolic Basis of Inherited Disease. 5th ed. New York: McGraw-Hill, 1983:655-71.

106. Morganroth J, Levy RI, Fredrickson DS. The biochemical, clinical, and genetic features of Type III hyperlipoproteinemia. Ann Int Med 1975; 82:158-74.

107. Fredrickson DS, Goldstein JL, Brown MS et al. The familial hyperlipoproteinemias. In: Stanbury JB, Wyngaarden J, eds. The Metabolic Basis of Inherited Disease. 4th ed. New York: McGraw Hill, 1978:604-55.

108. Roberts WC, Levy RI, Fredrickson DS. Necropsy observations in familial type III hyperlipoproteinemia. Circulation 1969; 40 Suppl 3:172.

109. Roberts WC, Levy RI, Fredrickson DS. Hyperlipoproteinemia. Arch Pathol 1970; 90:46-56.

110. Amatruda JM, Margolis S, Hutchins GM. Type III hyperlipoproteinemia with mesangial foam cells in renal glomeruli. Arch Pathol 1974; 98: 51-4.

111. Cabin HS, Schwartz DE, Virmani R et al. Type 111 hyperliproteinemia: Quantification, distribution, and nature of atherosclerotic coronary arterial narrowing in five necropsy patients. Am Heart J 1981; 102:830-5.

112. Gown AM, Hazzard WR, Benditt EP. Type III hyperlipoproteinemia and atherosclerosis: a case report and re-evaluatzion. Human Pathol 1982; 13:506-10.

113. Shore VG, Shore B, Hart RG. Changes in apolipoproteins and properties of rabbit very low density lipoproteins on induction of cholesteremia. Biochemistry 1974; 13:1579-85.

114. Mahley RW, Weisgraber KH. Canine lipoproteins and atherosclerosis I. Isolation and charac-

terization of plasma lipoproteins from control dogs. Circulation Res 1974; 35:713-21.

115. Mahley RW, Weisgraber KH, Innerarity T et al. Swine lipoproteins and atherosclerosis. Changes in the plasma lipoproteins and apoproteins induced by cholesterol feeding. Biochemistry 1975; 14:2817-23.

116. Mahley RW, Holcombe KS. Alterations of the plasma lipoproteins and apoproteins following cholesterol feeding in the rat. J. Lipid Res 1977; 18:314-24.

117. Mahley RW, Weisgraber KH, Innerarity T. Atherogenic hyperlipoproteinemia induced by cholesterol feeding in the Patas monkey. Biochemistry 1976; 15:2979-85.

118. Lees RS, Wilson DF, Schonfeld G et al. The familial dyslipoproteinemias. Progr Med Genet 1973; 9:237-90.

119. Nikkilä EA. Familial lipoprotein lipase deficiency and related disorders of chylomicron metabolism. In: Stanbury JB, Wyngaarden JB, Fredrickson DS et al. Eds. The Metabolic Basis of Inherited Disease. 5th ed. New york: McGraw Hill, 1983:622-42.

120. Malmros H, Swahn B, Truedsson E. Essential hyperlipaemia. Acta Med Scand 1954; 149: 91-108.

121. Goodman M, Shuman H, Goodman S. Idiopathic lipemia with secondary xanthomatosis, hepatosplenomegaly, with lipemic retinalis. J Pediat 1940; 1:596-605.

122. Roberts WC, Ferrans VT, Levy RI et al. Cardiovascular pathology in hyperlipoproteinemia. Am J Cardiol 1973; 31:557-70.

123. Chapman FD, Kinney TD. Hyperlipemia. "Idiopathic lipemia". Am J Dis Child 1941; 62:1014-24.

124. Poulsen HM. Familial lipemia. A new form of lipoidosis showing increase in neutral fats combined with attacks of acute pancreatitis. Acta Med Scand 1950; 138:413-20.

125. Nikkilä EA, Aro A. Family study of serum lipids and lipoproteins in coronary heart-disease. Lancet 1973; 1:954-9.

126. Fredrickson DS, Levy RI, Lees RS. Fat transport in lipoproteins—an integrated approach to mechanisms and disorders, New Engl J Med 1967; 276:32-44, 94-103, 148-56, 215-26, 273-81.

127. Bhattacharyya AK, Connor WE. Familial diseases with storage of sterols other than choles-

terol. In: Stanbury JB, Wyngaarden JB,eds. The Metabolic Basis of Inherited Disease. 4th ed. New York: McGraw Hill, 1978:656-69.

128. Salen G, Shafer S, Berginer VM. Familial diseases with storage of sterols other than cholesterol: cerebrotendinous xanthomatosis and sitosterolemia with xanthomatosis. In: Stanbury JB, Wyngaarden JB, Fredrickson DS et al. eds. The Metabolic Basis of Inherited Disease. 5th ed.New York: McGraw Hill, 1983:713-30.

129. Salen G. Cholestanol deposition in cerebrotendinous xanthomatosis. A possible mechanism. Ann Int Med 1971; 75:843-51.

130. Stahl WL, Sumi SM, Swanson PD. Subcellular distribution of cholestanol in cerebrotendinous xanthomatosis. J Neurochem 1971; 18:403-13.

131. Shulman RS, Bhattacharyya AK, Connor WE et al. ß-Sitosterolemia and xanthomatosis. New Engl J Med 1976; 294:482-3.

132. Miettinen TA. Phytosterolaemia, xanthomatosis and premature atherosclerotic arterial disease: A case with high plant sterol absorption, impaired sterol elimination and low cholesterol synthesis. J Clin Invest 1980; 10:27-35.

133. Kottke BA, Cornicelli JA, Didisheim P et al. Phytosterolemia, xanthomatosis, and acquired aortic valve stenosis. Arteriosclerosis 1958; 1:58.

134. Bevans M, Mosbach EH. Biological studies of dihydrocholesterol. Arch Pathol 1956; 62:11 2-7.

135. Herbert PN, Gotto AM, Fredrickson DS. Familial lipoprotein deficiency. (Abetalipoproteinemia, hypobetalipoproteinemia, and Tangier disease). In: Stanbury JB, Wyngaarden JB, Eds. The Metabolic Basis of Inherited Disease. 4th ed. New York: McGraw Hill, 1978:544-88.

136. Herbert PN, Assmann G, Gotto AM et al. Familial lipoprotein deficiency: hypobetalipoproteinemia, and Tangier disease. In: Stanbury JB, Wyngaarden JB, Fredrickson DS et al. eds. The Metabolic Basis of Inherited Disease. 5th ed. New York: McGraw Hill, 1983:589-621.

137. Schaeffer EJ, Zech LA, Schwartz DE et al. Coronary heart disease prevalence and other clinical features in familial high-density lipoprotein deficiency (Tangier disease). 1980; 93:261-6.

138. Fredrickson DS, Ferrans VJ. Acid cholesterylester hydrolase deficiency. (Wolman's disease and cholesteryl ester storage disease). In: Stanbury JB, Wyngaarden JB, eds. The Metabolic Basis of Inherited Disease. 4th ed. New York: McGraw Hill, 1978:670-87.

139. Lake BD, Patrick AD. Wolman's disease: deficiency of E600-resistant acid esterase activity with storage of lipids in lysosomes. J Pediat 1970; 76:262-6.

140. Marshall WC, Ackenden BG, Fosbrooke AS et al. Wolman's disease. A rare lipidosis with adrenal calcification. Arch Dis Child 1969; 44:331-41.

141. Lowden JA, Barson AJ, Wentworth P. Wolman's disease: a microscopic and biochemical study showing accumulation of ceroid and esterified cholesterol. Canad Med Ass J 1970; 102:402-5.

142. Assmann G, Fredrickson DS. Acid lipase deficiency: Wolman's disease and cholesteryl ester storage disease. In: Stanbury JB, Wyngaarden JB, Fredrickson DS et al. eds. The Metabolic Basis of Inherited Disease. 5th ed. New York: McGraw Hill, 1983:803-19.

143. Sloan HR, Fredrickson DS. Enzyme deficiency in cholesteryl ester storage disease. J Clin Invest 1972; 51:1923-6.

144. Beaudet AL, Ferry GD. Nichols et al. Cholesterol ester storage disease: clinical, biochemical, and pathological studies. J Pediat 1977; 90:910-4.

145. Talmud PJ, Humphries S. Molecular genetic analysis of coronary artery disease: an example of a multifactorial disease. In: McGee JO'D, Isaacson PG, Wright NA et al. eds. Oxford Text Book of Pathology. Vol 2b. Oxford:Oxford Univ Press, 1992:126-38.

146. Factor SM, Biempica L, Goldfisher S. Coronary intimal sclerosis in Morquio's syndrome. Virch Arch Pathol Anat 1978; 379:1-10.

CHAPTER 3

BASIC SCIENTIFIC PRECEPTS IN THE EPIDEMIOLOGY OF CORONARY HEART DISEASE AND ATHEROSCLEROSIS

Epidemiology is the scientific study of community medicine or of health and disease in populations, its aim being to determine factors which may facilitate prevention and control of diseases. Of particular value when dealing with infectious and occupational diseases, it has limited applicability to chronic degenerative diseases especially those that are ubiquitous and when five to seven decades elapse between initiation and death from the complications. Much research in support of the lipid hypothesis depends on the epidemiology of risk factors in coronary heart disease (CHD) with the results then being extrapolated to the cause of atherosclerosis.

It is a basic scientific precept that the terminology used must be precise and unambiguous and words must be used in their correct lexical sense to avoid confusion and misrepresentation. Words are the basis of communication and the tools of logical exposition. Their correct usage is essential to scientific exactitude and the pursuit of truth. As a scientific discipline, epidemiology must also adhere to these fundamental principles. Communication and indeed rational debate of the lipid hypothesis is impossible without uniform terminology and correct usage of words. Concepts and definitions are formulated to facilitate understanding and to distinguish one concept from all other concepts. Giving words arbitrary meanings is misrepresentation, precludes all meaningful communication and is resorting to the logic of Pooh Bear. If science is to progress there must be uniform terminology that is intelligible for all disciplines. Causal knowledge is indispensable to science[1] with medical science no exception. Several basic precepts have been established to facilitate the logical discussion of causality.[2]

SPECIFIC DISEASE ENTITIES

"Disease" should be restricted in usage to indicate a specific malady and not used loosely or synonymously with (a) symptoms, signs or laboratory findings, e.g., headache, pyrexia, hypertension, angina pectoris, hypercholesterolemia, etc.; (b) nonspecific complications of other diseases, e.g., embolism, suppuration, hemorrhage, ischemia, necrosis, edema, etc.; and (c) a group or class of pathological states such as stroke, dermatitis, subarachnoid hemorrhage, myocardial infarction or ischemia and CHD. Each is a manifestation of several specific disease entities and not a final diagnosis despite being often regarded as such clinically and even included as disease categories in the International Classification of Diseases (ICD). In clinical practice such terms are merely the starting point for investigation to determine the specific disease responsible for diagnostic accuracy and successful clinical management. This concept must apply to medical science including epidemiology. Because symptoms, signs, laboratory findings, and nonspecific complications and pathological states have multiple causes, it is alleged that specific diseases also have multiple causes.

Atherosclerosis is a specific disease of blood vessels but CHD is an imprecise clinical diagnosis comprising several clinical syndromes of myocardial ischemia attributable to insufficient coronary artery blood flow from any disease whatsoever. It is a nonspecific complication of many diseases.[3] Not being a specific disease, CHD is a misnomer. It is synonymous with myocardial ischemia but certainly not pathognomonic of coronary atherosclerosis, nor indicative of any specific degree of coronary involvement, although in practice it is usually assumed to represent a "severe" grade of coronary atherosclerosis. This anomalous situation was aggravated by a panel of experts of the National Institutes of Health (NIH) that incorrectly defined CHD as coronary atherosclerosis.[4]

In 1963 Dawber and Kannel[5] considered CHD was not a definable epidemiological disease entity and that therefore the use of CHD vital statistics was unwarranted. They also appreciated the fact that their Framingham data could not be used for the epidemiology of atherosclerosis or even of coronary atherosclerosis being valid with only an estimated 5 to 10% of the coronary atherosclerosis "iceberg" appearing as overt clinical CHD.[5,6] They decided it was legitimate to define CHD in terms of clinical syndromes which were considered to be reasonably specific viz angina pectoris, myocardial infarction and sudden death.[5] However even using these independently, as will be explained later, is associated with considerable error. Furthermore these syndromes are no more specific for atherosclerosis than CHD and congestive cardiac failure which can be due to the present or past complications of coronary atherosclerosis is not included in the term. Despite the opinions expressed by Dawber and Kannel it has become common practice to use CHD synonymously with coronary atherosclerosis in the Framingham Study and in epidemiology generally.

1. THE EPIDEMIOLOGICAL ENDPOINT OR PARAMETER

It is axiomatic in science that the desired parameter should be carefully and precisely defined and measured. In epidemiology the desired parameter or the specific endpoint should also be defined and concisely measured.[3] This is not done in the case of CHD and atherosclerosis.

In an epidemiological study of an infectious or occupational disease, population groups are divided into those with and those without the disease. In the case of CHD, the population groups are again divided into those with and those without CHD, which is being used as a surrogate monitor for atherosclerosis of undetermined severity. In reality those with and those without CHD all have atherosclerosis and as revealed pathologically there is moderately severe atherosclerosis in all adults over the age of 50 years[8] and once a certain degree of severity is reached, there is difficulty in comparing severity except for the degree of narrowing.

It is true that in an occupational disease such as lead poisoning, the blood lead level may be determined but this parameter is an indicator of the quantity of lead absorbed or the degree of exposure. In atherogenesis the correct and desired parameter to be sought and measured is the severity of atherosclerosis. There is currently no satisfactory method of measuring the severity of atherosclerosis during life and it is difficult enough to assess at autopsy. In any case there is difficulty in determining which parameter of atherosclerosis should be measured. Planimetric measurements of lipid-staining areas or of fibrous plaques are crude and unsatisfactory. The tendency of the wall to tear or ulcerate with secondary thromboembolism or to yield to produce an aneurysm is nearer the desired parameter.

Using CHD as a surrogate monitor of atherosclerosis or as a distinguishing feature of the alleged "disease" group means inappropriate sampling and its use as an endpoint in clinical trials is scientifically misleading. The natural history and pathogenesis of atherosclerosis differ from those of CHD and they are not interchangeable.

Coronary atherosclerosis exhibits a continuous range of severity from mild or minimal to severe but without tears, ulcers or stenoses sufficient to compromise flow. These severer grades overlap with clinically manifest disease and are variations in degree not differences in kind. An uncertain number of cases of myocardial ischemia and infarction are symptomless and unrecognized.

In epidemiological studies CHD does not indicate the severity of atherosclerosis and cannot be used as a surrogate monitor of severe coronary artery atherosclerosis when many other nonatherosclerotic factors can determine whether an atherosclerotic lesion with or without a tear will become manifest clinically or even lead to a fatal outcome.[2,3] Other problems consequent upon the use of CHD as a marker include subjects with congestive cardiac failure when attributable to chronic myocardial ischemia and severe atherosclerosis. Some of these subjects may die of bronchopneumonia. There are many diseases that can cause myocardial ischemia apart from atherosclerosis and its sequelae[3,9] particularly diseases that narrow the coronary ostia (syphilis, FH and other hereditary metabolic disorders), coronary artery embolism, bacterial endocarditis, chest trauma, small vessel disease, arteriovenous shunt, aortic valve stenosis, coronary arteritides (including polyarteritis nodosa, Takayasu's arteritis, Kawasaki's disease), various types of coronary artery aneurysms, illicit drug usage, thrombotic diathesis, oral contraceptives and hypotensive crises, etc. Buja and Willerson[10] stressed the low correlation between atherosclerosis severity and the clinical severity of CHD and in recent years vasospasm of intramyocardial arteries with ischemia and electrocardiographic evidence but without angiographic supportive evidence has attained considerable prominence as a cause of cardiac ischemia.[11]

The incidence of CHD as a monitor of "severe" atherosclerosis has additional confounding errors for it is not pathognomonic of atherosclerosis and on pathological grounds it has been estimated that only 90% are due to atherosclerosis.[12] One coronary artery has been found to have more than 70% lumen reduction in 66% of noncardiac atherosclerotic patients and in 39% of normal victims of accidental deaths but without other significant disease.[13] The prevalence of coronary stenosis was less than in CHD patients but too high for inclusion of such patients in a control sample of the population. In another study of 965 autopsies, 221 adults died of CHD (22%). An additional 136 patients had significant myocardial ischemia but died of other causes. At least one coronary artery exhibited 25 to 100% narrowing in 74% of adult autopsies[14] and Rodda[15] found total or near total occlusion in one or more main arteries of one leg in 42% of adult persons at autopsy. Lindbom[16] reported occlusion of large lower limb arteries was twice as common as coronary occlusions and since they are mostly symptomless, many more patients have significant atherosclerosis with occlusion than is indicated by CHD mortality rates or its clinical incidence. This is complicated by the substantial diagnostic error for clinical CHD which exceeds ± 30%.[17]

Angiographic assessments of the degree of narrowing of arteries are subjective, open to observer error and underestimate the severity of atherosclerosis because the lumen can remain relatively circular despite severe mural involvement. At the first clinical episode of CHD most cases already exhibit chronic and even multiple symptomless stenoses preexisting the clinical event by months or years. This indeterminate overlap in the two groups is never taken into account in statistical analyses of epidemiological studies. It is apparent that control samples of the population are all atherosclerotic and there is considerable but undetermined overlap in severity with the CHD population. In subjects with angina pectoris, it has been found that at least 20% have normal or near normal coronary angiograms[18,19] and up to 70% of ischemic episodes are symptomless in continuously monitored subjects.

The epidemiology of atherosclerosis is in practice the epidemiology of CHD as the two terms are used synonymously. It is now widely acknowledged that atherosclerosis commences as fibromusculoelastic intimal thickenings particularly about arterial branching sites and these commence early in fetal life although some believe they commence in infancy. Atherosclerosis progresses slowly and insidiously through a clinically quiescent phase to the stage of complications in the sixth decade or beyond (Fig. 2.2). CHD may or may not be due to atherosclerosis but if so, it is usually initiated by intimal tears or ulcerations followed by secondary thromboembolic phenomena and tertiary complications viz myocardial ischemia or infarction. CHD therefore usually does not manifest itself until the sixth decade and it is mostly evident thereafter. Death results then from cardiac insufficiency, arrhythmias, or even peripheral embolism, there being many factors that can provoke a fatal outcome independently of atherosclerosis, e.g., blood pressure, the cardiac status, cardiac workload, electrical instability or anemia, thrombotic diathesis, etc., and hemorheological factors particularly the tendency to red cell aggregation which is associated with increased varicosity. Yet some myocardial infarcts are clinically silent. On the other hand there could be many factors that affect the rapidity of progress of atherosclerosis or the likelihood of an intimal tear developing and these may be genetic, hemodynamic, environmental or due to stress and quite unrelated to diet or blood cholesterol levels. This emphasizes the inappropriate use of CHD as a surrogate of atherosclerosis and certainly the lack of validity of any extrapolation whatsoever from CHD epidemiology to the etiology of atherosclerosis.

It may be argued that the concern of the clinician is myocardial ischemia and not atherosclerosis. Under such circumstances the scientific approach is not to relate data, therapy or management to a diagnosis of a nonspecific pathological state (such as stroke, subarachnoid hemorrhage, dermatitis, etc.) caused by many specific diseases. The modern scientific approach is to determine the cause of each and then to investigate each such disease individually. Grouping all lipid dystrophies together would

be unscientific but gathering them with all the other cases without a lipid dystrophy is quite unacceptable. An epidemiological study to determine the cause and management of CHD in a mixture of cases of Kawasaki's disease, pseudoxanthoma elasticum, FH and congenital origin of the left coronary artery from the pulmonary artery would be avoided by any scientific assessing committee unless each disease category was dealt with separately. No knowledgeable physician in modern times would place all cases of stroke or even of subarachnoid hemorrhage in the same category and treating them all in the same manner would be malpractice. Yet the epidemiological approach is to classify all cases of CHD together, and not to differentiate one from another. This is also often the case with cerebrovascular disease (CVD) or stroke. The philosophy underlying this approach is equivalent to determining statistical associations with an imprecise clinical diagnosis (viz CHD) of a nonpathognomonic complication of end-stage atherosclerosis whilst ignoring (i) the lack of validity in considering the incidence of CHD as a surrogate monitor of the indeterminate severity of atherosclerosis, (ii) clinical diagnostic error for CHD, (iii) the presence of other diseases caught in the epidemiological dragnet, (iv) the fallacy of assuming a cause and effect relationship with CHD and (v) the lack of validity of any extrapolation from CHD to the etiology of atherosclerosis.

The correct correlation that should be sought is the severity of atherosclerosis with the duration and severity, grade or blood level of a factor suspected of involvement in the pathogenesis of atherosclerosis. If the relationship is biologically plausible and significant, the next procedure is to determine its role if any in the natural history of the disease and to assume nothing.

In epidemiology the inability to measure a necessary and specific parameter during life (viz the severity of atherosclerosis) can under no circumstances condone the use of an inappropriate surrogate monitor (incidence of CHD). The serious fallacy in this approach is displayed by the absurdity of equating "severity" with "incidence" in a ubiquitous disease (atherosclerosis) when most men and women over 50 years of age in the USA and no doubt other western countries have moderately advanced atherosclerosis.[3,4]

2. EVERY DISEASE MUST HAVE A CAUSE

It is a self-evident truth that every disease must have a cause and the most effective management, therapy and even prevention of any illness is dependent on the true or specific cause. When they are based on symptoms and clinical manifestations, treatments at best are palliative and nonspecific but extinction of a disease, e.g., small pox, would be a remote if not impossible goal. Definition of a disease on the basis of symptoms and clinical manifestations has been considered an option in epidemiology.[20] This is inconsistent with the basic logic of clinical science and classification of diseases is recognized as logically dependent on etiology, the elucidation of which is the major goal in research of any disease. This concept has pervaded the evolution of medical knowledge and science. Logically it follows that cause must be clearly defined.

At any particular time symptoms, signs and the natural history of an illness may suggest a syndrome or a specific disease but with further clinico-pathological study of many cases it may become apparent that the cause can be divided into several distinct categories each of which may have a specific genetic cause and distinctive phenotypic manifestations metabolically though with some overall similarities. It must always be remembered that knowledge is continuously evolving and the specific genetic defect must be sought for each category in the group. For each disease the underlying biochemical, physical and pathological disturbances together with the secondary factors participating in the pathogenesis must be elucidated.

3. SPECIFICITY OF EFFECT

All pathological manifestations or multiple organ involvement in a specific disease cannot be regarded as multiple separate effects of the specific cause. Sartwell[21] argued that a cause can have multiple effects, citing alcohol as a cause of acute alcoholic gastritis, hepatic cirrhosis and Korsakoff's syndrome. These are recognized pathological manifestations or components of alcoholic poisoning (acute or chronic) and do not negate the specificity of effect of the causative agent. Tuberculosis occurs in various sites dependent on the portal of entry and the vagaries of spread of the tubercle bacillus resulting in multiple tuberculous foci and Friedman[22] is incorrect in alleging that the tubercle bacillus has multiple effects and therefore its effect is nonspecific. It would also be inappropriate to consider osteoarthritis as having multiple effects because many joints are affected independently of one another. Likewise atherosclerosis is currently a specific disease despite its protean clinical manifestations and multiple organ involvement.

4. THE SUBJECT OF A CAUSAL RELATIONSHIP IS NOT A CAUSE

Since the cause produces an effect on the subject or object, it is illogical to confuse the subject of the relationship or its inherent characteristics with the cause itself. It is incorrect to consider the vermiform appendix as a cause of appendicitis and a man cannot be a cause of his own mugging because he exists nor can trees be a cause of forest fires.[23] If one species of tree is more flammable than another the genetic individuality of that species is not a cause of a forest fire. Different metals and timbers have different levels of fatigue endurance and it is still the repetitive or vibratory stress to which the metals and timbers are subjected that causes the fatigue failure. Variation in the subject or object and in conditions prevailing at a particular time can affect the response but this does not negate specificity of effect whether in biology or the physical sciences.

Common sense must prevail and variability of biological reactions to causative agents makes studies of causality more complex than in physical sciences. Latitude must be allowed because experimental conditions cannot be reproduced exactly even within one species. Species and individual susceptibility to a disease (infectious and noninfectious) is understandable in view of (i) the individualistic (genetically determined) anatomical, physico-chemical, physiological and metabolic characteristics even within the one species, (ii) the evolutionary development of variability of pathogen and host and (iii) the heterogeneous background experiences and exposure to noxious agents during an individual's lifetime.[2] Therefore it would be wrong to suggest that any variation in response must be due to yet another cause. Such factors may be important in affecting the inception and progression of the disease but they are not causes in the scientific sense. These secondary factors may explain why and how the disease developed as it did but the prime interest is what was the crucial factor that occasioned such specific effect on the individual without which the disease would not have occurred and when the exposed subjects are dissimilar in so many ways. The effect on the arteries and veins of an experimental arteriovenous shunt, allowing for a certain amount of leeway, is basically similar in rabbits, sheep and humans even though there are differences in genetics, vessel size, the architecture of the artery, size and site of shunt and hemodynamics. The term "specificity of response" implies a precision of which it is impossible to be certain, but if it became possible in the one species to duplicate all conditions exactly, there is no reason for believing that the results would differ. All factors pertaining to the subject (age, sex, hair or skin color), biochemical features, immune status, etc.) are individual characteristics of the subject and therefore cannot be regarded as causes and do not reflect on the adequacy of the cause even though they may affect the likelihood of development and the pathogenesis of the disease.

It must be appreciated that we may not always be able to explain the vagaries of racial or national occurrence and severity of every disease because of insufficient information at a particular time even if the available data are valid. Nor can any disease be expected to behave in an identical manner from population to population when we are dealing with such heterogeneous individuals.

CAUSALITY

Etiology comes from the Greek *aitiologica*, the science or doctrine of causation, especially the cause of disease. It is likely that the word may have had a somewhat different connotation in Aristotle's time for his four *aitia* when translated literally meant "answers or responses to questions" to provide an explanation or description of the nature of objects.[24]

1. What is it? The *what* is the *formal* cause

2. Out of what is it made? The *from what* is the *material* cause
3. By what agent? The *by what* is the *efficient* cause
4. For what end? The *for what* is the *final* cause

The answers to these fundamental questions do not provide four causes in the modern lexical usage of "cause". It is probably because of the restricted vocabulary of Latin in which *causa* meant both cause and reason that there has been subsequent philosophical confusion, debate and misuse of cause. The epidemiological use of "cause" is concerned more with the reasons or why an effect occurs rather than what specifically caused the effect. Why an effect occurs is not one of Aristotle's four aitia from which etiology is derived. Only the "efficient" cause can be a cause in the current lexical and popular usage if cause is to have a clear unambiguous meaning in medical science.

Cause is something that produces, occasions or effects a disease or a uniform antecedent of a phenomenon.[25] It does not mean to affect, influence, predispose to or aggravate the disease or its complications nor does it refer to the conditions under which the disease is produced or why. The epidemiological meaning of cause is nearer to, though often used in an even broader sense than pathogenesis which is the mode of origin and development of a disease. There is confusion between etiology and pathogenesis in epidemiology.

Nevertheless cause is often used loosely in general parlance and philosophers use it in the sense of the reason for events, actions and behavior. John Stuart Mill[26] wrote the "cause of a phenomenon is the assemblage of its conditions" but added "we have, philosophically speaking, no right to give the name of cause to one of them exclusively of the others". He acknowledged an effect can be the consequence of a single specific antecedent or that positive and negative conditions could account for an event, but it would be illogical to regard each such factor as a cause, as is current practice in epidemiology, particularly since the role of negative factors would be one of abatement—the very antithesis of causation.

Claude Bernard[27] emphasized that the metaphysical, spiritual and linguistic arguments of philosophers regarding the diverse use of "cause" are not applicable to biological sciences. He disagreed with the common medical practice of considering disease states as having many causes and philosophers such as Spinoza,[28] David Hume[29] and John Stuart Mills[26] stressed specificity of both cause and effect, which was also the crux of the Henle-Koch postulates. Bertrand Russell[30] confirmed that in the physical sciences, causation was explained only in terms of the efficient cause and if medicine is to be a scientific discipline in which diseases are to be explained ultimately by physical and chemical changes, then cause must have the same specific meaning in all scientific endeavors in which precision and exactitude are essential.[23] Unquestionably at present causation in reference to diseases has this same restricted usage accorded by the general public which is being misled by epidemiological misuse of cause.

In the late 19th century tuberculosis was believed to have many causes and had even been considered a nutritional deficiency. Such concepts were dependent on anecdotal experiences and assumption, not on scientific analysis and investigation. When Robert Koch identified the tubercle bacillus as the cause of tuberculosis in 1882, his discovery,[31] not surprisingly, met with skepticism and hostility despite eventual acceptance. However a present day school of epidemiology contests this concept believing that the tubercle bacillus is but one of many causes of tuberculosis and not necessarily the most important. Furthermore it is contended that the tubercle bacillus should not be singled out by any specific title such as cause because it could then be considered more important than the other factors participating in causation.[20] This concept of cause is contrary to the fundamental basis of modern medical science in which the specific cause of the ailment is the basis of diagnosis, clinical investigation, therapy, management and prevention. Antibiotic therapy for instance is based on knowing the specific causative organism.

Robert Koch, appreciating that there were at that time many spurious causes that had to be excluded, enunciated the famous Henle-Koch postulates with the express purpose of excluding such spurious causes and because of the need for rigorous proof of cause and effect.[31]

The work of Pasteur and Koch supported the monocausal concept of disease and cause became accepted as the sole prerequisite without which the disease cannot occur. It followed that the cause of the disease including atherosclerosis must be present in each individual and animal with the disease irrespective of its severity assuming that the disease is continuously progressive and all the evidence favors such a concept.

These postulates have been accepted as the epitome of scientific logic and firmly established the concept of one cause for one disease, i.e., the specificity of cause and effect. Within less than a century these postulates are regarded by many epidemiologists as outmoded.[32,35] It is now common epidemiological practice to regard causation of all diseases as an ecological system, a web or a constellation of interconnected determinants or links with each link itself the result of a complex genealogy of antecedents, with the complexity and origins of the web of causation beyond our understanding and awareness.[36,37] Such concepts lack common sense and the multitudinous factors or causes of any disease would date back to antiquity and comprise more than pathogenetic factors. Such causes are not necessary, not sufficient, nonspecific, noncausative and nonsensical.[2]

In a more restricted approach such factors as age, sex, race, living conditions, social networks, behavioral characteristics and socioeconomic factors are sought as statistical associations with CHD (social epidemiology). These may be contributing, predisposing, conditional, aggravating or even ameliorating factors and should be so labeled. Many epidemiologists prefer not to use "cause" because of the uncertainty of their results.[32,35,38] Instead they use the term "risk factor" but in practice this is equated with cause. The multicausal approach is thought to be sophisticated and basic to the epidemiological approach to disease prevention.[34] It has not been explained how this multicausal approach assisted in the eradication of small pox.

It serves no useful purpose to label multiple nonspecific factors as causes without determining their biological relevance and significance in the disease. If epidemiology is to be a scientific discipline, then determining the true relationship of these secondary factors to the disease and classifying them accordingly is a matter of scientific exactitude. Not to differentiate the tubercle bacillus for example from all the other pathogenetic and secondary sociological factors, as recommended by MacMahon,[20] is not only irrational but exaggerates the importance of the latter and denigrates the importance of the true cause whilst burying it in a morass of irrelevant genealogical, conditional and sociological data. To then propagate such information to the general public as the causes of specific diseases is quite misleading.

CAUSAL SUFFICIENCY

The logician's definition of cause is said to be a factor that is both necessary and sufficient[39] and philosophers and epidemiologists discuss cause in terms of being necessary and sufficient. The epidemiologists widened and instituted a less rigorous concept of causality. Most of their causes are certainly not necessary and sufficiency is interpreted as indicating that clinical disease must inevitably follow. In the case of tuberculosis such an interpretation is based on hypothetical situations, or lack of knowledge of tuberculosis and the primary tuberculous lesion.[40] In our present state of knowledge it is probably incorrect to allege that even one viable tubercle bacillus inoculated satisfactorily is insufficient or unable to cause a tuberculous response in a susceptible animal under controlled conditions as would be the case in physical sciences.[2]

To suggest that the cause must inevitably and unconditionally produce an effect is unrealistic and scientifically untenable. In both physical and biological sciences, under uncontrolled conditions, the number of contingencies that can interfere with, modify or prevent the cause from producing an effect, are prolix. If "sufficient" is interpreted in the epidemiological way, there is no cause that can invariably and unconditionally produce any effect in either medical science or the physical sciences. "Sufficient" must be interpreted as "able to produce the effect".[40]

RISK FACTORS AND CAUSALITY

Pathologists have long recognized that many factors participate in the pathogenesis of disease and when the etiology is unknown, such factors are eagerly sought. Recognition of these

factors was once dependent on astute observation and anecdotal experience which cannot always be relied upon. In more recent times statistical associations with CHD are sought and these factors may reveal only a small fraction of secondary factors participating in the pathogenesis of atherosclerosis and some no doubt are irrelevant or of no biological significance. However these factors, judged to be of biological significance, are considered to participate in the overall causation, development and progression of the disease and are thus called risk factors.

As previously indicated epidemiologists prefer to use risk factors rather than cause because of the uncertainty of their results but also because this is allegedly a more enlightened and sophisticated approach to the ecology of disease. Hence all diseases are regarded as being multifactorial in etiology and risk factors are in practice considered to be causative. The etiology of atherosclerosis is thus considered to have multiple causes which are the risk factors associated with CHD rather than with the etiology of atherosclerosis. Whilst epidemiologists and other protagonists of the lipid hypothesis may consider this approach to be sophisticated, the logical and scientific approach particularly in such a chronic life-long ubiquitous disease as atherosclerosis is to seek clues to the etiology by investigating the earliest pathological stages of the disease rather than by studying the clinical manifestations of one nonpathognomonic complication of end-stage atherosclerosis. It is quite apparent that many such risk factors may be totally unrelated to atherogenesis and even if they aggravate the development of atherosclerosis this cannot be interpreted as indicating it has multiple causes.

The widely accepted concept that atherosclerosis has multiple causes is based on the epidemiology of CHD but as yet no specific disease has been shown to have more than one cause.[3] For this reason McCormick considers multicausal etiology as a euphemism for ignorance or a synonym for unknown etiology.[41]

Currently no specific disease has more than one cause but atherosclerosis is regarded as being due to a variable mix of risk factors. Such a multicausal approach inhibits the establishment of testable hypotheses.[42] Under such circumstances it is impossible to prove or disprove the causal role of any risk factor. This in itself is not necessarily reason for abandoning the multicausal approach but until there is adequate evidence of multiple causes, the concept remains conjectural.

Risk means hazard, danger or exposure to some ill-effect and implies only the possibility or chance not the certainty of development or ability to cause the effect (myocardial ischemia). Not all individuals at risk will be affected and in this sense risk factors can in no way be regarded as a cause because exposure to a risk does not denote causality. The possibility of a factor being involved in the development of atherosclerosis is quite different from being the essential causal prerequisite which has a very specific meaning in causality.

To some epidemiologists a causal relation of a statistical association is demonstrated when alteration of one factor is followed by a change in frequency or quality of the other,[43] and Riegelman[44] also stipulated that the alleged cause should precede the effect and some CHD risk factors can hardly precede the development of atherosclerosis with the exception of hereditary metabolic disorders. Some epidemiologists have admitted that this did not meet the strict rules of logic[44,45] and I concur. Epidemiological criteria of causality for risk factors include the strength, consistency, plausibility and specificity of the association and covariance with the factor together with appropriate temporal relationships and supportive evidence. Even though these criteria for causality have been softened and lack Koch's rigorous logic, Kleinbaum et al[42] regarded none of the criteria were necessary or sufficient to indicate a causal relationship and they lack the specificity of cause and effect, establishing less rigid standards than for the physical sciences or for the precedence set for science and medical science by Gallileo,[46] Claude Bernard,[27] Robert Koch[31] and others.[2] Even so Kannel[47] admitted that none of the major CHD risk factors complies with even these less rigorous epidemiological criteria of causality and indicated the need to seek additional risk factors to clarify many of the inconsistencies in epidemiological studies of some populations.

The epidemiologists' criteria of causality include the following:

(I) STRENGTH OF THE ASSOCIATION

It is maintained that a strong association is more likely to be causative than a weak one. This association presupposes the factor is not an essential prerequisite in the lexical and scientific sense and so no current risk factor need be considered causative.

(II) CONSISTENCY OF THE ASSOCIATION

Confirmation of an association is essential but studies of risk factors abound with inconsistencies which necessitate revision by the CHD epidemiologists to review the premises on which their hypothesis stands.

Kleinbaum et al[42] admitted to inconsistencies and concluded that epidemiologists may have to resort to subjective judgment and rely on findings they believe to be more valid but the relative importance of risk factors varies between populations[48,49] and with the clinical manifestations of atherosclerosis. Moreover the serum cholesterol level varies in its relationship with the syndromes of CHD and CVD.

(III) SPECIFICITY

Risk factors are not present in every individual and animal with the disease and are therefore not essential, nor are they specific to atherosclerosis but are each features of many diseases. Epidemiologists are content to acknowledge that risk factors are nonessential and nonspecific.[32,42,50] In this event they must also be noncausal.

(IV) CHRONOLOGICAL RELATIONSHIP

Causes must precede the effects. Yet most risk factors are statistical correlations with CHD which is a monitor of end-stage disease in the middle-aged or elderly. The alleged causal risk factors may precede clinical manifestations of CHD and angina is actually a symptom of CHD, but they have a different temporal relationship to atherosclerosis (Fig. 2.2). Consequently CHD risk factors cannot be considered causes of atherosclerosis, since no CHD risk factor regularly precedes the initial lesions of atherosclerosis. Inherited metabolic disorders precede the initial lesions of atherosclerosis but there are other reasons for excluding them as causes of atherosclerosis.[51,52] Other genetic factors in humans are most likely to be predisposing or aggravating factors rather than causal.

(V) BIOLOGICAL GRADIENT

The disease must be of increased severity or incidence if the causal agent or exposure to the agent is increased, thus emphasizing the inappropriateness of using CHD incidence instead of the severity of atherosclerosis.

(VI) PLAUSIBILITY

The risk factor with the greatest "strength" viz hypercholesterolemia can no longer be regarded as plausible on pathological and experimental grounds.[51-54] No risk factor is present in every individual and animal with the disease. No CHD risk factor can be regarded as the cause of atherosclerosis on the criteria herein expounded.

(VII) COHERENCE

This criterion overlaps with consistency and biological plausibility and implies consistency with the known history of the disease and its epidemiology. Since risk factors relate to CHD they cannot be regarded as consistent or plausible in the etiology of atherosclerosis (Fig. 2.2).

(VIII) EXPERIMENTAL CONFIRMATION

Chapter 2 indicates that CHD risk factors are not confirmed as causal in experimental atherosclerosis and dietary induced hypercholesterolemia does not reproduce atherosclerosis and its complications.

(IX) ANALOGY

There appears to be no valid analogy in the relationship between risk factors and atherosclerosis in reference to causation. More than 270 risk factors have been reported[55] including gray hair,[56] premature baldness, snoring,[57] wifely love and even secondary manifestation of an underlying metabolic disorder, or an early symptom (angina pectoris) or electrocardiographic evidence of myocardial ischemia. This variable usage of the term and the inevitable surfacing of strong but irrelevant statistical associations emphasize the need for proof of causality which is generally assumed in epidemiology. Most can have no biological significance to atherogene-

sis, though some play a role in the pathogenesis and are pathogenetic factors rather than causes. Some may aggravate the secondary complications of intimal tears, ulceration or aneurysm formation as indicated. To conclude that CHD risk factors are causes of atherosclerosis, when even epidemiological causes must precede the development of the disease, is invalid.

This loose usage of cause, CHD, and risk factor underlies the epidemiological evidence for the lipid hypothesis and leads to the inevitable surfacing of irrelevant statistical associations, indicating the need for proof of causality which is usually assumed.[37,48] Such an assumption is allegedly justifiable because of the difficulty in providing proof and because current epidemiological methods have provided much "useful information",[48] but the alleged value of the data obtained can never be used to validate the methodology. With current epidemiological methods and assumed causation the conclusions reached cannot be classified as science. Some risk factors and essential metabolites are classified as "atherogenic" and an atherogenic index has been devised and programmed pocket calculators have been provided for determining individual risk based on risk factors, thus promulgating the causal role of cholesterol and the validity of edicts from the CHD school of epidemiology.

Whilst many authors have acknowledged that epidemiological studies cannot prove a cause and effect relationship, the use of "risk factors" instead of "cause", the multicausal concept of disease, the assumed causal role of risk factors[37,48] and the softened epidemiological criteria for causality have led to misrepresentation of the role and limitations of epidemiology by falsely inflating its capabilities. As a consequence this epidemiological approach would dispense with the need for accuracy and rigorous scientific evidence for proof of causality. Yet in epidemiological circles the notion of causality has been considered abstract,[36] an artifact of the processes of thought[58,59] and dependent on utility rather than truth.[60] MacMahon[20] considered absolute proof of causation to be unrealistic whilst others have considered causation to be a matter of judgment after weighing up the available evidence.[61,62] Causal inference is said to "depend on human insight, intuition, and imagination as links in the process connecting observational theory.[42] Distinction between causes and contributing factors has been said to be arbitrary and often meaningless,[37] but lack of such differentiation diminishes the importance of the cause and exaggerates the role of secondary "noncausative" factors. Espousing another opinion Renwick[63] thinks it more important to prevent or abate the disease than to seek its cause. Friedman[22] regarded the benefits of finding the true cause to be more philosophical or psychological than practical. This latter view would not apply to a disease like smallpox at all and indicates ignorance of modern medical practice, the basis of prevention and management of infectious diseases. As we approach the 21st century there is difficulty in reconciling such views with scientific thinking and logic.

The concepts of cause and reason are different. One answers what and the other why, but epidemiologists label as causes not only the answers to what and why but also when, where and how. They trivialize cause and appear to be disinterested in determining what is the true or specific cause of atherosclerosis and its underlying mechanisms.

Some epidemiologists view causation in chronic diseases quite differently. Yerushalmy and Palmer[64] contended the cause must be present in every case of the disease and that nonspecificity indicates that the factor under suspicion is unlikely to be the cause. They likened the current status of the search for the cause of many chronic diseases including atherosclerosis to the situation prior to the discovery of specific bacteria when the problem of multiple causation must have been more disturbing than later when the specific causal organism had been identified. Risk factors statistically associated with the imprecise clinical diagnosis of CHD, even if they really do participate in the development or outcome of CHD, cannot be assumed to be either a predisposing factor or to play a causal role in the etiology of atherosclerosis. The so-called risk is also relative and its duration and severity can rarely be evaluated. The endpoint that should be determined is not the prevalence of CHD but the severity of atherosclerosis which cannot be assessed satisfactorily during life. Until the etiol-ogy and pathogenesis of atherosclerosis are more fully elucidated and general accepted, invocation of risk factors as causative agents in atherogenesis is unacceptable.

Another reason for abandoning the use of "risk" in science is that in epidemiology and in clinical trials "relative risk" and "risk reduction" have been given in mathematical terms as if to infer validity and to grossly inflate the dangers of a specified blood cholesterol level or the benefit of a reduction in blood cholesterol levels, without explaining the significance of the means by which the figures are derived. The calculations in fact are dependent on the ratio of numerators without considering the denominators which are needed to interpret the true significance of the epidemiological data.[65,66] Such creative statistical manipulations degrade science. The terms risk and risk factor serve no useful purpose in science and should be abandoned because of their misusage and misrepresentation regarding the causal role of cholesterol in CHD and atherogenesis.

THE ULTIMATE TEST OF CAUSALITY

The critical test of causality is its experimental reproduction and Koch's postulates[31] were designed specifically to provide criteria, compliance with which would preclude spurious causes from consideration. These postulates served medicine well in respect of infectious diseases although some modifications were required for very chronic infections due to long-acting viruses and also to incorporate immunological techniques. Several authors (lipid protagonists) have alleged that cholesterol complies with unmodified Koch's postulates[67-70] and that cholesterol is just as assuredly the cause of atherosclerosis as the tubercle bacillus is the cause of tuberculosis.[67] Common sense dictates that Koch's postulates were for infections and that specific criteria are required for non-infectious diseases and for the experimental production of atherosclerosis in particular. The specific amended criteria that have been proposed[53] are: (i) The experimental procedure must reproduce or be comparable to those conditions existing in man. (ii) The sequence of pathological changes in the vessel wall must be similar to that in man. (iii) The experimental lesion must be similar to human atherosclerosis morphologically and topographically. (iv) The complications of the disease, i.e., intimal tears, mural dissection, thrombosis and aneurysmal dilatation must result when lesions are produced. Application of such criteria will help maintain scientific standards.

The essence of these modified postulates is that the experimental procedure must reproduce the disease, its pathogenesis and its complications under conditions analogous to those prevailing in man. However a chronic degenerative disease that is ubiquitous in man has special considerations for its experimental reproduction.[2] (i) In view of the prolonged quiescent stage of atherosclerosis (Fig. 2.2), experimental atherosclerosis must be accelerated for logistic reasons. The initial proliferative lesion must be fibromusculoelastic intimal thickening and the gamut of changes both histological and ultrastructural that characterize atherogenesis (Chapter 2) must be reproduced. (ii) If the definition of atherosclerosis includes nonlipid containing intimal proliferation in the aorta and about arterial forks as many now contend, then the disease is even more widespread than previously believed. It is ubiquitous at least in sizable mammals so far examined and more than possibly in other genera also. Arteries of man and most experimental animal species contain the same types of cellular and noncellular connective tissues and are architecturally similar except for size and age. This means that the cause of the proliferative lesions must pertain to lower animals so affected and that experimental atherosclerosis should also be applicable to man. If atherosclerosis already occurs in such animals in its early intimal proliferative form, then the experimental production of advanced disease has to be one of causation or aggravation. If intimal pads at arterial forks can be induced to progress to the stage of atheroma and thrombosis, it could be argued that the experimental procedure merely aggravates the already preexisting early lesion. However if even mild but accelerated atherosclerosis can be induced experimentally in a vein or an artery where there was no preexisting intimal proliferation then this would be convincing evidence of both initiation and progression.[2] (iii) Degenerative diseases such as atherosclerosis or osteoarthritis involve localized regions of the

body in isolation without any tendency to spread as occurs with infections and tumors. The topography of atherosclerosis suggests the dominating influence of local factors which localize and govern the severity of the disease at that site independently of a possible circulating pathogenetic human factor in the blood.[71] These local factors make the site susceptible to the accumulation of lipid and each lesion may develop, extend and become confluent with neighboring lesions. Eventually the disease becomes diffuse though generally remaining most severe at sites of initiation. By virtue of the chronicity and slow, inexorable progression of the disease, it is highly likely that the cause is present throughout life. Lesions that distort the lumen or induce tortuosity may be associated with secondary pathological changes in the vessel wall as has been demonstrated experimentally.[71] Nor is it necessary to reproduce all clinical and pathological manifestations (CHD, stroke, gangrene of the limbs) seen in man as these are secondary or tertiary complications of the disease.

Since these various aspects of the proliferative lesions can be induced experimentally in herbivorous animals on a stock diet, our experiments are consistent with the criteria or modified postulates proposed above.[71,72] These experiments provide strong support for an alternative and viable theory to the lipid/cholesterol hypothesis and after all the ultimate proof of causality is its experimental reproduction. Furthermore they provide additional reasons why the lipid hypothesis is an inadequate explanation for the etiology of atherosclerosis.

COMMENTARY

Epidemiology has much to offer medical science particularly in infectious and occupational diseases. By means of well conducted and critical appraisal of the incidence or prevalence of specific diseases with accurate diagnosis primarily based on objective or reliable laboratory data, epidemiology places population-based diseases on a more reliable basis than anecdotal experiences. Furthermore by similar techniques monitoring programs can be implemented. However in the field of chronic ubiquitous degenerative diseases epidemiology has limitations which have been recognized.[73] Unfortunately those who established the current CHD school of epidemiology have not served their discipline well.

Epidemiologists, like those in any other field of endeavor wishing to be scientific in their approach, must adhere to the basic tenets of scientific research, viz precision, logic and truth. Inherent in these requirements is the need for precise, unambiguous and accurate usage of words in particular avoiding the misusage of cause which lies at the very crux of the cholesterol controversy. Without clear, specific meanings to words "neither critical judgments nor thinking of any kind is possible".[74] Giving "cause" a vague meaning, at variance with its lexical and scientific use, decrying its use and importance and preferentially using risk factors and at the same time assuming a causal role has had a detrimental effect on atherosclerosis research, and has misled the public and governmental health agencies. The greatest danger of risk factors is that the readers are at risk of believing whatsoever they read. Scientists however have a moral responsibility not to mislead and not to misrepresent their subject.

CHD is an unfortunate and undesirable term being a misnomer. As indicated, the inability to measure the desired and essential parameter, viz the severity of atherosclerosis, does not condone using vague nonpathognomonic surrogates that have little relevance to the basic quest, viz the etiology of atherosclerosis. CHD is not the desired endpoint in clinical trials and its use in epidemiological studies is a basic flaw in the data of any investigation. No adjustment can compensate for such an error and to extrapolate from CHD risk factors to the etiology of atherosclerosis is scientifically invalid.

Cause must have the same specific meaning for medical science and the physical sciences reaffirmed by famous scientists (Gallileo, Bernard, Pasteur, Koch).[2] Terms such as CHD and risk factor are inappropriate and misleading. Vague, imprecise and ambiguous terminology has provided unreliable data, the validity of which has not been demonstrated because the CHD school assumed causality. This is not a semantic argument but a reaffirmation of the need for precision, logic and truth in CHD epidemiology as in science in general. The evolution and intellectual achievements of *Homo*

sapiens revolve about causal enquiry. It is from seeking the cause of all things and events together with the power to reason logically that knowledge has been developed. To denigrate cause or to misuse cause to exaggerate the capabilities of epidemiology threatens the survival of logic and science in medicine.[2] The implications of misrepresenting cause has implications far wider than CHD epidemiology and though it occurs frequently in public life, there is no excuse for any aspiring or alleged scientist to be guilty of such misusage.

In conclusion, cause must be used as the sole prerequisite without which the disease cannot occur. Such terms as CHD and risk factors should be abandoned for more explicit terminology. These faults have contributed substantially to the CHD lipid/cholesterol dogma which had its genesis in vague generalizations, misusage of words, and imprecise and ambiguous terminology.[2]

References

1. Mackie JL. Causes and conditions. Am Philosoph Quart 1965; 2:245-64.
2. Stehbens WE. Causality in medical science with reference to coronary heart disease and atherosclerosis. Perspect Biol Med 1992; 36:97-119.
3. Stehbens WE. Basic precepts and the lipid hypothesis of atherogenesis. Med Hypoth 1990; 31:105-13.
4. National Heart, Lung and Blood Institute. Arteriosclerosis. The Report of the 1977 Working Group to review the 1971 Report by the National Heart and Lung Institute Task Force on Arteriosclerosis. Washington, 1977:DHEW Publ No (NIH) 78-1526.
5. Dawber TR, Kannel WB. Coronary heart disease as an epidemiology entity. Am J Pub Health 1963; 53:433-7.
6. Kagan A, Dawber TR, Kannel WB et al Framingham study: A prospective study of coronary heart disease. Fed Proc 1962; 21 Suppl 11:52-7.
7. Spain DM, Bradess VA. The relationship of coronary thrombosis to coronary atherosclerosis and ischemic heart disease. Am J Med Sc 1960; 240:701-10.
8. Strong JP, McGill HC. The national history of coronary atherosclerosis. Am J Pathol 1962; 40:37-49.

9. Cheitlin MD, McAllister HA, de Castro CM. Myocardial infarction without atherosclerosis. JAMA 1975; 231:951-9.

10. Buja LM, Willerson JT. The role of coronary artery lesions in ischemic heart disease: Insights from recent clinicopathologic, coronary arteriographic, and experimental studies. Human Pathol 1987; 18:451-61.

11. Gutstein WH, Anversa P, Guideri G. Coronary artery spasm: Involvement of small intramyocardial branches. Atherosclerosis 1987; 67:1-7.

12. Robbins SL, Angell M, Kumar V. Basic Pathology. 3rd ed. Philadelphia: W B Saunders, 1981: 289-99.

13. Baroldi G. Coronary stenosis: Ischemic or nonischemic factor? Am Heart J 1978; 96:139-43.

14. Spiekerman RE, Brandenburg JT, Achor RWP et al. Incidence of coronary artery disease at necropsy in a community of 30,000. Circulation 1060; 22:816-7.

15. Rodda RA. Arteriosclerosis in the lower limbs: A pathological study of fifty cases with no ischaemia. MD Thesis, Dunedin: Univ of Otago, 1950.

16. Lindbom Å. Arteriosclerosis and arterial thrombosis in the lower limb. A roentgenological study. Acta Radiol 1950; Suppl 80:1-80.

17. Stehbens WE. An appraisal of the epidemic rise of coronary heart disease and its decline. Lancet 1987; 1:606-11.

18. Cohn PF. Asymptomatic coronary artery disease Pathophysiology, diagnosis, management. Mod Concepts Cardiovasc Dis 1981; 50:55-60.

19. Gazes PC. Angina pectoris: Classification and diagnosis. Part 2. Mod Concepts Cardiovasc Dis 1988; 57:25-7.

20. MacMahon B. Causes and entities of disease. In: Clark DW, MacMahon B, eds. Preventative and Community Medicine, 2nd ed. Boston: Little Brown & Co, 1981: 17-22.

21. Sartwell PE. On the methodology of investigations of etiologic factors in chronic diseases— further comments. J Chron Dis 1960; 11:61-3.

22. Friedman GD. Primer of Epidemiology. 2nd ed. New York: McGraw Hill, 1980.

23. Stehbens WE. The concept of cause in disease. J Chr Dis 1985; 38:947-50.

24. Randall JH. Aristotle. New York: Columbia Univ Press, 1960.

25. Simon HA. Causation. In: International Encyclopedia of the Social Science. Vol 2. 1968; 2: 350-6.

26. Mill JS. A System of Logic In: Ratiocinative and Inductive. Toronto: Univ of Toronto, 1973.

27. Bernard C. Lectures on the Phenomena of Life common to Animals and Plants. Vol 1. Trans by Hoff HE, Guillemin R, Guillemin L. Springfield: CC Thomas, 1974.

28. de Spinoza B. In: Spinoza's Ethic. Trans by White WH. London: Trübner & Co, 1883.

29. Hume D. In: Enquiries Concerning the Human Understanding and Concerning the Principles of Morals. Selbe-Bigg LA, ed. 2nd ed. Oxford: Clarendon Press, 1963.

30. Russell B. In: Wisdom of the West. Foulkes P, ed. London: Rathbone Books, 1959: 88.

31. Rivers TM. Viruses and Koch's Postulates. J Bacteriol 1937; 33:1-12.

32. Dawber TR. The Framingham Study. The Epidemiology of Atherosclerotic Disease, Cambridge: Harvard Univ Press, 1980.

33. Morris JN. Uses of Epidemiology. 3rd ed. Edinburgh: Churchill Livingstone, 1975.

34. Leavell HD, Clark EG. Preventive Medicine for The Doctor in his Community. New York: McGraw Hill, 1958.

35. Lave LB, Seskin EP, Epidemiology, causality and public policy. Am Scientist 1979; 67:178-86.

36. MacMahon B, Pugh TF. Epidemiology. Principles and Methods. Boston: Little Brown & Co, 1970.

37. MacMahon B. Pugh TF. Ipsen J. Epidemiological Methods. London: J & A Churchill, 1960.

38. Le Riche WH, Milner J. Epidemiology as Medical Ecology. Edinburgh: Churchill Livingstone, 1971.

39. Lilienfeld AM. Lilenfeld DE. Foundations of Epidemiology. 2nd ed. Oxford: Oxford Univ Press, 1980.

40. Stehbens WE. On the "cause" of atheroclerosis. Pathology 1987; 19:115-9.

41. McCormick J. The multifactorial aetiology of coronary heart disease: A dangerous delusion. Perspect Biol Med 1988; 32:103-8.

42. Kleinbaum DG, Kupper LL, Morgenstern H. Epidemiological Research: Principles and Quantitative Methods. Belmont: Wadsworth Inc, 1982.

43. Simpson J. An Introduction to Preventive Medicine. London: William Heinemann, 1970.

44. Riegelman R. Contributory cause: Unnecessary and insufficient. Postgrad Med 1979; 66:177-9.

45. Lilienfeld AM. Epidemiological methods and inferences in studies of noninfectious diseases. Pub Health Rep 1957; 72:51-60.

46. Bunge M. Causality. The Place of the Causal Principle in Modern Science. Cambridge: Harvard Univ Press. 1959.

47. Kannel WB. Recent highlights from the Framingham Study. Aust NZ J Int Med 1976; 6:373-86.

48. Epstein FH. The epidemiology of coronary heart disease. J Chron Dis 1965; 18:735-74.

49. Walker ARP. Studies bearing on coronary heart disease in South African populations. SA Med J 1973; 47:85-90.

50. Ahlbom A. Criteria of causal associations in epidemiology. In: Nordenfelt L, Lindahl BIB, eds. Health, Disease and Causal Explanations in Medicine. Dordrecht: Reidel Pub, 1984: 93-8.

51. Stehbens WE, Wierzbicki E. The relationship of hypercholesterolemia to atherosclerosis and with particular emphasis on familial hypercholesterolemia, diabetes mellitus, obstructive jaundice, myxedema and the the nephrotic syndrome. Progr Cardiovasc Dis 1988; 30: 289-306.

52. Stehbens WE, Martin M. The vascular pathology of familial hypercholesterolemia. Pathology 1991; 23:54-61.

53. Stehbens WE. An appraisal of cholesterol-feeding in experimental atherogenesis. Progr Cardiovasc Dis 1986; 29:107-28.

54. Stehbens WE. Vascular complications in experimental atherosclerosis. Progr Cardiovasc Dis 1986; 29:221-37.

55. Hopkins PN, Williams RR. Identification and relative weight of cardiovascular risk factors. Cardiovasc Clinics 1986; 4:3-31.

56. Gould L. Reddy CVR, Oh KC et al. Premature hair graying: A probable coronary risk factor. Angiology 1978; 29:800-3.

57. Koskenvuo M, Kaprio J, Telakiri et al. Snoring as a risk factor for ischaemic heart disease and stroke. Br Med J 1987; 294:16-19.

58. Kolenda K. Philosophy's Journey: A Historical Introduction. Philadelpha: Addison-Wesley, 1974.

59. Murphy EA. The Logic of Medicine. Baltimore: Johns Hopk Univ, 1976.

60. Knox EG. Epidemiology in Health Care Planning. New York: Oxford Univ Press, 1979.

61. Susser M. Causal Thinking in the Health Sciences. London: Oxford Univ Press, 1973.

62. Beaglehole R. Does passive smoking cause heart disease? Br Med J 1990; 301:1343-4.

63. Renwick JH. Analysis of cause—long cut to prevention? Nature 1973; 246:114-5.

64. Yerushalmy J, Palmer CE. On the methodology of investigations of etiologic factors in chronic diseases. J Chron Dis 1959; 10:27-40.

65. Weissler AM, Miller BI, Boudoulas H. The need for clarification of percent risk reduction data in clinical cardiovascular trial reports. J Am Coll Cardiol 1989; 13:764-6.

66. Smith RL, Pinckney ER. The Cholesterol Conspiracy. St Louis: Warren H Green, 1991.

67. Dock W. Atherosclerosis. Why do we pretend the pathogenesis is mysterious? Circulation 1974; 50:647-9.

68. Katz LN, Stamler J. Experimental Atherosclerosis. Springfield: C C Thomas, 1953.

69. Leary T. The genesis of atherosclerosis. Arch Pathol 1941; 32:507-55.

70. Stamler J. Shekelle R. Dietary cholesterol and human coronary heart disease. Arch Pathol 1988; 112:1032-40.

71. Stehbens WE. The lipid hypothesis and the role of hemodynamics in atherogenesis. Progr Cardiovasc Dis 1990; 33:119-36.

72. Stehbens, WE. Experimental induction of atherosclerosis associated with femoral arteriovenous fistulae in rabbits on a stock diet. Atherosclerosis 1992; 95:127-35.

73. Rand A. Philosophy: Who Needs It? Indianapolis: Bobbs-Merril, 1982.

CHAPTER 4

DIAGNOSTIC ERROR AND THE VALIDITY OF VITAL STATISTICS

In the preceding chapter it was argued that coronary heart disease (CHD) is an inappropriate monitor of severe atherosclerosis. Notwithstanding this contention and other deficiencies in the epidemiological approach, further problems require consideration.

Epidemiological investigations involve community groups or whole populations and no matter whether epidemiologists rely on the diagnosis of a clinical endpoint or on vital statistics, the validity of the results and conclusions derived therefrom depend on accuracy of the diagnosis, this being a basic requirement of any clinical scientific investigation. It is particularly important if the results of such investigations influence governmental and public health policies and pronouncements affecting communities and populations. As this is the current state of affairs the accuracy of clinical diagnoses and the validity of vital statistics pertaining to atherosclerosis and its manifestations warrant review.

CLINICAL DIAGNOSTIC ERROR FOR CORONARY HEART DISEASE

The most dependable means of determining the accuracy of serious fatal diseases is to compare the final clinical diagnosis or death certificate with the results of a well conducted autopsy. Historically this type of clinicopathological correlation has contributed much to modern medicine. Questioning the accuracy of death certificates by this method, in 1912 Cabot[1] found that for 28 disorders the accuracy varied from 16 to 95%. Medical advances have effected only marginal improvement for a similar rate of error was reported[2] in 1937 and again in 1960, due to inadequate identification of new diseases and related problems. Disagreement between ante- and postmortem diagnoses at two United Kingdom (UK) hospitals[3] between 1959 and 1972, varied from 20 to 23%. Findings of similar concern were reported[4] in the United States of America (USA) between 1960 and 1980. In 1985 approximately 33.8% of 2067 autopsies from 32 teaching and nonteaching hospitals in the USA had major discrepancies between clinical and autopsy diagnoses. Prominent amongst the errors were myocardial and cerebral infarcts.[5] In a review of the rate of disagreement between clinical and autopsy diagnoses in different countries,[6] the rate varied from 6% to 68%. In 75 British hospitals there was agreement between clinical and autopsy diagnoses in only 49.5% of 9,501 necropsies.[7]

Errors tend to be more frequent in the elderly, in those hospitalized for less than 24 hours or for very protracted periods of time and, as one might expect, when the clinical diagnoses are uncertain. The diagnostic error continues to be substantial even with modern ancillary aids. It is well to remember that this type of monitoring of diagnostic errors occurs primarily in teaching and major general hospitals and it is a safe assumption that the error is probably substantially lower there than in provincial hospitals and in general practice.[3,7]

Errors are made in determining both the primary cause of death and contributory causes. Britton[8] reported that 15% of contributory causes diagnosed clinically had been disproved at autopsy and 46% of contributory causes found at autopsy were overlooked antemortem. When acute myocardial infarction was considered a contributory cause of death, it was missed clinically in 93% of cases.[9] When CHD, CVD and other vascular diseases were diagnosed clinically as contributory causes of death, 13.2% were not confirmed at autopsy, but when 319 causes were so diagnosed at autopsy 134 were unrecognized clinically (42%).[9] In a prospective study of 1152 hospital autopsies the major underlying clinical cause of death was not confirmed in 39% of cases, in 66% of conditions resulting from the main disease but which were ultimately responsible for death, and in 81% of additional lesions which may or may not have contributed to death.[10] When Cameron and McGoogan[11] included acute myocardial infarction as the principal or contributory cause of death, together with coexisting significant infarcts, 198 clinical diagnoses were confirmed at autopsy, 51 were first discovered at autopsy and another 58 were over-diagnosed.

Gittelsohn[12] reported an increased tendency in the USA for usage of nonspecific terminology. Standardized mortality rates for some specific diseases varied geographically by a factor of 20. Inaccuracies in the underlying cause of death at times resulted from recording and coding mistakes. Gau and Diehl,[13] testing 97 general practitioners on 10 case histories, found 90% agreement on the cause of death when diagnoses were grouped into broad International Classification of Diseases (ICD) categories and only one organ system was involved in the history. With more than one organ system involved agreement was less than 50%. With the least complicated there was agreement amongst only 90% of general practitioners. Walford[14] estimated that in death certificates from general practice giving coronary occlusion as the cause of death, approximately 20% were based mainly on guesswork.

Differences in reported mortality rates between countries or populations may be due to variation in national custom in diagnosis, classification and coding of causes of death. For example Reid and Rose[15] circulated full case histories to hospital doctors in Bergen, Boston and London requesting death certificates on the cause of each death. More deaths were attributed to CHD by doctors in the USA and to emphysema and bronchiectasis by British doctors in the UK, tendencies according with reported mortality differences from specific diseases.

Autopsies are certainly not infallible and are performed mostly by trainees under variable supervision. The interpretation of results may be deficient and may require confirmatory discussion with the clinician in charge of the patient. However they still provide more reliable information on the cause of death and diseases contributing to death than clinical diagnoses. At autopsy death may be attributed to CHD as a last resort if the coronary arteries are moderately atherosclerotic. Within the same country differences in pathological findings and assessments of the severity of atherosclerosis are reported from different institutions and sometimes from within the one institution.[16] Nevertheless autopsies are a better gauge for auditing death certificates than retrospective clinical appraisals which while still quite revealing, tend to underestimate diagnostic error. The value of the autopsy however is partially negated if the results are not used to correct the death certificate or are improperly recorded. This occurred in 42% of autopsied cases in the study by Engel et al.[17]

Of 3,900 death certificates 57% were defective, almost half were incomplete, 24% used obsolete terminology and 28% were frankly inaccurate.[18] Moriyama et al[19] considered the cause of death on only 79% of 1837 death certificates in Pennsylvania was probably correct or reasonable on available evidence. When studying 191 death certificates at the Royal College of Physicians of London,[20] (autopsy rate of 48%), agreement on the cause of death was found in only 51.3%: discrepancies were major in 20.4% and minor in 28.3%, but in 25% the disagreement was epidemiologically misleading.

In a comparison of the principal clinical diagnosis in hospital with the underlying cause of death on 1216 death certificates, there were discrepancies in 39%, more often with certain diseases.[21] Discrepancies were least common with malignant tumors and frequent among the aged and in some specialties. There were coding differences in 18% of cerebrovascular diseases, 18% for CHD and 75% for "other diseases of the heart". In 105 random cases the original codes for hospital diagnoses and death certificates differed in 40%, most errors being due to mistaking a complication or an associated illness for the principal diagnosis or underlying cause of death. Such errors on a national scale seriously reduce the value of death certificates and are particularly frequent when death is sudden such as with CHD and CVD.[22,23]

DIAGNOSIS OF CHD AS THE CAUSE OF DEATH

In 1919 the chance of a correct diagnosis of diseases of the heart and pericardium[24] was only 47% and for blood vessels 42%. Such accuracy is probably exaggerated because coronary occlusion and myocardial infarction became widely recognized only in the late 1920s. Diagnostics of CHD have improved since then and pathologists are more familiar with the pathology of CHD but the diagnostic error is still substantial as seen in Table 4.1. It is usually greater for old healed infarcts: Levine and Phillips[47] reported that 75% of acute infarcts were recognized clinically but only 20% of old infarcts, this no doubt being a reflection of the cases missed clinically. Johnson et al[33] reported that 61% of acute infarcts were clinically diagnosed whereas in two series of old infarcts 50% had been recognized.[33,48] In a recent report from the USA, 28.3% of clinical diagnoses of acute myocardial infarction were not confirmed at autopsy.[49]

Gover[50] reported that in 1940 in the USA, heart disease as the primary cause of death (161 per 100,000) was little more than the rate as a contributory cause (121 per 100,000), indicating that an additional 75% of cases were not included in vital statistics which could be radically altered by a shift in status from contributing to underlying cause or the reverse without real change in the incidence of CHD at death. Beadenkopf et al[51] compared death certificates with autopsy data and found diagnostic specificity of atherosclerotic heart disease was 82% but sensitivity was only 50%. CHD was present in 25% of patients classified as not having CHD, CVD, hypertension or diabetes mellitus.

CHD mortality in Scotland is said to be higher than in England and Wales but when samples of death certificates were appraised, diagnostic accuracy was greater by 33% in the English sample[52] but this is partly due to differences in legal practice.[53] Keys[54] said CHD was underestimated in Norway in 1964 by 15% whilst in premenopausal Australian women, myocardial infarction was diagnosed clinically 3.4 times more often than at autopsy.[55] In Japan the incidence is considered low but the autopsy rate for all deaths[56] is only 4.4% with the possibility of considerable but undetermined diagnostic error. Approximately half the larger infarcts in a Japanese autopsy study were found initially at necropsy and all small infarcts less than 5 cm in the greatest dimension were missed clinically.[57] In the larger infarcts typical cardiac pain was present in only 50%.

In comparing CHD mortality rates or prevalence in many underdeveloped countries the validity of the data must first be assessed. In 1954 no vital statistics for the Bantu of South Africa existed and knowledge of disease pattern was dependent on clinical impression and examination of hospital material which is selected. Even today many still have a tribal lifestyle, thus precluding reliable vital statistics. Atherosclerosis is "common" in the Bantu[58] but its severity is less than in the USA and other western countries. Personal experience of senior pathologists confirms the lesser severity.[59,60] This experiential evidence has led to speculative causal relationships but the degree of severity is difficult to quantitate. Becker[61] considered the severity to be little different at autopsy from that in the West and admitted difficulty in comparison without detailed age distribution

Table 4.1. Diagnostic errors for CHD as reported in the literature

Authors	Study period	Type of lesion	No. of cases diagnosed clinically and confirmed at autopsy	No. of cases diagnosed clinically but not confirmed at autopsy (False +ve)	No. of cases diagnosed at autopsy but undiagnosed clinically (False -ve)
Bean[25]	1922–36	acute MI	114	–	62 (35.2)
Swartout & Webster[26]	1933–37	disease of coronary arteries	145	74 (33.8)	–
		arteriosclerosis	56	29 (34.1)	–
Wallgren[27]	1934–39	coronary thrombosis	6	20 (76.9)	–
Feil et al[28]	1938	recent MI	28	6 (17.6)	6 (17.6)
Yater et al[29]	W.W.II	CHD	116	–	87 (42.9)
Munck[30]	1940–49	coronary thrombosis	26	14 (35)	7 (21.2)
Gould & Cawley[31]	1945–55	Old MI	277	–	175 (38.7)
James et al[18]	1951–52	arteriosclerotic heart disease	201	75 (27.2)	66 (24.7)
Friedberg et al[32]	1952–56	coronary occlusion	73	14 (16.1)	68 (48.2)
Johnson et al[33]	1953–54	acute or healed MI	57	–	86 (60.1)
Paton[34]	1954–55	recent MI	118	96 (44.9)	52 (30.6)
Registrar General[35]	1955	arteriosclerotic heart disease	93	65 (41.1)	69 (42.6)
Lee et al[36]	1957	acute MI	403	–	97 (19.4)
Heasman & Lipworth[7]	1959–60	CHD	552	443 (44.5)	513 (48.2)
Melichar et al[37]	1959–60	recent and old MI	365	–	398 (52.2)
Mitchell et al[38]	1959–71	acute MI & arteriosclerotic heart disease	60	–	15 (20)
Abramson et al[39]	1960–63	CHD	98	–	35 (26.3)
Goldman et al[4]	1960–80	MI	28	–	13 (31.7)
Engel et al[17]	1970	vascular heart disease	64	14 (17.9)	7 (9.9)
		acute MI	16	12 (42.9)	8 (33.3)

Table 4.1. Diagnostic errors for CHD as reported in the literature (continued)

Authors	Study period	Type of lesion	No. of cases diagnosed clinically and confirmed at autopsy	No. of cases diagnosed clinically but not confirmed at autopsy (False +ve)	No. of cases diagnosed at autopsy but undiagnosed clinically (False –ve)
Britton[8,9]	1970–71	acute MI	74	11 (12.9)	30 (28.8)
		chronic ischemic heart disease	20	36*(64.3)	4 (16.7)
Hartveit[40]	1975	arteriosclerotic heart disease	300	49 (14.0)	50 (14.3)
Waldron & Vickerstaff[3]	1975–76	isechemic heart disease	128	39 (23.4)	118 (48.0)
Cameron & McGoogan[10,11]	1975–77	cardiovascular disease	276	117 (29.8)	137 (33.2)
		acute MI	188	55 (22.6)	42 (18.3)
Sandritter et al[41] & Drexler et al[42]	1976–77	MI	114	44 (27.9)	41 (26.5)
Asnaes & Paaske[43]	1980	CHD (medicolegal examination)	333	143 (30)	30 (8.3)
Zarling et al[44]	1983	acute MI	53	–	47 (47.0)
Stevanovic et al[45]	1981–84	MI	258	56 (17.8)	83 (24.3)
Longoni et al[46]	1982–84	MI	13	3 (18.8)	7 (35.0)
McGoogan[22]	1984	acute MI	198	58 (22.7)	51 (20.5)

*Unless recent infarct was diagnosed clinically, old infarcts were not included.
False positive and false negative rates are given in parenthesis as percentages.
(Adapted from Stehbens WE, Lancet 1987; 1:606–11)

of autopsies. The nature of the selection and availability for autopsy is also unknown and variation within African countries has not been studied despite variation in environment, diet and lifestyle. Meyer[62] confirmed the lesser severity of coronary atherosclerosis in the Bantu but no difference in cerebral atherosclerosis was found between white and Bantu populations. Nigerian Negroes have less severe cerebral atherosclerosis[63] and Ugandans have the same severity of cerebral atherosclerosis as American Caucasians.[64]

Yater et al[29] reported a series of 203 cases of CHD at autopsy and death occurred before a doctor could see the patients in an additional 247 cases. These sudden deaths are often accepted as due to CHD but Lundberg and Voigt[65] found only 49% of 100 cases of sudden death that conformed to diagnostic criteria of CHD in the USA were confirmed at autopsy. Schottenfeld et al[23] reported concordance between death certificate and autopsy in 87% of cases. When the certificate was prepared prior to autopsy, agreement was only in 69% for CHD.

Cardiovascular diseases present clinicians with considerable difficulty. Moriyama et al[19] considered absolute accuracy for cause-of-death statements unattainable. In 1966 Moriyama et al[66] considered only 70 to 75% of certified deaths classified as cardiovascular disease and 54% of cerebrovascular disease as reasonable inferences. Even so, these figures may have been vastly different if each case had been autopsied. Najem et al[67] assessing reliability of death certificate diagnoses of ischemic and hypertensive heart disease according to predetermined diagnostic criteria, found agreement in 49% of cases of ischemic heart disease and in 47% of hypertensive heart disease. Reliability was greater for hospital rather than nonhospital patients and significantly in the elderly, all ischemic heart disease and 80% of hypertensive heart disease diagnoses from nursing or convalescent homes were classified as wrong or doubtful. The greater inaccuracy in the elderly is important because most CHD deaths occur in those of 65 years and over (Table 4.2).

In the USA where some natural deaths are assessed by "external medico-legal examination" alone, 807 cases were autopsied to monitor validity of the external examination. The cause of death differed in 35.4% of females and 33.9% of males with considerable over-diagnosis of CHD.[43] In a further 87 medically unattended deaths, autopsies were performed after medico-legal certification and the cause of death differed in 30% mostly due to over-diagnosis of CHD. Acute myocardial infarction was correctly assigned as the cause of death in 50% of cases.[69] Vanatta and Petty[70] reported that 29% of 89 natural deaths with medico-legal death certification had an incorrect cause of death following autopsy, mostly due to over-diagnosis of CVD.

It is apparent that the diagnostic accuracy of death certificates leaves much to be desired. Briggs[71] considered death certificates to be valid only for cases that were autopsied. Rose and Barker[72] suggested errors cancel each other out even with this alarming inaccuracy. Table 4.1

Table 4.2. Combined male and female mortality of some vascular diseases in the USA, 1988

	Total number of deaths in specified age groups					
Cause of Death	1-34	35-44	45-54	55-64	65-74	75+
Acute myocardial infarction and ischemic heart disease	1,316 (0.26)	6,793 (1.3)	20,380 (4.0)	58,267 (11.4)	121,112 (23.77)	301,643 (59.2)
Hypertension	269 (0.85)	735 (2.3)	1,810 (5.7)	41,64 (13.1)	7,287 (23)	17,420 (55)
Atherosclerosis	10 (0.05)	54 (0.24)	176 (0.8)	787 (3.56)	2,699 (12.2)	18,356 (83.1)
Cerebrovascular disease	1,362 (0.9)	2,423 (1.6)	4,630 (3.1)	11,196 (7.5)	27,694 (18.4)	10,3051 (68.5)

Figures obtained from the World Health Statistics Annual,[68] excluding neonates (age 0) and those of unspecified age. Percentages are given in parenthesis.

Table 4.3. Mortality from vascular diseases in the USA, 1984

Diagnosis on death Certificate	No. of deaths	Percentage for which diagnosis was causal	Percentage for which diagnosis was contributory
Diseases of the heart	1,163,586	65.8	34.2
Hypertension	88,571	8.8	91.2
Arteriosclerosis	120,639	20.3	79.7
Diabetes mellitus	144,548	24.8	75.2
Cerebrovascular disease	262,508	58.8	41.2

Figures obtained from Puffer.[73]

refutes this. In the example given, the overlap in cases and noncases was unacceptably large and would be increased when the error in contributing diseases is included (Table 4.3). Waldron and Vickerstaff[3] confirmed the clinical diagnosis of CHD in 167 patients in only 128 (76.6%) but CHD cases found at autopsy numbered 246, an increase of 1.4 times in males and 1.7 times in females. False negatives were approximately three times more frequent than false positives. When contributory causes were taken into account, these rates increased to 1.5 (males) and 1.9 (females) respectively. Moreover deaths in 34.5% of patients incorrectly diagnosed as malignant disease were attributed to CHD though most (89.3%) were unsuspected clinically. Scientists should not rely on hoped for coincidences with vital statistics when the diagnostic error is of a magnitude similar to that pertaining to CHD.

IMPRECISION IN THE CLINICAL DIAGNOSIS OF CHD

Traditionally physicians have viewed diagnosis as an intuitive art, based upon background knowledge and personal experience. The clinical diagnosis is dependent on powers of observation and the objectivity and ability of the physician to elicit relevant facts. Progressive increase in knowledge and ancillary aids has improved the diagnostic capability of the physician but the variability in observer error and the clinical picture remains. The clinical diagnosis is ultimately based on probabilities and perhaps the clinician becomes accustomed to the lack of precision. There was concern in the Framingham study that "nondiseased" persons placed in the "diseased" category might so dilute the sample as to mask a significant characteristic.[74] The reverse might also hold true. In addition the fact that the nondiseased (a misnomer) are not nondiseased was ignored. The degree of overlap varies from study to study and Copeland et al[75] consider that if misclassification is large but equal, the estimate of risk is more likely to be of null value. Reference to Tables 4.1 and 4.3 demonstrates that overlap could be considerable but that in most instances the misclassification would be unequal. In nonblind clinical studies when so many investigators appear to be utterly convinced of the

validity of the lipid hypothesis, the possibility of investigator bias in determining a clinical endpoint is possible. Moreover the variable overlap or misclassification may contribute to the inconsistent results of clinical studies.

Many epidemiological studies have involved a population sample manifesting one or other of the clinical syndromes seen in CHD viz (i) angina pectoris, (ii) myocardial infarction, (iii) sudden death. In other cases with CHD the diagnosis is made coincidentally or at autopsy often with congestive cardiac failure. An essential feature in subject selection is reliable detection of the chosen endpoint of the disease. The possibility of misdiagnosis exists in each syndrome.

(1) ANGINA PECTORIS

Typical anginal pain is considered to be due to myocardial ischemia occasioned by insufficient blood flow through severely narrowed coronary arteries most often due to atherosclerosis. Corroborative physical findings of cardiac disease may be lacking and anginal pain may be atypical. Myocardial damage is not the only cause of chest pain which can be due to psychoneurotic, neurological, pulmonary, musculoskeletal and gastrointestinal disturbances. The prevalence of noncardiac chest pain erroneously diagnosed as angina is uncertain. In a study of 57 men who reported chest pain, all were interviewed for 15 minutes by each of three physicians who attempted to determine whether or not they had angina pectoris. Agreement was found in 55%. Koran[76] declared that physicians studied for reliability of clinical methods, data and judgments, almost always disagreed with one another in at least 10% and often 20% of cases. Such margins of disagreement are not inconsequential and given the already documented diagnostic variability amongst all practitioners, probably compound the rate of disagreement to a level in excess of 20%. The reliability of patients' information is also questionable. For example, patients' statements regarding circumcision differed from physical findings in 34.4% of cases and a similar percentage of wives were unable to provide accurate information about this aspect of their husbands anatomy.[77] The reliability of reporting physicians' diagnoses by patients is poor and only 60% reported diagnosed heart disease.[78] Work histories obtained by interview were incorrect in 18% of cases.[79] Even a slight lack of standardization may introduce major bias in the answer to questionnaires and differences in culture and language often leads to different interpretations. Self-administered questionnaires double the number of positive answers when compared with those administered by interviewers.[80]

Angiographic evidence of CHD was found in 88.9% of patients with typical angina but only 49.9% of those with atypical angina had CHD angiographically.[81] There is wide variation in severity of involvement according to age and sex. The predictive value of angina, the electrocardiographic stress test, and other aids vary with the subject's age and sex and are aids only to physician judgement.[81] Coronary angiography cannot be performed on all suspected cases of CHD. Typical angina can be readily recognized as can myocardial infarction but coronary artery insufficiency and frank infarction occur in the absence of significant coronary artery atherosclerosis or occlusion[82] and may be asymptomatic.[83] Pain associated with tissue damage is a primordial warning system and why transient myocardial ischemia may be painless is unknown. The hemodynamic profile associated with spontaneous and reversible electrocardiographic evidence of transient ischemia may be the same whether accompanied or unaccompanied by pain[84] and even extensive frank infarction can be painless.

Cohn[85] estimated that there could be four to five million patients with silent myocardial infarction in the USA. This includes 50,000 asymptomatic patients who have had myocardial infarction, one to two million asymptomatic patients with no history of myocardial infarction or angina and three million patients with angina. The diagnosis depends on fortuitous exercise testing[85] and routine electrocardiography or autopsy. Approximately 70% of ischemic episodes are asymptomatic in patients that are continuously monitored.[86] Of 1583 subjects with more than 70% coronary artery narrowing, 70.2% had developed angina pectoris or ST depression during exercise testing but in all 56.6% had no pain, 44.4% had no ST de-

pression and 29.8% had neither.[87] The prevalence of unrecognized ischemia or infarction is considerably higher than usually appreciated and freedom from severe coronary disease in those with angina is not uncommon and may be as high as 20 or 30%.[88-90] Malliani and associates[91] concluded that myocardial ischemia most often does not produce pain, but it may also be delayed.[91] Sigwart et al[92] considered silent ischemia may be found in every CHD patient at some stage and that the prevalence of angina pectoris should be regarded merely as the tip of the iceberg. Since severe coronary atherosclerosis is extraordinarily common in unselected autopsies and an appreciable number of subjects with severe coronary atherosclerosis have normal electrocardiographs despite exercise testing,[93,94] there is no indisputable method of determining the frequency of CHD by clinical means. Ischemic attacks can be triggered by daily activities[95] including strain such as mental computation, cold exposure and even mastication. These patients tend to develop clinical CHD with time.[96] The presence of clinical angina considerably underestimates the incidence of cardiac ischemia. In studies reviewed by Cohn[85] asymptomatic myocardial ischemia was found in 2.5% to 10% of adults tested which represents a great number of individuals in the population at large. In patients with CHD monitored and found to have multiple episodes of ischemic type S-T segment depression, Schang and Pepine[95] found only 25% were associated with angina. Most occurred at rest or during very light activity.

Not everyone with anginal pain has CHD and the likelihood varies with age and sex. No definite syndrome heralds the onset of significant CHD and this makes the diagnosis on clinical grounds uncertain, and hints at a broad transition zone with considerable overlap of those with and those without clinical disease.[97] Goodale et al[98] contend that the greater clinical suspicion of CHD in men than in women is likely to be operative when the disease is mild, nonfatal and difficult to diagnose. There are patients with angina and myocardial infarction with angiographically normal coronary arteries[82] and others with only minimal disease. The clinical diagnosis depends ultimately on probabilities with the magnitude of diagnostic error or omission considerable but unquantifiable.

(2) MYOCARDIAL INFARCTION

Clinical presentation of myocardial infarction can vary widely. The classical acute form is readily diagnosed but prolonged and persistent angina may simulate frank infarction. Other patients may present primarily with dyspnea or congestive cardiac failure. Sudden death is common with asymptomatic infarction more frequent than is generally recognized, particularly in diabetics.[99] Silent infarctions pose a major diagnostic problem of uncertain magnitude.

Myocardial infarction was rarely diagnosed before 1920 and Table 4.1 indicates the considerable diagnostic error reported in fatal cases in the literature since then. Boyd and Werblow[100] reported that 29.3% of their myocardial infarcts at autopsy were clinically undiagnosed.

In 1960 it was stated "Even with modern diagnostic methods, the vast majority of completed certifications of death with the primary cause as "acute coronary thrombosis" or "acute myocardial infarction", are, at best, educated guesses.[98] It would be expected that within the past 20 or so years advances in diagnostic technology for CHD would suggest increased sensitivity and specificity in the diagnosis of acute myocardial infarction but in 1983 Zarling et al[44] reported that only 53% of autopsy proven acute myocardial infarctions were correctly diagnosed clinically. Half of their cases were managed by cardiologists. Goldman et al[4] studying autopsy diagnoses in the academic years 1960, 1970 and 1980 at one university teaching hospital, found 32% of patients coming to autopsy with myocardial infarction in the three years were missed clinically with an actual increase in the 20 year period. The difficulty in diagnosing myocardial ischemia is not widely appreciated and diagnosis remains largely subjective. Even in institutions with modern ancillary aids, it is not possible to employ the facilities in every case. The reliability of clinical diagnoses varies within institutions, from hospital to hospital, country to country, and from decade to decade and as indicated earlier, in general practice the diagnosis is often guesswork.[14]

Reviews in the 1930s recorded history of no pain in 33-39% of patients with myocardial infarction.[100,101] In 200 consecutive autopsied cases of myocardial infarction, Kennedy[101] reported that 22% of old infarcts were painless but only 4% of those dying within eight weeks of the infarct had experienced no pain. In about one-third of acute infarctions, an adequate history is impossible to elicit, often because of such interventions as sudden death, coma, surgical anesthesia and complicating cerebrovascular accidents.[102] In other patients various chest sensations have been misinterpreted, often as indigestion. Melichar et al[37] considered only 10% of 398 unrecognized myocardial infarcts found at autopsy could have been deduced because in 87.6% of recent infarcts both onset and course were painless. Old age, rapid death (53%), encephalomalacia (17%), and coincidental pulmonary embolism (11%) can be responsible for nonrecognition. Some old infarcts were found in patients dying of congestive cardiac failure or other serious noncardiac pathology but rapidly progressive cardiac failure can complicate a recent massive septal infarct particularly with a perforated septum. In one clinical series of patients with myocardial infarction, 20% were admitted with no symptoms referable to the heart[103] but in autopsy-proven infarcts, many subjects die before a history can be obtained. Clinical diagnosis of myocardial infarction is particularly variable in the elderly. In patients aged 65 years and over only 19.4% presented with the classical onset.[104] An equal number presented with sudden dyspnea or an exacerbation of heart failure. Most other forms of presentation were not directly referable to the heart. On the other hand Yater et al[29] found that half of the fatal nonsudden cases of myocardial infarction (males aged 18 to 39 years) had no known symptoms prior to the fatal attack. In a series of patients with pathologically proven myocardial infarction,[105] only 47% presented with characteristic pain, 38% with dyspnea and in 11% the clinical picture was obscure and diagnosis made only at autopsy.

Myocardial infarction can occur as the first indication of ischemic heart disease in patients with severe or minimal coronary atherosclerosis[106] with sudden unexpected death one of the manifestations of such ischemia. Associated embolic phenomena may lead to cerebrovascular disease (CVD) as the mode of clinical presentation but the diagnosis of myocardial infarction is often made on insufficient evidence. Paton[34] reported that in a group of subjects diagnosed clinically to have myocardial infarction with electrocardiography but not dying suddenly, only 35% were confirmed at autopsy.

Electrocardiographic evidence has varied in its reliability over the years and with observer error.[107,108] The electrocardiogram, rarely normal in acute myocardial infarction, was atypical in 32% of 215 patients[109] and was therefore open to variable interpretation. In a review of the literature[110] only 63% of infarcts at autopsy had electrocardiographic evidence of infarction and in 306 infarcts with adequate antemortem studies, more than 20% were unrecognized by any clinical means. In a more recent study[111] the diagnosis of acute recurrent infarction was made electrocardiographically in only 81% of patients.

Woods et al[112] found the accuracy rate of electrocardiography fell from 82% when infarction was acute to 27% with a single old infarct. Where multiple old infarcts were found at autopsy the accuracy rate rose to 58% but the overall accuracy rate was only 48%. Unequivocal electrocardiographic signs of myocardial infarction were found in 81.5% of cases by Weiss and Weiss[113] and in 35% by Skjaeggestad and Molne[114] who found equivocal signs in 34% and no evidence at all in 31%.

According to Cox[115] 10.9% of middle aged men with myocardial infarction had a normal electrocardiogram after one year and 20.0% at four years, thus allowing silent and misdiagnosed cases to remain undetected. In another 128 patients with previous myocardial infarction 31% failed to show electrocardiographic evidence of old infarction.[116] This variability in diagnostic value of the electrocardiograph may be partially due to observer error as Davies[107] reported disagreement of surprising magnitude between cardiologists with agreement in only one-third and, when retested they disagreed with their own interpretations in 12%. Segall[117] reported 90 to 100% agreement in only 44% of electrocardiographs. Acheson[118] reported 50% disagreement for myocardial infarction and 26%

for ischemia alone. Such discrepancies in the interpretation of this important clinical investigation add yet another serious dimension to the question of reliability or otherwise of clinical epidemiological studies of CHD.

In 1959 at Framingham 21% of myocardial infarcts had gone unrecognized.[105] In 1984 more than 25% of myocardial infarctions were detected during routine biennial electrocardiographic examinations[119] and almost half of these were silent. Moreover 30.1% of all initial infarcts were unrecognized and it was concluded that the "frequency of unrecognized infarctions reported here underestimates the true incidence, since it excludes persons with electrocardiographic findings that were not persistent and those whose unrecognized infarctions resulted in out-of-hospital death". Of their out-of-hospital "heart attacks", 34% had unrecognized infarcts[120] (more frequent in diabetics and hypertensives). Considerable overlap between "cases" and controls must have occurred and the inference is that much of the early Framingham literature is in need of review.

In a five-year follow-up of subjects over 40 years of age 39.8% of myocardial infarcts were unrecognized[121] and the rate rose steeply with increasing age. In a *Lancet* editorial[122] it was estimated that for every clinical infarct detected there is probably at least one unrecognized infarct in the same population and even this may be an underestimate.[123] There are many factors other than the severity of atherosclerosis that affect detection and survival. Outcome of an infarct and therefore the likelihood of detection is dependent on infarct size, left ventricular functional impairment, the severity of atherosclerosis in collateral arteries supplying the viable muscle, arrhythmias and the presence of other concomitant diseases such as diabetes mellitus, hypertension, the functional state of the cardiac valves and obesity.

(3) SUDDEN DEATH

Kuller et al[124] attributed 61.4% of sudden deaths to CHD and 9.2% to CVD and considered 60% of all deaths from atherosclerotic heart disease between 40 and 60 years of age were sudden. Sudden death was thought to be the first manifestation of CHD in 20 to 25% of patients but these appraisals were unconfirmed by autopsy.

Noncardiac causes[125] and even cardiac causes independent of severe coronary atherosclerosis can be responsible for sudden death.[126,127] These include glue sniffing[128] and cocaine usage.[129] It has been suggested that sudden death may be due to ventricular fibrillation mediated by the autonomic nervous system due to emotional stress.[130] The evidence may be anecdotal but dysrhythmias appear to be an important factor and the tendency may be enhanced by smoking[131] possibly mediated by pharmacological agents absorbed from the inhaled smoke. Enhanced cardiac irritability associated with smoking, psychological stress[132] or primary (unexplained) "electrical" instability[133] could conceivably occur with less severe grades of coronary atherosclerosis than would otherwise be the case. It has been suggested that hearts with less extensive ischemia are more prone to fibrillate and cause sudden death than those with extensive myocardial involvement.[134] Hypertensive and diabetic patients are particularly prone to sudden death[99] and the syndrome with ventricular fibrillation can be artificially produced by severe experimental myocardial ischemia.[135]

The definition of sudden death varies but in those attributable to CHD, myocardial infarction is unlikely to be demonstrable if death occurred within six hours although it may have been pre-existing. If no other cause of death is demonstrable at autopsy and coronary atherosclerosis is severe, death will usually be attributed to CHD especially in the presence of left ventricular hypertrophy. A mural thrombus in a coronary artery with transient myocardial ischemic attacks could be overlooked producing a variable clinical picture[136] with ample opportunity for cardiac dysrhythmia precipitated by ischemia. It is estimated that 15 to 30% of patients with acute myocardial infarction die within an hour of its onset,[137] whereas Rosenberg and Malach[102] reported sudden death in 60% of patients dying of acute myocardial infarction. However 6 of the 29 patients (21%) with ventricular fibrillation who were successively resuscitated had normal coronary arteries angiographically.[138] While not excluding the possibility of ulceration and mural thrombosis with embolism of coronary arteries,[136] this indicates the fallacy of assuming that clinical CHD can always be

equated with a severe grade of atherosclerosis.

In 500 consecutive cases of sudden death autopsied at the coroner's office and ascribed to CHD, 184 (36.8%) had either a recent coronary artery thrombosis, acute myocardial infarction or both to explain the event.[139] The remainder had coronary atherosclerosis of a very variable degree of involvement and healed infarcts in 275 hearts (55%). It was believed[139] that differential oxygenation of various portions of the myocardium caused cardiac electrical instability resulting in dysrhythmia.

Gould and Cawley[31] reported old healed myocardial infarcts in 3.5% of autopsies at a county hospital and cited studies in which an old infarct was found in 25 to 32% of persons dying suddenly and unexpectedly without a previous history of CHD. One of the most important studies was that of Lundberg and Voigt[65] who found CHD postmortem in only 49% of 100 cases of sudden death selected to conform to the diagnosis of ischemic heart disease in the USA.

A cardiac cause of sudden death is probably assumed too often and since about two-thirds of coronary deaths occur outside hospital[137] and often suddenly, there is the potential for considerable error since few would come to autopsy. A cardiac cause is often one of convenience based only on the history of heart disease, the suddenness of death or the absence of other known possible causes. This, allied to the clinical diagnostic error when clinical information is available, casts further doubt on the validity of the clinical diagnosis of CHD.

MALDIAGNOSIS OF CHD

Clinical medicine is not an exact science and diagnoses are subjective and based on probabilities and often recognition of a clinical syndrome of history, symptoms, age and possibly a family history. The purpose of this review is not to be critical of physicians and cardiologists but to explain how readily maldiagnoses occur. The accuracy of the diagnosis of CHD both clinically and as a cause of death is unquantifiable because of variation in the mode of presentation, reliability of the patient, diagnostic fashions, observer error clinically and electrocardiographically and the experience and training of the physician. Chest pain often masquerades as other syndromes (congestive cardiac failure, neurological defects, indigestion, cholecystitis, apprehension, syncope) giving ample opportunity for misdiagnosis. Cardiologists are familiar with the diagnostic difficulties and the number of patients with silent ischemia and infarction remains unknown but is very substantial.[85] Therefore in clinical epidemiological studies the reliability of the division of a population into two groups, viz an experimental and control, is suspect. Many more subjects have severe atherosclerosis than those with symptoms.[106] Added to this is the possibility of up to 12% of patients with angina or myocardial infarction having minimal coronary atherosclerosis,[106] the silent nature of 70% of ischemic episodes in continuously monitored patients and the inappropriateness of using CHD to monitor the severity of atherosclerosis.

From the review of clinical diagnosis and CHD mortality rates (Table 4.1), a conservative estimate is that clinical epidemiological reviews can have an overlap (misclassification) of 30 to 40% in each group and the Framingham study is no exception. In trials which compare clinical manifestations of the pathological vagaries of atherosclerosis and its complications in two population samples this degree of maldiagnosis is scientifically unacceptable.

Some epidemiologists have allegedly validated clinical diagnoses of CHD in the epidemiological community studies by the use of WHO criteria for CHD. There is no reason to believe that epidemiologists trained in epidemiological and statistical methods and not in clinical medicine are more reliable diagnostically than cardiologists and internists. Validation must be by autopsy but unfortunately autopsy rates worldwide are in decline. Autopsies are a better gauge for auditing death certificates than retrospective reappraisal without the benefit of autopsies.

NATIONAL CHD MORTALITY RATES

Epidemiologists, lacking alternative data on causes of death, have relied heavily on national mortality statistics. Collected and published by the World Health Organization (WHO), they are the only source of national and geographic mortality rates of CHD. The rates are based on death certificates which are important legal and social requirements but are not specifically designed for scientific purposes. The published data are restricted to countries with adequately reported data, which are used to demonstrate age, sex, annual, geographic, national, racial and community differences in death rates in the hope that possible clues to the etiology or to the factors assisting in disease prevention will become apparent. Vital statistics for CHD (and to a lesser extent stroke) have been widely used for this purpose. The value of such investigations depends on input accuracy and valid interpretation. Sophisticated statistical techniques are used and numerical data are often assumed to be as absolute as grams and centimeters used in laboratories.[140] The validity of these vital statistics has been criticized by many authors.[6,140-143] The diagnostic accuracy in death certification is far from satisfactory as indicated and additional features contribute to their lack of reliability.

(1) CENSUS DATA

Population censuses need to be accurate to determine mortality rates but standards are variable. Census counts tend to be low due to illegal immigration, transients and especially children under five years. In one Irish study[144] not all births were registered. In the 1950 USA census,[144] the population was considered to be underestimated by 1.4% with about 10% of Negroes not included.[145]

Age-corrected mortality rates are essential for geographic comparison of mortality rates but the ages of death have significant error. In 1941 in the USA, 25% of ages for whites obtained from hospital or physician notes did not fall in the same five-year age group recorded on the death certificates. There was agreement for colored subjects in only 66%. The percentage agreement was greater for males than for females.[146] Such inaccuracies can mislead.

(2) REGISTRATION OF DEATHS

Not all deaths are registered and this is particularly so during wars.[144] In a survey of Irish parish burial records, 14% of 2000 deaths were unregistered[144] though census data and death registrations have improved immensely since 1900.

(3) MEDICAL CERTIFICATION OF DEATHS

In some countries not all deaths are medically certified[140,144] and this confounds the already unreliable mortality data. In the late 1940s the percentage of deaths not medically certified varied in French geographic regions[147] from 10 to 54%. Laymen signed 20% of death certificates in Sweden and senility and uncertain causes still constituted about 20% of the causes of death.[148] In 1952 since only 43% of ill people in Japan were treated by physicians,[140] the medical certification rate must have been low. Also CHD was regarded as socially unacceptable on a death certificate.[149] Likewise not all deaths were certified in Ireland,[144,150] with up to 9.2% of deaths uncertified in 1954, dropping to 3.3% in 1965. The prevalence of this problem in most western countries is lower now but was probably significant in earlier years.

In France the custom has been to attribute death to CHD if closely related in time to a recognizable infarct but when cardiac failure sets in after a lag period, death is attributed to chronic myocarditis[151] which is often mistaken for CHD.[152] Some intentionally incorrect diagnoses are thought to be due to the physician's desire to protect a family from adverse publicity.

Diagnostic fashions or customs bestow derogatory implications which are not intentional but associated with the circumstances prevailing at a particular time and place. Mortality rates in wartime are recognized as less reliable than they would otherwise be. France was said to have a rise in CHD during the Second World War[147] despite food restrictions, which were incriminated in the alleged decrease in CHD in Norway during the same period.[140] Since 1947 the variation between geographic regions in percentage of deaths not medically certified ranged from 10 to 54%. Robb-Smith[140] attributed the low French CHD mortality to certification habits rather than to nutritional deficiencies.

In Japan the low CHD incidence is inconsistent with the allegedly high incidence of CVD, but the necropsy rate has always been low. In 1952 Japan supposedly had the highest rate of cerebral hemorrhage in the world, but the high incidence is now attributed to diagnostic fashion.[143,153]

(4) USE OF AUTOPSY RESULTS

Autopsy results are often not incorporated in death certificates.[17,26,154] In one Scottish study 23.6% of death certificates did not accord with pathologists' conclusions.[154] Engel et al[17] found that the cause of death was improperly recorded on the death certificate in 42% of autopsies and in 46% of acute myocardial infarcts, a problem obviously requiring rectification. As autopsy rates decline the validity of the death certificates will inevitably suffer and this does not augur well for future mortality statistics. Only about 9% of cardiovascular deaths have an autopsy. Validation of clinical diagnoses by autopsies is desirable but they too have inherent limitations.[48]

The autopsy is usually performed by trainees under variable supervision and sometimes by nonpathologists. Its value depends on the ability of the prosector and the severity of atherosclerosis is usually greater than is recognized in angiograms but the lumen may appear smaller at autopsy. The degree of stenosis is usually only a subjective estimate and a mural thrombus may be overlooked. Difficulty also arises when atherosclerosis is severe and no occlusion or acute coronary lesion accounting for death is found. Cardiac dysrhythmia is assumed to be the cause of death particularly in the presence of left ventricular hypertrophy and hypertension. On other occasions when no other explanation for death is available severe coronary atherosclerosis becomes a diagnosis of convenience rightly or wrongly. Hypertrophic obstructive cardiomyopathy continues to be missed by pathologists as might myocarditis or coronary arteritis without histological examination. When other causes of death have been excluded, consultation with the clinician and review of the electrocardiograph may reveal abnormalities of relevance.[155] Small vessel disease, conduction defects and concealed suicide should be considered.

A major problem is severe atherosclerosis even with myocardial scarring with congestive cardiac failure in the presence of other lesions, e.g., calcific aortic stenosis, pulmonary emphysema, bronchopneumonia or even cardiac amyloidosis making a clear cut answer impossible. The final interpretation is subjective and can be a cause of controversy. The diagnosis will be less reliable or the cause missed more often by trainees than by experienced physicians. Any pathologist with a specialty interest will attest to frequent autopsy errors and omissions by general pathologists in that specialty.

(5) Medical Nosology and Technology

These have changed considerably due to advances in medical science and ancillary aids with inevitable changes in diagnostic accuracy which vary within and between countries. The alterations in terminology and the introduction of CHD as a cause of death in the 1930 revision of the International Classification of Diseases (ICD) makes comparison of causes of death during this century difficult in retrospective analyses quite apart from the errors associated with the use of the term CHD and its diagnosis.

Substantial differences in mortality rates follow changes in the ICD. Radical changes introduced in 1949 in procedures and classification of causes of death invalidate direct comparison of CHD death rates before and after 1949. Following the 8th Revision (1969) of the ICD, about 15% more deaths were assigned to CHD from other categories[144] with a reduction of 43% in the age-adjusted death rate for arteriosclerosis.[156] The 9th Revision of the ICD about 1979 may also have affected comparability of mortality rates for CHD. Adjustments for such changes remain subjective and can cause substantial error,[157] leading to speculation on the reasons for such fluctuations.

(6) The Human Factor

A precise diagnosis cannot always be made and there will always be variation in the physician's education, experience and ability, observer error, diagnostic standards and care taken in death certification and conscientiousness in adapting to ICD changes. Certifying practices or fashions can affect most death certificates substantially from country to country and certifying practices accord well with the mortality differences from specific diseases.[15] Individual differences occur even within the same institution. For example, three physicians trained in death certification prepared death certificates for each of 768 deaths from a Hypertension Detection and Follow-up program.[158]

Relevant information was available including additional hospital or autopsy information. Certificates were then coded by three nosologists who had also dealt with the original certificates. The procedures agreed in only 60.1% of cases using the three digit ICD with an increased agreement (72.5%) when diseases were classified only in broad disease categories.

(7) Death Certificates

As previously indicated the use of CHD deaths to monitor the severity of atherosclerosis is inappropriate but even so CHD mortality rates have other flaws. The attending physician is the best person to complete death certificates which are often incomplete (up to 20%). The diagnostic accuracy is unsatisfactory as demonstrated (Table 4.1) and autopsy confirmation of every death is logistically impossible. Traditionally one cause of death is used in vital statistics although death certificates in most countries request the listing of other contributory diseases. Multiple diagnoses are more likely in the elderly in whom diagnostic errors are also more frequent. More than half of the death certificates in the USA contain two or more diagnoses[23] but this has not always been the case in some other countries. Such errors are also prevalent with secondary diagnoses, e.g., almost half of the contributory causes in Britton's study[8] were not recorded and in another series,[39] CHD was confirmed at autopsy as a contributory cause of death in only 65.3% of subjects.

Difficulty arises in listing which of two or several diagnoses is the primary cause of death for death certificates but the greatest source of error is the use of only the cause of death in national mortality statistics. Contributory causes are never taken into account even though they appear on the death certificate as contributing to death. Guralnick[159] reported that coding all diagnoses on death certificates (assuming the diagnoses were correct) would demonstrate an additional 30% arteriosclerotic heart disease (including CHD), 75% CVD, 65% general arteriosclerosis and another 150% hypertensive disease.

Of all contributory diseases on death certificates in the USA[145] in 1955, CHD was cited in 30% but in 1940 heart disease as a contributing disorder would have added an additional

75% to the death rate. Dorn and Moriyama[160] reported the number of deaths for which death certificates indicated vascular diseases as either causal or contributory to death in 1955. Similar but more recent figures are tabulated in Table 4.3. A substantial increase in the incidence of diseases would be recognized if contributory diseases were included. However a significant number of subjects with hypertension, arteriosclerosis, diabetes mellitus and CVD would also have severe coronary atherosclerosis but such cases would be excluded from consideration using monocausal death certificates.

Wiener et al[161] indicated that in 2,587 death certificates, 10.4% were attributed to hypertension, whereas with contributory causes also considered, 22.1% had hypertension, an increase greater than 100%. Markush and Seigel[162] showed the prevalence of CHD varied with age when contributory causes were included, increasing by 12.5% for males 35 to 44 years of age to 27.6% for men 65 to 74 years, whereas for CVD the prevalence increased by more than 100% for each sex and age group.

It is mechanically cumbersome to tabulate and publish combinations of "causes of death"[159] and the above reveals yet another reason for the gross inaccuracy of the incidence of severe grades of these vascular diseases when relying on monocausal mortality statistics. Assuming the diseases listed were present in any one case physicians may not agree on which is the primary cause of death and which is contributory.

(8) CODING OF DEATH CERTIFICATES

This can also be a source of considerable error and contribute to the lack of comparability within and between countries. A study of national coding practices in 1935 revealed differences so great as to largely nullify comparability of national mortality statistics of several countries.[160] Errors (4%) were found in coding a series of death certificates[67] in 1975 and in a later study three nosologists,[163] agreed in 90.2% of cases for three digit ICD categories and two agreed in 99.7%. When CVD, CHD, myocardial infarctions and neoplasms were examined, full agreement among the three and between two of the three was lowest for myocardial infarction viz 86.5% and 88.0% respectively. Intranosonologist disagreement varied from 2.6% to 5.2%.

In a review of 110 patients coded as having acute myocardial infarction, there was no indication of myocardial infarction in 39.1%. This high false positive coding rate could contribute to wide fluctuations in assigned causes of death in mortality statistics.[164]

To assume that coding of death certificates is irreproachable in any country would be unwise and international variability is unknown.

COMMENTARY

Investigations and the reporting of flaws in mortality statistics are valuable contributions to medical science and the overall need for improvement in the quality of data pertaining to causes of death is well recognized. Unfortunately publication of mortality rates by national and international organizations leads many to believe that the figures are accurate and reliable. The use and alleged reliability of these statistics is deeply ingrained in our societies. Yet it is apparent that errors of variable magnitude are present at all steps in the development of vital statistics, and wide national and geographic variabilities of nomenclature, technology and criteria in diagnostics should continue in the foreseeable future. Errors vary with time making retrospective comparisons or adjustments futile speculations and no country can assume that its mortality rates are free of such errors. CHD mortality rates are too inaccurate for scientific use and it cannot be assumed that inherent errors will be similar from country to country nor that statistical analyses can launder the data. Unfortunately with further decline in the autopsy rate in many countries national mortality statistics are unlikely to improve in the foreseeable future.

THE EPIDEMIC RISE OF CHD AND ITS DECLINE

Epidemiologists have used mortality statistics to demonstrate a sharp rise in the incidence of CHD since the turn of the century in many western countries and a decline in some countries since about 1968. It was explained (Chapter 1) how information on the clinicopathological knowledge of myocardial ischemia, although known, had not percolated into either the general medical literature or the awareness of general practitioners until the 1920s. Such a category was not included in the ICD until 1930 and so CHD was assigned to other categories and attributed to other pathological states. With the substantial changes in longevity, population and ICD there has been undoubtedly an increase in the prevalence of the disease which has been misused or mistaken for an increase in age and sex specific mortality rates. This view has been expressed by other authors reviewed briefly in Chapter 1. However in view of the vagaries of death certification, the undefinable diagnostic error in domiciliary and institutional care, the inappropriate use of CHD as a surrogate of atherosclerosis and the many deficiencies in monocausal mortality rates, the only scientific conclusion that can be reached is that the vital statistics are too unreliable to determine whether there has been an epidemic increase in CHD mortality rates or more appropriately the severity of atherosclerosis. On scientific grounds the epidemic of CHD must be regarded as fictitious rather than artifactual and it is unscientific to make unfounded assumptions. Therefore it becomes apparent that the CHD school of epidemiology has been seeking environmental reasons for an epidemic for which there is no evidence.

In epidemiology of infectious diseases, an increase in prevalence irrespective of the size and age of the population would constitute an epidemic. However when a chronic degenerative ubiquitous disease such as atherosclerosis is considered, it is not increased prevalence of CHD deaths that determines the presence of an epidemic. An increase in the rate of progression of atherosclerosis or substantially increased severity of the disease would need to be demonstrated, and I can see no way of ever demonstrating such a phenomenon or fluctuations in severity of atherosclerosis retrospectively until it is possible to assess its severity.

Robb-Smith[140] reviewed the evidence for an increase in severity of atherosclerosis during this century rightly concluding that such retrospective studies were too unreliable for serious consideration. He also refuted allegations by Morris[165] that the severity of coronary atherosclerosis had decreased while the incidence of CHD had increased sevenfold between 1907 and 1949. Few pathologists conversant with vari-

ability in autopsy quality would accept retrospective estimates of severity of coronary atherosclerosis from necropsy reports over such a time range, in view of the known unreliability of visual appraisals of severity of this disease in on-going studies, the inexplicable variation in incidence and severity of diseases even within the same institute and the growth in knowledge of and familiarity with the disease over the same period.

Epidemics of infectious diseases are known for some inexplicable reason to decline possibly because the critical level of immune people in the community is exceeded or perhaps due to a change in the pathogen. In the late 1960s a decline in the CHD morality rate was reported first in the USA and subsequently in several other western countries. Speculations regarding possible explanations were rife. Correlations were alleged with changes in diet, lifestyle and particularly risk factors.[166] Changes in medical education brought about the dramatic increase in CHD mortality rates about 1930 and likewise may again be responsible for some decline as the result of better diagnoses notwithstanding the other defects in national vital statistics. Levy[167] considered that primary prevention was not necessarily the major cause of the decline. Stallones[168] doubted that any risk factors accounted for the mortality variation and Burrows[169] attributed the decline to improved diagnostic accuracy.

It has been suggested that technological advances and improved management contributed to the decline[166] especially hypertension therapy.[170] The decline in mortality for influenza and pneumonia which are believed to enhance CHD mortality was also advanced as being partly responsible.[170] The influence of such factors is difficult to quantify and is conjectural. However at the same time, other countries reported an increase of from 10 to 85% (Austria, West Germany, France, Denmark and Eastern European countries) without satisfactory explanations being offered for the different mortality rates. Sweden, Poland, Italy and Spain experienced an increase for males[171-174] while the female rate declined, remained unchanged or showed a small rise. These changes in national CHD mortality rates were not consistent with changes in dietary consumption of saturated fat and cholesterol and other lifestyle events.[172] Such unexplained inconsistencies are themselves suspicious although the validity of the decline has been virtually unquestioned and its magnitude and consistency were thought to preclude artifacts.[175]

Since previously the CHD mortality rate for the USA was substantially higher than in the UK, and differences in mortality rates and in certifying practices between USA and the UK exist,[15] the difference in CHD rates between the two countries may be fictitious. A fall could denote change in diagnostic accuracy possibly associated with technological advances. Goldberg et al[176] considered the decline in the USA reflected out of hospital coronary deaths and improved hospital survival rates for acute myocardial infarction. Since 60 to 70% of CHD in the USA occurs outside hospital,[177] diagnostic error is likely to be higher than in hospitals where specialists are available and diagnoses are likely to be monitored and influenced by greater experience and continuing education. The variation is difficult to monitor but errors in diagnosis of acute myocardial infarction at a Boston hospital[4] increased between 1960 and 1980. Allegations that differences in such unreliable mortality rates are attributable to greater adherence to beneficial life styles are unfounded and unscientific.

Other causes of death including the overall mortality rate for the USA are declining simultaneously at a rate comparable with CHD[178] and this is consistent with the concept that CHD mortality is a general average cause of death.[179,180]

Strong et al[181] concluded from comparison of coronary arteries from necropsies in New Orleans 10 years apart that there was a reduction in the severity of coronary atherosclerosis amongst white but not black males. The racial difference raises suspicions regarding the reliability of comparison of small samples of arteries a decade apart but even so this does not validate CHD mortality rates which provide "defective data and fallacious science"[141] a fact not appreciated but perhaps ignored by most users of these statistics.

Implicit faith in mortality statistics in general and CHD in particular is unwarranted. The error in vital statistics for CHD is of such un-

certain magnitude that when superimposed on other deficiencies already indicated, the concept of an epidemic rise and decline in many countries must be regarded as unproven in the absence of reliable data. Governmental and health policies based on such data are untenable.[6]

CEREBROVASCULAR MORTALITY RATES

Cerebrovascular disease (CVD) mortality rates are used increasingly to establish a relationship with CHD risk factors. CVD is a nonspecific term comprising (i) cerebral softening due to thrombosis or embolism, (ii) cerebral hemorrhage and (iii) subarachnoid hemorrhage. Stroke is a nonspecific term indicating an abrupt onset of a neurological deficit irrespective of the cause and is therefore often used synonymously with CVD or to encompass cerebral hemorrhage and thromboembolic infarction. Each is an imprecise diagnosis as is CHD. Such diagnoses could include an unknown number of cases in which the lesions are secondary and not primarily due to degenerative vascular disease.[153] Use of CVD as a surrogate marker of the severity of atherosclerosis is more inappropriate than using CHD because of the wide variation in age and severity of proliferative atherosclerosis in the subdivision of CVD. They are often thought to represent (i) atherosclerotic cerebral softening due to thrombosis superimposed on an atherosclerotic ulcer or alternatively atheroembolism, (ii) primary hypertensive intracerebral hemorrhage and (iii) primary (aneurysmal) subarachnoid hemorrhage respectively. Whilst there may be increasing evidence for considering primary instances of these lesions as due to atherosclerosis,[153,182,183] they are usually said to have very different etiologies. The severity of atherosclerosis tends to be less in primary intracerebral hemorrhage than with infarction or embolism and is least severe with berry aneurysms.[153] The ICD also includes under CVD, spasm of the cerebral arteries and unspecified strokes[184] although these are in the minority.

A complicating factor is the difference in atherosclerosis with transient ischemic attacks between Japan and western countries.[153] Small intracranial arteries are more often affected in Japanese than the extracranial arteries (carotid sinus) suggesting possible different etiologies. Cerebral arteritis may also be more prevalent in some Asian countries,[153] thereby affecting the use of CVD as a surrogate of atherosclerosis.

Attempts have been made to verify the relevance of CHD risk factors for CVD but death certificates and hence mortality rates for CVD or stroke and its subdivisions have a large and variable diagnostic error generally considered to be greater than that for CHD.[143,153] It has been estimated that deaths for subdivisions of CVD are incorrectly differentiated in 30 to 80% of cases[184] and differentiation between cerebral hemorrhage and thrombosis was considered to be hazardous, so not surprisingly CVD is not usually subclassified. Combining all CVD in this way masks possible significant differences in national, geographic or racial mortalities. Hartveit[40] considered the CVD accuracy rate to be about 50%. There is considerable evidence of over-diagnosis of CVD (24%) by clinicians in the study by Heasman and Lipworth[7] and particularly of cerebral hemorrhage (43%). They reported that 10% of patients diagnosed as having cerebral tumor were found to have cerebral hemorrhage at autopsy. As in CHD, many patients with deaths due to other causes also have CVD and consequently the mortality rates even if correct, indicate only a percentage of those afflicted.

Errors are frequent as with CHD because of relatively sudden unexpected deaths from the fifth decade onwards. Abramson et al[39] reported an autopsy confirmation rate of clinical diagnoses of CVD of 82.2% as a cause of death and 78.7% as a contributing factor. CVD was underestimated by a factor of 2.5 as a cause of death and 1.9 when contributory. Ratios were higher for those of 65 years of age and born in Europe or America (3.2 and 2.4 respectively). According to Table 4.3 death certificates in which CVD was contributory could add 70% to the mortality rate for CVD.

Britton[8] found 38% of clinically diagnosed circulatory diseases (including CHD and CVD) were incorrect after autopsy and of cases in which clinicians considered CVD was contributory 16% were disproven at autopsy. When CVD was contributory at autopsy, 51% were unrecognized clinically. Cameron and McGoogan[11] reported that CVD at autopsy was contributory

in a further 77.3%. Schottenfeld et al[23] reported that only 75% of clinical diagnosis of CVD were confirmed at autopsy. It is quite apparent that CVD vital statistics must also be regarded as too unreliable for scientific purposes.

In the Framingham study[185] approximately 40% of stroke diagnoses were incorrect and of 196 persons dying of stroke, the diagnosis was not on the death certificate in 35%. A later report[186] from Framingham gave the false positive rate as 21% and the false negative rate as 40% without even taking into account the diagnostic error for subclassification of subtypes. Only 18% of these subjects were autopsied and in 40% of those confirmed at autopsy, stroke was not entered on the death certificate. Diagnostic accuracy varies with clinical skill. Even modern ancillary aids, though useful, are a supplement to and not a substitute for correct clinical evaluation. The large proportion of strokes in general practice, where these aids are unavailable, will mask their effect.

There are of course errors involved in the compilation of national mortality rates. The quality of data in such vital statistics would be unacceptable in any experimental animal project. Treating all cerebrovascular diseases as one cannot provide significant epidemiological findings and no deductions can be made from the relationship of environmental factors using such data. Yet based on such diagnostic inaccuracy, an association of blood lipids and lipoproteins has been sought with CVD as with CHD even though their mortality rates have not paralleled each other this century. The evidence for a relationship has been found inadequate.[184,187] Diabetes mellitus, hyperlipidemia, obesity and smoking have been considered of less relevance to stroke than to CHD.[188] This is probably the reason for the concentration of effort on lipids in CHD although in recent years the interest has increased.

To Stallones[189] the most remarkable finding in the comparison of CVD mortality rates between countries was the wide disparity between different areas without a meaningful pattern and he thought it may well be spurious. The geographic distribution of CVD deaths did not resemble that for CHD and in a comparison of CHD and CVD mortality rates for Ireland and the USA there was little agreement and time trends diverged. He concluded that the determinants of CVD for these two countries differed and, contrary to expectation, were independent of coronary atherosclerosis or hypertension. Tunstall-Pedoe[190] agreed that international mortality rates showed no good correlation between CVD and CHD, men showing a weak positive and women a weak negative correlation.

For the elderly afflicted with strokes due to atherosclerosis, serum cholesterol levels are generally normal and paradoxically the Framingham study recorded an increased risk for stroke in women with low blood LDL levels.[191] A significant correlation between blood cholesterol levels and stroke has not been found.[192] Yano et al[193] found an inverse association between serum cholesterol levels and the risk of intracerebral hemorrhage but a positive correlation with nonhemorrhagic stroke. This reveals the fallacy of combining all types of stroke in epidemiological studies.

The substantial geographic and national variation in CVD death rates has interested epidemiologists but the peculiarly high and low rates have not been explained. Kurtzke[184] stressed the similarity in age-specific annual death rates within Denmark, Eire, England and Wales, Norway, Sweden and the United States where medical and reporting standards were reliable. For CHD the evidence is to the contrary and the diagnostic error for CVD is even greater regardless of the other problems in the compilation of vital statistics within countries. The frequency of CVD in the USA is related to availability of medical services[194] and inversely proportional to the physician population[184] suggesting that some degree of skepticism is warranted.

In Japan, CVD mortality (especially cerebral hemorrhage) is peculiarly high,[184] constituting 59% of all cardiovascular deaths.[153,189] That this was due to diagnostic artifact was strengthened by studies of atomic bomb survivors from Hiroshima and Nagasaki, where only 10% of deaths diagnosed clinically as CVD were confirmed at autopsy and on considering both false positive and negative diagnoses, clinical estimates were six times the number confirmed at autopsy.[195] The death rate was high in the northeast of the main island where hypertension was attributed to a high intake of dietary salt. In 1952, 92% of all cerebrovascular deaths in Japan were classified as cerebral hemorrhage ad in 1962 they comprised 71%, whilst deaths due to cerebral thromboembolism rose from four to 28 per 100,000 in the same interval.[184] Autopsy material provides evidence that cerebral thrombosis is more prevalent than cerebral hemorrhage.[196,197] The high mortality for cerebral hemorrhage and CVD in general is now regarded as due to diagnostic fashion,[195,198] cerebral hemorrhage being a status symbol, an honorable cause of death and indicative of superior intellect in the deceased. This is consistent with (i) Schroeder's findings[199] that cerebral hemorrhage was higher in rural areas where medical services were less developed than in urban districts and (ii) in 1952 the majority of people were cared for by acupuncturists, judo-orthopedists or folk medicine.[140] From 1975 to 1979 cerebral infarction was more common than cerebral hemorrhage.[200]

Variation in incidence of CHD and CVD in Japanese men in Japan, Hawaii and California has led to the conclusion that migration associated with Westernization of lifestyle is accompanied by an increased frequency of these disorders.[201] This interpretation does not take into account natural and geographic variation in diagnostic error and practices which may explain differences rather than the adoption of different lifestyles.

Listing all types of CVD as one will not provide significant epidemiological findings. Even in the UK and North America where physicians attend most people when ill, the reliability of mortality rates for CVD is less than that for CHD. Many cases of stroke (major and minor) which are not considered to have been the cause of death will be excluded. Autopsies cannot be performed on everyone even though they provide a better incidence of stroke on the nonrepresentative population and they can reveal small and perhaps silent lesions not otherwise taken into consideration. It must be concluded that CVD vital statistics contain errors of such magnitude as to make epidemiological conclusions concerning CVD unacceptable. However when the incidence of clinical CVD is used as a nonpathognomonic surrogate for atherosclerosis of variable and uncertain severity rather than measuring the severity of ubiquitous atherosclerosis, the use of such data must be regarded as futile speculation.

Stroke is the third most common cause of death in the western world and a decline in stroke incidence is generally conceded.[202,203] This trend has been said to be evident for 50 years, preceding the advent of hypotensive therapy and the alleged decline in CHD and to have accelerated.[202] Antihypertensive drug therapy appears to have had a pronounced effect on primary cerebral hemorrhage and in major hospitals its incidence at autopsy has declined markedly in the last 20 years.[153] It is highly probable that antihypertensive therapy will reduce the rapidity of progression of atherosclerosis with the effect difficult to measure, less pronounced, and consequently later in appearance than with primary cerebral hemorrhage. Cerebral thrombosis and infarction do not parallel the mortality rate for CHD and are said to be less dependent on environmental factors than CHD.[204] Mortality rates for stroke have declined in several countries preceding the alleged decline of CHD by at least a decade.[205] This disparity in trends between CHD and CVD may be attributed to greater imprecision in the term CVD and the variability and inexactitude of the data.

There is evidence that CVD survival may have improved but comparability of cases and their incidence over a time span of 10 years and more is fraught with insurmountable methodological problems. Contrary to expectations the decline does not affect the sexes simultaneously.[206] Improved CVD mortality data would be needed before there can be any certainty about a decline,[207] or fluctuations in the incidence of CVD and the severity of atherosclerosis.

OTHER VASCULAR DISEASES

The coexistence of CHD and CVD is well recognized and they too may be the cause of death in subjects suffering from peripheral vascular disease (PVD) and aortic aneurysm. In severe aortic, iliac and femoral atherosclerosis aortic aneurysm and thromboembolic phenomena are the two most likely complications. The latter is less often fatal because of the enormous potential for compensatory collateral circulation in the lower limbs. There may be multiple occlusions without clinical evidence of ische-

mia and massive destruction of the arterial tree before gangrene ensues.[208] Intermittent claudication and gangrene may eventuate but such severe involvement of coronary or cerebral arteries is more prone to a fatal outcome.

It is not possible to identify fatal aortic aneurysm from vital statistics but in recent years detection, diagnosis and therapy of aortic aneurysms and their rupture have improved. Death, when not the result of a surgical complication of the prosthesis, is more likely to be due to CHD, CVD or rupture of a second aneurysm elsewhere. The deduction is that severe asymptomatic atherosclerosis of the aorta and large peripheral vessels is much more frequent than CHD or CVD incidence would indicate. This is substantiated by the finding of occlusion of one or more of the main arteries in 42% of 50 left legs studied at routine unselected autopsies (24 to 82 years of age). None had clinical history of ischemia and if all subjects had been over 50 years of age, the incidence would have been higher.[208] Even so this incidence of occlusion of lower limb vessels is higher than that of coronary arteries as Lindbom[209] confirmed.

In one autopsy series,[210] arteriosclerotic heart disease and acute myocardial infarction accounted for 49.9% of 1000 deaths whereas aortic aneurysm was the cause of death in 4.5%. Lower limb vessels were not mentioned. Deaths from aortic aneurysms did not parallel the increase in CHD early in the century but poor differentiation of syphilis and atherosclerosis of the aorta have undoubtedly been a confounding factor. Yet recently ruptured abdominal aortic aneurysm is said to be increasing in incidence[211,212] whilst CHD and CVD have allegedly declined. This, of course, is inconsistent with the lipid hypothesis.

There have been few studies of the diagnostic accuracy for aortic aneurysms and PVD but Table 4.4 indicates the substantial but variable diagnostic error reported for vascular diseases other than CHD and CVD. McGoogan[22] reported that in addition to ruptured and dissecting aortic aneurysms, almost half of which were not diagnosed clinically, the majority of intact saccular aortic aneurysms found incidentally at autopsy even though large was missed clinically. Intermittent claudication, being a symptom of transient ischemia, increases in frequency with age and clinicians seem more inclined to accept symptoms referable to the lower limbs as claudication in patients with known vascular disease.[214] Observer error in recording the presence of peripheral pulses is well recognized and whilst some may consider the results reasonably reproducible,[215] others assert that inability to detect an ankle pulse by one observer is of little significance.[216] Diagnostic error for lower limb ischemia may be low but for other manifestations of severe aortic atherosclerosis the error has been considerable despite epidemiologists neglecting these manifestations of atherosclerosis. The important conclusions are that vital statistics related to clinically manifest aortic atherosclerosis and PVD grossly underestimate the severity of involvement of these arteries by atherosclerosis and to divide a population sample into those with and those without such clinically overt disease is unscientific. The overlap between these categories is unquantifiable and such invalid sampling cannot substitute for grading the severity of aortic and peripheral atherosclerosis.

CONCLUSION

Dawber[214] indicated that CHD, CVD and PVD could be used as syndromes in the study of environmental factors that may influence atherosclerosis. Aortic atherosclerosis with aneurysmal dilatation and PVD are serious complications but their course appears chronic and often insidiously silent and clinically less frequent than the other two syndromes. The diagnostic error associated with these syndromes is very substantial but variable and their incidence clinically underestimates the severity, especially in the lower limbs. The errors are greater than most investigators concede and are not taken into account in evaluating results. It cannot be assumed that such errors are static in time or location and if such an allegation is made evidence for its validity must be provided.

Epidemiologists depend heavily on CHD mortality rates and require an accurate clinical diagnosis of CHD as a surrogacy of atherosclerosis and as endpoints in clinical trials. Apart from the inappropriate use of CHD as previously indicated, the inaccuracy of the data thus provided is substantial and unquantifiable. It

Table 4.4. Tabulation of diagnostic error for noncardiac and noncerebral vascular disease

Authors	Study period	Type of lesion	No. of cases diagnosed clinically and confirmed at autopsy	No. of cases diagnosed clinically but not confirmed at autopsy (False +ve)	No. of cases diagnosed at autopsy but undiagnosed clinically (False −ve)
Karsner et al[24]	1919	Disease of blood vessels (minor errors only)	24	15 (38.5)	21 (46.7)
Mitchell et al[38]	1956–69	Vascular disease (not CHD or CVD)	12	–	10 (45.5)
Engel et al[17]	1970	Vascular disease	64	14 (17.9)	5 (7.2)
Waldron & Vickerstaff[3]	1975–76	Diseases of arteries	29	15 (34.1)	15 (34.1)
Cameron & McGoogan[11]	1975–77	Arterial embolism & thrombosis	10	2 (16.7)	10 (50)
		Aortic aneurysms	14	1 (6.7)	13 (48.2)
Kircher et al[213]	1980	Circulatory disease	59	13 (18.1)	20 (25.3)

Percentage errors (false positive and false negative) are provided in parentheses must be concluded from this review of the nature and quality of CHD and CVD vital statistics that Feinstein[141] was correct when he stated that "no knowledgeable clinician or pathologist in the second half of the 20th century believes that single choices of death certificate diagnoses can indicate specific causes of death and that those choices represent the actual occurrence of the specified diseases". He also said that to use vital statistics for analysis of rates of specific disease and then "to speculate uninhibitedly about genetic or environmental causes of change in these rates, and to initiate elaborate new epidemiological projects based on the unproved causal speculations are activities that seem as strange in modern medical science as would the methods of alchemy applied to molecular biology".[217]

In the use of clinical CHD or CVD in clinical studies of determinants of atherosclerosis and in clinical trials as endpoints to study treatment or regression of atherosclerosis, epidemiologists must take into account and justify not only the inappropriate use of these diagnostic categories but also the substantial and indeterminate diagnostic errors that are known to exist. In such epidemiological investigations the quality of the data is defective and fallacious.

Statistical analyses cannot convert bad data into good data. The unavailability of reliable vital statistics and the inability to measure the severity of atherosclerosis do not excuse the current use of defective and fallacious data but indicate the need to seek better data or more worthwhile avenues of research. Epidemiological conclusions related to the cause and pathogenesis of CHD, CVD and PVD and reached on the basis of such fallacious data are scientifically unacceptable. To use these rates as monitors of the severity of atherosclerosis is worse.

REFERENCES

1. Cabot RC. Diagnostic pitfalls identified during a study of three thousand autopsies. JAMA 1912; 59:2295-8.
2. Gall EA. The necropsy as a tool in medical progress. Bull N Y Acad Med 1968; 44:808-29.
3. Waldron A, Vickerstaff L. Intimations of Quality. Ante-mortem and post-mortem diagnosis. London: Nuffield Provincial Hospital Trust, 1977.
4. Goldman L, Sayson R, Robbins S et al. The value of the autopsy in three medical eras. New Engl J Med 1983; 308:1000-5.
5. Battle RM, Anderson RE, Key CR et al. Factors influencing discrepancies between pre- and post-mortem diagnoses. Lab Invest 1985; 52:5A-6A.
6. Stehbens WE. An appraisal of the epidemic rise of coronary heart disease and its decline. Lancet 1987; 1:606-11.
7. Heasman MA, Lipworth L. Accuracy of certification of cause of death. London: HMSO, 1966.
8. Britton M. Diagnostic errors discovered at autopsy. Acta Med Scand 1974; 196:203-210.
9. Britton M. Clinical diagnostics: Experience from 383 autopsied cases. Acta Med Scand 1974; 196:211-9.
10. Cameron HM, McGoogan E. A prospectove study of 1152 hospital autopsies: I. Inaccuracies in death certification. J Pathol 1981; 133:273-83.
11. Cameron HM, McGoogan E. A prospective study of 1152 hospital autopsies: II. Analysis of inaccuracies in clinical diagnosis and their significance. J Pathol. 1981; 133:285-300.
12. Gittelsohn AM. On the distribution of underlying causes of death. Am J Pub Health 1982; 72:133-40.
13. Gau DW, Diehl AK. Disagreement among general practitioners regarding cause of death. Br Med J 1982; 284:239-41.
14. Walford PA. Sudden death in coronary thrombosis. J Roy Coll Gen Pract 1971; 21:654-6
15. Reid DD, Rose GA. Assessing the comparability of mortality statistics. Br Med J 1964; 2:1437-9.
16. Jacob W. On quality control and standardization of pathoanatomic findings within the framework of an epidemiological pathology. Pathol Europ (Lond) 1973; 8:253-8
17. Engel LW, Strauchen JA, Chiazzel L et al. Accuracy of death certification in an autopsied population with specific attention to malignant neoplasms and vascular diseases. Am J Epidemiol 1980; 111:99-112.
18. James G, Patton RE, Heslin AS. Accuracy of cause-of-death statements on death certificates. Publ Health Rep 1955; 70:39-51.
19. Moriyama IM, Baum WS, Haenzel WM et al. Inquiry into diagnostic evidence supporting medical certifications of death. Am J Publ Health 1958; 48:1376-87.
20. Royal College of Physicians' Medical Services

Study Group. Death certification and epidemiological research. Br Med J 1978; 2:1063-5.

21. Alderson MR, Meade TW. Accuracy of diagnosis on death certificates compared with that in hospital records. Br J Prev Soc Med 1967; 21:22-9.

22. McGoogan E. The autopsy and clinical diagnosis. J Roy Coll Phys Lond 1984; 18:240.

23. Schottenfeld D, Eaton M, Sommers SC et al. The autopsy as a measure of the death certificate. Bull N Y Acad Med 1982; 58:778-94.

24. Karsner HT, Rothschild L, Crump ES. Clinical diagnosis as compared with necropsy findings. JAMA 1919; 73:666-9.

25. Bean WB. Infarction of the heart.II Symptomatology of acute attack. Ann Int Med 1938; 11:2086-108.

26. Swartout HO, Webster RG. To what degree are mortality statistics dependable? Am J Publ Health 1940; 30:811-5.

27. Wallgren I. Obduktionsfyndet och de klinska diagnoserna. Nord Med 1945; 26:1311-6.

28. Feil H, Cushing EH, Hardesty JT. Accuracy in diagnosis and localization of myocardial infarction. Am Heart J 1938; 15:721-38.

29. Yater WM, Traum AH, Brown WG et al. Coronary artery disease in men 18 to 39 years of age. Report of 866 cases, 450 with necropsy examinations. Am Heart J 1948; 36:334-72, 481-526, 683-722.

30. Munck W. Autopsy finding and clinical diagnosis. A comparative study of 1000 cases. Acta Med Scand 1952; Suppl 266:775-81.

31. Gould SE, Cawley LP. Unsuspected healed myocardial infarction in patients dying in a general hospital. Arch Int Med 1958; 101:524-7.

32. Friedberg R, Dybkaer R, Poulsen H. The epidemiology of coronary occlusion in Denmark. Dan Med Bull 1960; 7:1-8.

33. Johnson WJ, Achor RWP, Burchell HB et al. Unrecognized myocardial infarction. Arch Int Med 1959; 103:253-61.

34. Paton BC. The accuracy of diagnosis of myocardial infarction. Am J Med 1957; 23:761-8.

35. Registrar General's Statistical Review of England and Wales for the year 1956. Part III Commentary. London: HMSO, 1958.

36. Lee KT, Thomas WA, Rabin et al. Clinical and anatomic features in five hundred patients with fatal acute myocardial infarction. Circulation 1957; 15:197-202.

37. Melichar F, Jedlicka V, Havlík L. A Study of undiagnosed myocardial infarctions. Acta Med Scand 1963; 174:761-8.

38. Mitchell RS, Maisel JC, Dart GA et al. The accuracy of the death certificate in reporting cause of death in adults with special reference to chronic bronchitis and emphysema. Am Rev Resp Dis 1971; 104:844-50.

39. Abramson JH, Sacks MI, Cahana E. Death certificate data as an indication of the presence of certain common diseases. J Chr Dis 1971; 24:417-31.

40. Hartveit F. Clinical and post-mortem assessment of the cause of death. J Pathol 1977; 123:193-210.

41. Sandritter W, Staeudinger M, Drexler H. Autopsy and clinical diagnosis. Path Res Pract 1980; 168:107-14.

42. Drexler H, Staeudinger M, Sandritter W. Autopsie and klinische Diagnose Med Welt 1979; 30:1177-83

43. Asnaes S, Paaske F. Uncertainty of determining cause of death in a medico-legal material without autopsy. an autopsy study. Forens Sc Internat 1980; 15:103-14.

44. Zarling EJ, Sexton H, Milner P. Failure to diagnose acute myocardial infarction The clinicopathologic experience at a large community hospital. JAMA 1983; 250:1177-81.

45. Stevanovic G, Tucakovic G, Dotlic R et al. Correlation of clinical diagnoses with autopsy findings: A retrospective study of 2,145 consecutive autopsies. Human Pathol 1986; 17:1225-30.

46. Longoni P, Ruggeri R, Terni E et al. Confronto tra diagnosi clinica e anatomopathologica. Il contributo dell'autopsia per il clinico. Medicina 1985; 76:305-8.

47. Levine HD, Phillips E. An appraisal of the newer electrocardiography: Correlations in one humdred and fifty consecutive cases. New Engl J Med 1951; 245:833-42.

48. Edwards JE. The value and limitations of necropsy studies in coronary arterial disease. Progr Cardiovasc Dis 1971; 13:309-23.

49. Battle RM, Pathak D, Humble CG et al. Factors influencing discrepancies between premortem and postmortem diagnoses. JAMA 1987; 258:339-44.

50. Gover M. Statistical studies of heart disease. III. Heart disease associated with other major causes of death as primary or contributing cause.

Publ Health Rep 1949; 64:104-8.

51. Beadenkopf WG, Abrams M, Daoud A et al. An assessment of certain medical aspects of death certificate data for epidemiologic study of arteriosclerotic heart disease. J Chr Dis 1963; 16:249-62.

52. Phillips R, Carson P, Haites N et al. Variation in mortality from ischaemic heart disease between England and Scotland. Quart J Med 1987; 63:441-8.

53. Moulton C, Pennycook A. Coroners, procurators fiscal, and deaths from coronary heart disease. Lancet 1991; 338:1336-7.

54. Keys A. An epidemiological look at atherosclerosis. In: Brest An, Moyer JH, eds. Atherosclerotic Vascular Disease. New York: Meredith Publ, 1967:76-83.

55. Green A, Donald KJ. Necropsy as a control of death certification. Med J Aust 1976; 2:131-2.

56. Urano Y, Aizawa S, Baba K et al.In: Statistics of Intractable Diseases from the Autopsy Data in Japan. Tokyo: The Ministry Health and Welfare Japan, 1987.

57. Hiyoshi Y, Omae T, Hirota Y et al. Clinicopathologic study of the heart and coronary arteries of autopsied cases from the community of Hasayama during a 10 yr period. I. Ischaemic myocardial lesions. J Chr Dis 1978; 31:313-9

58. Laurie W, Wood JD. Atherosclerosis and its cerebral complications in the South African Bantu. Lancet 1958; 1:231-2.

59. Higginson J, Pepler WJ. Fat intake, serum cholesterol concentration, and atherosclerosis in the South African Bantu. Part II. Atherosclerosis and coronary artery disease. J Clin Invest 1954; 33:1366-71.

60. Strong JP, Wainwright J, McGill HC. Atherosclerosis in the Bantu. Circulation 1959; 20:1118-27.

61. Becker BJP. Cardiovascular disease in the Bantu and colored races of South Africa. S Afr J Med Sc 1946; 11:97-105.

62. Meyer BJ. Anatomical, chemical and physical aspects of atherosclerosis. S Afr Med J 1970; 44:1343-9.

63. Resch JA, Williams AO, Lemercier G et al. Comparative autopsy study on cerebral atherosclerosis in Nigerian and Senegal Negroes, American Negroes and Caucasians. Atherosclerosis 1970; 12:401-7.

64. Owor R, Resch JA, Loewenson RB. Cerebral atherosclerosis in Uganda. Stroke 1976; 7:404-6.

65. Lundberg GD, Voigt GE. Reliability of a presumptive diagnosis in sudden unexpected death in adults. JAMA 1979; 242:2328-30.

66. Moriyama IM, Dawber TR, Kannel WB. Evaluation of diagnostic information supporting medical certification of deaths from cardiovascular disease. Nat Cancer Inst Monog Jan 1966; 19:405-19.

67. Najem GR, Riley HD, Najem LI. Reliability of heart disease diagnoses. Oklahoma State Med J 1975; 68:452-7.

68. World Health Statistics Annual 1990. Geneva: World Health Organization, 1990.

69. Asnaes S. The uncertainty of determining the mode and time of death without autopsy. Forens Sci Internat 1980; 15:191-6.

70. Vanatta PR, Petty CS. Limitations of the forensic external examination in determining the cause and manner of death. Human Pathol 1987; 18:170-4.

71. Briggs RC. Quality of death certificate diagnosis as compared to autopsy findings. Arizona Med 1975; 32:617-9.

72. Rose G, Barker DJP. What is epidemiology? Br Med J 1978; 2:803-4.

73. Puffer RR. New Approaches for epidemiologic studies of mortality statistics. Bull Pan Am Health Org 1989; 23:365-83.

74. Dawber TR, Kannel WB. Coronary heart disease as an epidemiology entity. Am J Publ Health 1963; 53:433-7.

75. Copeland KT, Checkoway H, McMichael AJ et al. Bias due to misclassification in the estimation of relative risk. Am J Epidemiol 1977; 105:488-95.

76. Koran LM, The reliability of clinical methods, data and judgements. New Engl J Med 1975; 293:642-6, 695-701.

77. Lilienfeld AM, Graham S. Validity of determining circumcision status by questionnaire as related to epidemiological studies of cancer of the cervix. J Nat Cancer Inst 1958; 21:713-20.

78. Ludwig EA, Collette JC. Some measures of health statistics. JAMA 1971; 216:493-9.

79. Baumgarten M, Siamiatycki J, Gibbs GW. Validity of work histories obtained by interview for epidemiologic purposes. Am J Epidemiol 1983; 118:583-91.

80. Rose GA. Ischaemic heart disease. Chest pain questionnaire. Milbank Mem Fund Quart 1965; 43:32-9.

81. Diamond GA, Forrester JS. Analysis of probability as an art in the clinical diagnosis of coronary-artery disease. New Engl J Med 1979; 300:1350-8.

82. James TN. Angina without coronary disease (sic). Circulation 1970; 42:189-91.

83. Parmley WW. Silent ischemia. Tip of the iceberg. Am J Med 1985; 79 Suppl 3A:1.

84. Malliani A. The elusive link between transient myocardial ischemia and pain. Circulation 1986; 73:201-4.

85. Cohn PF. Silent myocardial ischemia: Classification, prevalence, and prognosis. Am J Med 1985; 79 Suppl 3A:2-6.

86. Maseri A, Chierchia S, Davies G et al. Mechanisms of ischemic cardiac pain and silent myyocardial ischemia. Am J Med 1985; 79(Suppl 3A):7-11.

87. Wiener DA, Ryan TJ, McCabe CH et al. Significance of silent myocardial ischemia during exercise testing in patients with coronary artery disease. Am J Cardiol 1987; 59:725-9.

88. Gazes PC. Angina pectoris: Classification and diagnosis. Part 2. Mod Concepts Cardiovasc Dis 1988; 57:25-7.

89. Maseri A. The changing face of angina pectoris: Practical implications. Lancet 1983; 1:746-9.

90. Mukerji V, Alpert MA, Hewett JE et al. Can patients with chest pain and normal coronary arteries be discriminated from those with coronary artery disease prior to coronary angiography? Angiology 1989; 40:276-82.

91. Malliani A, Lombardi F, Pagani M. Presence or absence of angina pectoris during myocardial ischemia. In: Rutishauser W. Roskamm H, eds. Silent Myocardial Infarction. Berlin: Springer-Verlag, 1984:7-13.

92. Sigwart U, Grbic M, Payot M et al. Ischemic events during coronary artery balloon obstruction. In: Rutishauser W. Roskamm H, eds. Silent Myocardial Infarction. Berlin: Springer-Verlag, 1984:29-36.

93. Friesinger GC, Smith RF. Correlation of electrocardiographic studies and arteriographic findings with angina pectoris. Circulation 1972; 46:1173-84.

94. Redwood DR, Epstein SE. Uses and limitations of stress testing in the evaluation of ischemic heart disease. Circulation 1972; 46:1115-31.

95. Schang JJ, Pepine CJ. Transient asymptomatic S-T segment depression during daily activity. Am J Cardiol 1977; 39:396-402.

96. Giagnoni E, Secchi MB, Wu SC et al. Prognostic value of excercise EKG testing in asymptomatic normotensive subjects. New Engl J Med 1983; 309:1085-9.

97. Epstein SE. Implications of probability analysis on the strategy used for noninvasive detection of cononary artery disease. Am J Cardiol 1980; 46:491-9.

98. Goodale F, Thomas WA, O'Neal RM. Myocardial infarction in women. A study of autopsy populations. Arch Pathol 1960; 60:599-604.

99. Nesto RW, Phillips RT. Asymptomatic myocardial ischemia in diabetes patients. Am J Med 1886; 80 (Suppl 4C):40-7.

100. Boyd LT, Werblow SC. Coronary thrombosis without pain. Am J Med Soc 1937; 194:814-24.

101. Kennedy JA. The incidence of myocardial infarction without pain in 200 autopsied cases. Am Heart J 1937; 14:703-9.

102. Rosenberg BA, Malach M. Acute myocardial infarction in a city hospital. IV. Clinical-pathological correlations. Am J Cardiol 1960; 6:272-80.

103. Baer S, Frankel H. Studies in acute myocardial infarction 1. The clinical picture and diagnosis. Ann Int Med 1944; 20:108-14.

104. Pathy MS. Clinical presentation of myocardial infarction in the elderly. Brit Heart J 1967; 29:190-9.

105. Stokes J, Dawber TR. The "silent coronary": The frequency and clinical characteristics of unrecognized myocardial infarction in the Framingham Study. Ann Int Med 1959; 50:1359-69.

106. Maseri A. Expanding views on ischaemic heart disease: A prospective for the 1980s. Clin Sc 1982; 62:119-23.

107. Davies LG. Observer variation in reports on electrocardiograms. Brit Heart J 1958; 20:153-61.

108. Epstein FH, Doyle JT, Pollack AA et al. Observer interpretation of electrocardiograms. JAMA 1961; 175:847-50.

109. Ericksen J, Müller C, Anderssen JN. Atypical case histories and electrocardiograms in myocardial infarctions. Acta Med Scand 1970; 138:95-102.

110. Zinn WJ, Cosby RS. Myocardial infarction. II. A reevaluation of the diagnostic accuracy of the electrocardiogram. Am J Med 1950; 8:177-9.

111. Merrill Sl, Pearce ML, An autopsy study of the accuracy of the electrocardiogram in the diagnosis of recurrent myocardial infarction. Am Heart J 1971; 81:48-54.

112. Woods JD, Laurie W, Smith WG. The reliability of the electrocardiogram in myocardial infarction. Lancet 1963; 2:265-9.

113. Weiss MM, Weiss MM. The electrocardiogram in myocardial infarction. Arch Int Med 1958; 101:1126-8.

114. Skjaeggestad Ö, Molne K. Electrocardiogram in patients with healed myocardial infarction disclosed at autopsy. Acta Med Scand 1966; 179:23-7.

115. Cox CJB. Return to normal of the electrocardigram after myocardial infarction. Lancet 1967; 1:1194-7.

116. Anderson N, Skjaeggestad Ö. The electrocardiogram in patients with previous myocardial infarction. Acta Med Scand 1964; 176:123-6.

117. Segall HN. The electrocardiogram and its interpretation. A study of reports by 20 physicians on a set of 100 electrocardiograms. Canad Med Ass J 1960; 82:2-6.

118. Acheson RM. Observer error and variation in the interpretation of electrocardiograms in an epidemiological study of coronary heart disease. Brit J Prev Soc Med 1960; 14:99-122.

119. Kannel W.B, Abbott RD. Incidence and prognosis of unrecognized myocardial infarction. New Engl J Med 1984; 311:1144-7.

120. Kannel WB, McNamara PM, Feinleib M et al. The unrecognized myocardial infarction. Geriatrics 1970; 25:75-87.

121. Medalie JH, Goldbourt U. Unreconized myocardial infarction: Five-year incidence, mortality, and risk factors. Ann Int Med 1976; 84:526-31.

122. Editorial: Unrecognized myocardial infarction. Lancet 1976; 2:449-50.

123. Todd JW. Unrecognized myocardial infarction. Lancet 1976; 2:569.

124. Kuller L, Anderson H, Peterson D et al. Nationwide cerebrovascular disease morbidity study. Stroke 1970; 1:86-90.

125. Randall B. Fatty liver and sudden death. Human Pathol 1980; 11:147-53.

126. Davis JH, Wright RK. The very sudden cardiac death syndrome—a conceptual model for pathologists. Human Pathol 1980; 11:117-21.

127. Goldschlager N, Pfeifer J, Cohn K et al. The natural history of aortic regurgitation. A clinical and hemodynamic study. Am J Med 1973; 54:577-88.

128. Wiseman MN, Banim S. "Glue sniffer's" heart? 1987; 294:739.

129. Cregler LL, Mark H. Medical complications of cocaine abuse. New Engl J Med 1986; 313:1495-500.

130. Lovell RHH, Prineas RJ. Mechanisms of sudden death and their implications for prevention and management. Progr Cardiovasc Dis 1971; 13:482-94.

131. Hallstrom AP, Cobb LA, Ray R. Smoking as a risk factor for recurrence of sudden cardiac arrest. New Engl J Med 1986; 314:271-5.

132. Lown B. Sudden cardiac death: The major challenge confronting contemporary cardiology. Am J Cardiol 1979; 43:313-28.

133. Buxton AE. Sudden cardiac death—1986. Ann Int Med 1986; 104:716-8.

134. Liberthson RR, Nagel EL, Hirschmen JC et al. Pathophysiologic observations in prehospital ventricular fibrillation and sudden cardiac death. Circulation 1974; 49:790-8.

135. Lee KT, Lie WM, Han J et al. Experimental model for study of "sudden death" from ventricular fibrillation or asystole. Am J Cardiol 1973; 32:62-73.

136. Stehbens WE. Relationship of coronary-artery thrombosis to myocardial infarction. Lancet 1985; 2:639-42.

137. Surawicz B. Sudden death: Pathogenesis and prevention. In: Likoff W, Segal BL, Insull W et al. eds. Atherosclerosis and Heart Disease. New York: Grune & Stratton, 1972:511-9.

138. Cobb LA, Baum RS, Alvarez H et al. Resuscitation from out-of-hospital ventricular fibrillation: 4 years follow-up. Circulation 1975; 51 and 52 Suppl III: III-222-8.

139. Adelson L, Hoffman W. Sudden death from coronary disease related to a lethal mechanism arising independently of vascular occlusion or myocardial damage. New Engl J Med 1961; 176:131-5.

140. Robb-Smith AHT. The Enigma of Coronary Heart Disease. London: Lloyd-Luke, 1967.

141. Feinstein AR. Clinical Epidemiology. The Ar-

chitecture of Clinical Research. Philadelphia: WB Saunders, 1985.

142. Stehbens WE. Review of the validity of national coronary heart disease mortality rates. Angiology 1990; 41:85-94.

143. Stehbens WE. Validity of cerebrovascular mortality rates. Angiology 1991; 42:261-7.

144. Alderson M. International Mortality Statistics. Bury St. Edmunds: St Edmundsburg Press, 1981.

145. Moriyama IM, Krueger DE, Stamler J. Cardiovascular Diseases in the United States. Cambridge: Harvard Univ Press, 1971.

146. Dorn HF, Horn JI. Reliability of certificates of death from cancer. Am J Hyg 1941; Sect A 34:12-23.

147. Moine M. Sur l'augmentation de quelques causes de décès. Bull l'Inst Nat Hyg 1952; 7:279-94.

148. Werkö L. Diet, lipids and heart attacks. Acta Med Scand 1970; 206:435-9.

149. Carruthers M. Fats on Trial. Tunbridge Wells: Butter Information Council, 1980.

150. Bourke GJ. "Accuracy of death certification". Irish J Med Sc 1969; 2:35-42.

151. McMichael J. French wine and death cartificates. Lancet 1979; 1:1186-7.

152. Riccitelli ML. Myocardial disease in the aged, including a review of the literature. J Am Geriat Soc 1968; 14:366-79.

153. Busuttil A, Kemp IW, Heasman MA. The accuracy of medical certificates of cause of death. Health Bull 1981; 39:146-52.

155. Davies MJ. Pathological view of sudden cardiac death. Br Heart J 1981; 45:88-96.

156. Klebba Aj, Maurer JD, Glass EJ. Mortality Trends for Leading Causes of Death: United States 1950-69. Rockville Md. U S Dept of Health, Education & Welfare. Series 20, No.16, National Center for Health Statistics, 1974.

157. Clarke C, Whitfield AGW. Deaths from rhesus haemolytic disease in England and Wales in 1977: Accuracy of records and assessment of ant-D prophylaxis. Br Med J 1979; 1:1665-9.

158. Davis BR, Curb JD, Tung B et al. Standardized physician preparation of death certificates. Controlled Clin Trials 1987; 8:110-20.

159. Guralnick L. Some problems in the use of multiple causes of death. J Chr Dis 1966; 19:979-90.

160. Dorn HF, Moriyama IM. Uses and significance of multiple cause tabulations for mortality statistics. Am J Publ Health 1964; 54:400-6.

161. Wiener L. Bellows MT, McAvoy GH et al. Use of multiple causes in the classification of deaths from cardiovascular-renal diseases. Am J Publ Health 1955; 45:492-501.

162. Markush RE, Seigel DG. Prevalence at death. 1. A new method for deriving death rates for specific diseases. Am J Publ Health 1968; 58:544-57.

163. Curb JD, Babcock C, Pressel S et al. Nosological coding of cause of death. Am J Epidemiol 1983; 118:122-8.

164. Kennedy GT, Stern MP, Crawford MH. Miscoding of hospital discharges as acute myocardial infarction: Implication for surveillance programs aimed at elucidating trends in coronary artery disease. Am J Cardiol 1984; 53:1000-2.

165. Morris JN. Recent history of coronary disease. Lancet 1951; 1:69-73.

166. Kannel WB. Meaning of the downward trend in cardiovascular mortality. JAMA 1982; 247:877-80.

167. Levy RI. Declining mortality in coronary heart disease. Atherosclerosis 1981; 1:312-25.

168. Stallones RA. The rise and fall of ischemic heart disease. Sci Am 1980; 243 (5):43-9.

169. Burrows S. The postmortem examination. Scientific necessity or folly? JAMA 1975; 233:441-3.

170. Editorial A decline in coronary mortality. Br Med J 1976; 1:58.

171. Alfredsson L, Ahlbom A. Increasing incidence and mortality from myocardial infarction in Stockholm county. Br Med J 1983; 286:1931-3.

172. Marmot MG. Interpretation of trends in coronary heart disease mortality. Acta Med Scand 1985; 701 Suppl:58-65.

173. Pyörälä K, Epstein FH, Kornitzer M. Changing trends in coronary heart disease mortality; possible explanations. Cardiology 1985; 72:5-10.

174. Welin L, Larsson B, Svärdsudd K, et al. Why is the incidence of ischaemic heart disease in Sweden increasing? Study of men born in 1913 and 1923. Lancet 1983; 1:1087-9.

175. Morgan PP, Wigle DT. Medical care and the declining rates of death due to heart disease and stroke. Canad Med Ass J 1981; 125:953-4.

176. Goldberg RJ, Gore JM, Alpert JS et al. Recent changes in attack and survival rates of acute myocardial infarction (1975 through 1981).

The Worcester Heart Attack Study. JAMA 1986; 255:2774-9.

177. Walker WJ. Changing United States life-style and declining vascular mortality: Cause or coincidence? New Engl J Med 1977; 297:163-5.

178. Havlik RJ, Feinleib M. Summary of the Conference. In: Havlik RJ. Feinlab M, eds. Proc. of the Conference on the Decline in Coronary Heart Disease Mortality. Bethesda: NIH Publication No.79-1610, 1979: XXIII-VII.

179. Jones HB. A Special consideration of the aging process, disease and life expectancy. Advances Biol Med Phys 1956; 4:281-337.

180. Blomqvist G, Biörck G. Coronary mortality in relation to total mortality. Acta Med Scand 1963; 173:229-33.

181. Strong JP, Guzman MA, Tracy RE et al. Is coronary atherosclerosis decreasing in the U.S.A.? Lancet 1979; 2:1294.

182. Stehbens WE. The lipid hypothesis and the role of hemodynamics in atherogenesis. Progr Cardiovasc Dis 1990; 33:119-36.

183. Stehbens WE. Experimental induction of atherosclerosis associated with femoral arteiovenous fistulae in rabbits on a stock diet. Atherosclerosis 1992; 95:127-35.

184. Kurtzke JF. Epidemiology of Cerebrovascular Disease. Berlin: Springer-Verlag, 1969.

185. Wolf Dr. Discussion. Advances Neurol 1978; 19:310-11.

186. Corwin LI, Wolf PA, Kannel WB et al. Accuracy of death certification of stroke: The Framingham Study. Stroke 1982; 13:818-21.

187. Kuller LH. Epidemiology of stroke. Advances Neurol 1979; 19:281-311.

188. Marquardsen J. Epidemiology of strokes in Europe. In: Barnett HJM, Stein BM, Mohr JP et al, eds. Stroke, Pathophysiology, Diagnosis and Management. New York: Churchill Livingstone. 1986:31-43.

189. Stallones RA, Epidemiology of cerebrovascular disease. A review. J Chr Dis 1965; 18:859-72.

190. Tunstall-Pedoe H. Stroke. In: Miller DL, Farmer RDT, eds. Epidemiology of Diseases. Oxford: Blackwell Scientific Publ, 1982:136-45.

191. Yatsu FM. Atherogenesis and stroke. In: Barnett HJM, Stein BM, Mohr JP et al, Stroke. Pathophysiology, Diagnosis and Management. New York: Churchill Livingstone, 1986:45-56.

192. Tell GS, Crouse JR, Furberg CD. Relation between blood lipids, lipoproteins, and cerebrovascular atherosclerosis. A Review. Stroke 1988; 19:423-30.

193. Yano K, Reid DM, MacLean CJ. Serum cholesterol and hemorrhagic stroke in the Honolulu Heart Program.Stroke 1989; 20:1460-5.

194. Health United States 1984. U.S. Department of Health and Human Services. Hyattsville Md: Publ no(PHS) 85-1232, 1984

195. Wylie CM. Epidemiology of cerebrovascular disease. Handbook Clin Neurol 1972; 11:183-207.

196. Katsuki S, Hirota Y. Current concepts of the frequency of cerebral hemorrhage and cerebral infarction in Japan. In: Milliken CH, Siekert RG, Whisnant JP, eds. Cerebral Vascular Diseases. New York: Grune & Stratton, 1966:99-111.

197. Otsu S. The incidence of cardio- and cerebrovascular diseases in autopsy cases. Jap Circul J 1969; 33:1459-65.

198. Kurtzke JF, Jurland LT. Epidemiology of cerebrovascular disease In: Siekert RG, ed. Cerebrovascular Survey Report for Joint Council Subcommittee on Cerebrovascular Disease. Nat Inst Neurol Dis and Stroke and Nat Heart and Lung Inst. 1970 163-75.

199. Schroeder HA. Degenerative cardiovascular disease in the Orient. 1.Atherosclerosis 1958; 8:287-333.

200. Komachi Y, Tanaka H, Shimamoto T et al. A collaborative study of stroke incidence in Japan: 1975-1979. Stroke 1984; 15:28-36.

201. Robertson TL, Kato H, Rhoads GG et al. Epidemiologic studies of coronary heart disease and stroke in Japanese men living in Japan, Hawaii and California. Am J Cardiol 1977; 39:239-43.

202. Levy RI. Stroke decline: Implications and prospects. New Engl J Med 1979; 300:490-1.

203. Wolf PA. Risk factors for stroke. Stroke 1985; 16:359-60.

204. Yablonski M, Behar A, Ungar H et al. Cerebral atherosclerosis among Israeli Jews of European and Afro-Asian origin. Neurology 1968; 18:550-8.

205. Editorial Why has stroke mortality declined? Lancet 1983; 1:1195-6.

206. Garraway WM, Whisnant JP, Drury I. The continuing decline in the incidence of stroke. Mayo Clin Proc 1983; 58:520-3.

207. Kramer S, Diamond EL, Lilenfeld AM. Patterns

of incidence and trends in diagnostic classification of cerebrovascular disease in Washington county—Maryland. 1969-71 to 1974-1976. Am J Epidemiol 1982; 115:398-411.

208. Rodda RA. Arteriosclerosis in the lower limbs: A pathological study of fifty cases with no ischaemia. Thesis, Doctorate of Med. Dunedin: Univ Otago, 1950.

209. Lindbom Å, Arteriosclerosis and arterial thrombosis in the lower limb. A roentgenological study. Acta Radiol 1950; Suppl 80:1-80.

210. Rosenblatt MB, Teng PK, Kerpe S et al. Causes of death in 1,000 consecutive autopsies. New York State J Med 1971; 71:2189-93.

211. Castleden WM, Mercer JC and the Members of the West Australian Vascular Service. Abdominal aortic aneurysms in Western Australia: Descriptive epidemiology and patterns of rupture. Br J Surg 1985; 72:109-12.

212. Allen PIM, Gourevitch D, McKinley J et al. Population screening for aortic aneurysms. Lancet 1987; 2:736.

213. Kircher T, Nelson J, Burdo H. The autopsy as a measure of accuracy of the death certificate. New Engl J Med 1985; 313:1263-9.

214. Dawber TR. The Framingham Study. The Epidemiology of Atherosclerotic Disease. Cambridge: Harvard Univ Press, 1980.

215. Meade TW, Gardner MJ, Cannon P et al. Observer variability in recording the peripheral pulses. Br Heart J 1968; 30:661-5.

216. Ludbrook J, Clarke AM, McKenzie JK. Significance of absent ankle pulse. Br Med J 1962; 1:1724-6.

217. Feinstein AR. Clinical Epidemiology. II The identification rates of disease. Ann Int Med 1968; 69:1037-61.

CHAPTER 5

LIPIDS AND CHOLESTEROL IN THE LIPID HYPOTHESIS

The concept that diet plays a pivotal role in atherogenesis was originally based on three observations, viz, (i) advanced atherosclerotic lesions contained both fat and calcium salts, (ii) administration of large quantities of cholesterol or egg yolk[1] and vitamin D[2] induces hypercholesterolemia and hypercalcemia and in turn lipid and mineral deposition respectively in experimental animals and (iii) both cholesterol and vitamin D occur in particularly large amounts in foodstuffs of animal origin (egg yolk, butter, animal fats). The simple deduction was that an elevated blood level of lipid or minerals would increase the accumulation in the vessel wall. Interest in vitamin D and arterial calcification waned as preoccupation with lipids and cholesterol strengthened and research on dietary-induced hypercholesterolemia in the rabbit intensified.

The concept's credibility was further strengthened by pathologists accepting the rabbit vascular lesions as atherosclerotic and their similarity to the vascular lesions of the rare cases of hereditary familial hypercholesterolemia and the insulin-untreated diabetic on a high fat diet. By the middle of the century dietary fat was suspect and considered responsible for the caseous lipid-rich material in the arterial wall and the fibrocellular component was regarded as a reaction to the deposition of lipid. The presence of cholesterol crystals in the caseous atheromatous debris reinforced the concept that dietary fat of animal origin was involved. The first "significant" study correlating CHD mortality rates with dietary fat was by Ancel Keys[3]. His biased selection of six countries demonstrated a truly remarkable correlation between CHD mortality rates and the dietary fat available for consumption expressed in calories. The serious flaws in this paper (Chapter 1) outlined by Yerushalmy and Hilleboe[4] were ignored but the fallacious results stimulated further research on dietary fat in atherogenesis. Most investigations on nutrition and atherosclerosis, disregarding other components of the atherosclerotic lesion, focused on dietary control of serum lipid and particularly serum cholesterol. Emphasis has been on a high dietary intake of animal fats. Saturated fatty acids (particularly stearic and palmitic acids) and cholesterol have been alleged to be responsible for unduly high blood levels of cholesterol, low density lipoprotein (LDL) and LDL cholesterol. Dietary cholesterol has been portrayed to the general public as not merely bad but as a toxin endangering the health of the nation. Misleading food advertisements are now permitted to portray calves as the only animals that should ever drink cows' milk whilst a manufacturer advertises its margarine product with the statement, "It's called Sunrise because with animal fats you may not see another". Yet the role of dietary cholesterol in spontaneous atherogenesis in captive wild animals appears to be unimportant and mammals (felines) with diets highest in animal (saturated) fats are said to be not vulnerable to spontaneous atherosclerosis.[5]

We are biologically omnivorous although Roberts,[6] editor of the *American Journal of Cardiology*, ignoring the existence of omnivores and on unsatisfactory anthropological grounds, has recently divided the animal kingdom into herbivores and carnivores, reclassifying *Homo sapiens* as a herbivore. The human diet is essentially dependent on socio-economic and cultural characteristics and has in the past remained relatively static for protracted time periods. In recent years with increased travel and transportation and the admixture of different racial and cultural groups into previously relatively static populations, dietary habits are changing rapidly. Nevertheless lipid protagonists continue to proclaim dietary animal fat and cholesterol as the major environmental agent responsible for elevated serum lipids and severe atherosclerosis in populations of technologically developed countries.[7,8]

The dietary approach in epidemiology has been based on the preconceived idea that the dietary factor has to be one of the primary dietary constituents, viz, fat, carbohydrate or protein, whereas it should have been conceded that deficiencies of secondary constituents (vitamins, minerals, etc.) or occasional or sporadic noxious ingredients might aggravate the disease but would not become apparent in national or short-term individual dietary surveys. Some noxious agents, unaccounted for in surveys, might affect some individuals more than others and could easily be ingested less than once monthly or be present in minute quantities, e.g., food additives. A semiscorbutic state for example in old individuals, by adversely affecting collagen metabolism, could well aggravate the severity of atherosclerosis and enhance the propensity to intimal tears. National or population food consumption estimates are unlikely to expose such factors or dietary deficiencies. Moreover the national consumption of some essential dietary constituent may suggest the average intake is above the daily requirement and mask the adverse effect of deficiency states in individuals or even toxic states from excessive intake in others within that population. Conversely occasionally ingested food items could have an ameliorating effect on atherosclerosis or thrombosis. Few attempts were made until recently to identify beneficial food constituents and now fish oils are considered to be possibly beneficial.

Diets relating nutrition to atherosclerosis in humans are mostly epidemiological or retrospective studies correlating nutrition to CHD mortality rates or to changes in serum cholesterol which are then deduced to be atherogenic if the serum cholesterol is elevated and beneficial if the serum cholesterol level falls—all decreed without ever determining an effect on atherosclerosis. This is called the "substitution game" and is a potential source of considerable error and an example of assumed causality.[9]

DIETARY ASSESSMENTS

Dietary assessments have been conducted for many types of epidemiological study and there are many reasons for mistrusting such surveys and the conclusions reached primarily because of defects in the methodology employed:[10]

(i) Some are based on the total quantity of food available for consumption nationally which when divided by the population census is supposed to indicate the *per capita* food available for consumption. The quantity of food produced nationally is adjusted for imports, exports, changes in stocks, and wastage up to the retail stage and represents the total food available for consumption. This is usually expressed in terms of calories, protein, fat and carbohydrates. The validity of the estimates depends on the reliability of national statistics on production, marketing and utilization, the accuracy of which is variable. In underdeveloped countries the estimates are rough being particularly weak for animal products.[4] This data obviously cannot provide consumption levels related to occupations, race, religion or income levels etc., and

therefore are of limited value. Completely dis-
regarded is the dictum of paramount importance that it is invalid to argue from the general to the particular and from the population
to the individual, the serious error that pervades CHD epidemiology. The correct correlation to be sought in epidemiology is a graded
relationship between individual fat consumption and severity of atherosclerosis but the lack
of reliable and valid methods for grading either
the severity of the disease in vivo or for taking
dietary histories is a major obstacle[11] precluding
satisfactory study of individual dietary intakes.

(ii) The food available does not equate with
food consumed and it is not possible to assess
accurately food wastage which varies with the
individual, the household and socioeconomic
status. Loss by cooking is an unknown but significant variable. The fat content of sausages,
some meats and bacon in the USA is higher
than in many other countries but much is lost
during cooking and heat-labile vitamins are
vulnerable to cooking. If food wastage is impossible to estimate correctly, the average food
consumption is also inexact.

(iii) Both dietary protein and carbohydrates
influence serum cholesterol levels[12,13] and therefore to focus on dietary fat alone is inappropriate. It is not possible to alter carbohydrate,
protein or fat content without effecting secondary influences on other dietary constituents (vitamins and minerals) and caloric intake as well,
one or more of which may be shown ultimately
to have a direct aggravating or ameliorating
metabolic effect on atherogenesis. Dietary interactions are not always apparent.[14]

(iv) Repeatedly in the literature the role of
nutrients or other factors on serum cholesterol
or lipoproteins is assumed to have a corresponding effect on the severity of atherosclerosis, yet
another example of the "substitution game".[9]

(v) Correlations of dietary data pertaining
to populations with other attributes such as
CHD mortality or blood cholesterol levels are
not always based on the same populations.[15]

(vi) It is "difficult to overcome the problems that exist with respect to the validity of
nutritional data collected on individuals, not
only because of limitations in techniques of
measurement, but also because of the varying
effects on the dietary patterns of individuals

caused by examinee awareness of being evaluated".[16] Stamler[16] acknowledged that the relationship of dietary lipid and serum cholesterol
of individuals showed a low order or no correlation and attributed this to (a) other unknown
nondietary factors contributing to interindividual differences in serum cholesterol, (b)
limitations in the techniques of measurement
in the face of examinee awareness and the lack
of validity of nutritional data collected on individuals, and (c) intraindividual variation often
being greater than the interindividual variability. The fact remains that individual food
consumption is extremely variable with time and
the quality of the nutritional data is low even
though CHD epidemiologists may be loath to
disbelieve results obtained by their methodology.

Individual dietary habits are assessed by
means of a food diary or a questionnaire and
recall of the diet during the preceding 24 hours
or a week or more, the quantities being assessed by illustrations or models and food
tables.[17] Alternatively identical portions may be
analyzed over a day or a week. This, obviously
the most accurate method, is logistically difficult for a large number of persons even for a
short period and reliability of assessments must
be low.

As an example in a seven-day prospective
dietary survey,[18] 113 men and women were
asked to record food intake for one week. The
method of cooking was recorded, plastic tea-
spoons and tablespoons were distributed to help
estimations of food quantities and a plastic
measuring cup was available only on request.
The difficulty in describing the food and then
estimating the quantity of fat, carbohydrate and
protein in stews, soups and takeaway fast food
commodities from individual reporting of food
consumed is considerable. When one apple was
recorded, an average weight was coded and the
authors clearly stated that "Measurement of all
food consumed was not required" and only a
minority of participants endeavored to do so.
The authors concluded that "The prospective
design of this study, the use of a seven day
diary and the use of measuring implements to
estimate the size of the food portions consumed
support the validity of assessing dietary intake".
The data was collated and converted to precise
quantities of primary food constituents (as g

per day), including of course the allegedly deleterious saturated fats and cholesterol. The results of this heart study and a comparison with other such dietary surveys led the authors to conclude that there has been "an apparent decrease in both the absolute amount and proportion of cholesterol and saturated fat" and to infer that the study was typical of the national adult diet. The possible effects of vitamins, food additives, minerals, contaminants and seasonal and geographic variation were ignored and the age group of consenting participants selected in one city is not representative of the national adult population.

Ancel Keys[17] was aware of the lack of reliability and poor reproducibility of such short-term studies of estimates or poorly measured food intake, there being detected an unintentional tendency to misrepresent dietary habits both qualitatively and quantitatively. The reliability of assessments by recall or dietary diaries will vary probably more than the 34% error demonstrated in Lilienfeld and Graham's survey of circumcision[19] or the 18% lack of concordance with employment records[20] reported by Baumgarten et al. Subtle differences in the wording of questionnaires led to substantial differences in results,[21] and there will always be considerable difficulty in obtaining accurate quantitative assessments when dealing with multiple continuous variables as in dietary estimations. Response error in questionnaires in general is high[22] varying from 14% to 36%. Even ignoring the omissions, recall of diet and quantities ingested would be far worse than a chemical assessment of duplicate helpings over days or a week, again logistically impossible for such large numbers.

Groover et al[23] found substantial inaccuracy in data derived from five different types of dietary survey. Inaccuracy is greater in field samples than in hospital samples, but institutionalization of subjects in dietary studies is not logistically possible for a substantial, representative sample of the population. Duplicate samples had errors greater than 100% for certain food constituents and only 11 fell within ± 20%. The appraisal of nutrient values for individual diets in a study by Eagles et al[24] was subject to considerable error which depended on the nutritionist's interpretation of the descriptive terms and approximate measurements. Both fat and protein were overestimated with deviations up to 85% and 34% respectively. Comparison of the food intake of a group of men revealed that 71% of those in an extreme third on the first day were in the same group by the average intake for six subsequent days, 24% were in the middle third and 5% in the opposite third.[25] Such errors and the degree of misclassification that would occur are unacceptable.

Nutritional status within a population is subject to much variation particularly with respect to individual likes and dislikes, food fads, affluence, habit, religion and geography. Comparison between populations exhibits even greater variability[26] whilst ignoring the heterogeneous nature of the population. Individual variability in man, his genetics, environment, experiences and diet over a life time, especially in the western world, is so great as to make international comparisons particularly with those in underdeveloped countries (with populations often on a subsistence diet with seasonal fluctuations in supply, and with stagnant dietary habits and unchanging cultural life styles) scientifically and logistically difficult. Assuming that variation in severity of atherosclerosis is due to variation only in fat content of diet is simplistic, tenuous and speculative.

The very high intraindividual variation seen for fatty acids, cholesterol and polyunsaturated to unsaturated fat ratios in a 24-hour dietary recall study by Beaton et al[27] was attributed to low precision of the methodology. Chappell[28] found that errors up to 25% of average nutrient values can be expected with dietary sampling of individuals for one week only and even greater errors for some vitamins. Intraindividual variation will bias estimates of correlation coefficients and regression slopes towards 0 and results in misclassification of subjects into ranges of usual dietary intakes. Block[29] alleged that accuracy of dietary data at an individual level is not essential to provide valid results and answer important questions. He admits misclassification is inevitable but deems it unimportant. Such a view is contrary to the basic philosophy of science.

In the International Atherosclerosis Project, Scrimshaw and Guzmán[30] revealed how preconceived ideas can bias attitudes. Despite the large amount of epidemiological and experimental evidence relating type and quality of dietary animal fat to hypercholesterolemia, the relationships in their investigation were not statistically significant and other factors contributed to the association. They found a strong positive correlation with animal protein consumption but ignored the relationship because of current "evidence" in support of dietary fat determining the serum cholesterol level.

In a review of dietary survey methods Keys[17] acknowledged that (i) many dietary surveys were unreliable, (ii) attempts to demonstrate repeatability were often lacking or poor, (iii) the validity of dietary recall was impossible to prove, (iv) mean values for families and populations did not indicate individual dietary intake and variability and (v) there was no way of correlating individual data with disease severity. To Keys reliability meant repeatability but accuracy of the data must also be considered. Whilst admitting that absolute validity was rarely attainable in dietary surveys, Keys considered this lack of certainty though unacceptable in a biochemistry laboratory, was of value for comparison with other data of similar uncertainty because errors would be random, not biased and of similar magnitude in the two population groups similarly assessed. This philosophy, so often reiterated in epidemiology, is at variance with scientific methods and seems to be fostered by the erroneous belief that a statistical program and a computer can launder the data. No reliance can be placed on conclusions derived from inaccurate and fallacious data. The concern is not merely a matter of bias between two population samples as Keys[17] infers. Significant differences determined by statistical analysis do not validate the data and do not in themselves indicate biological significance. The relevance of such studies to CHD and atherosclerosis is unproven. Conclusions require reliable and accurate evidence which is currently unavailable and furthermore dietary records of individuals developing chronic diseases are generally similar to those of their healthy peers.[31]

Bingham's[32,33] review of dietary assessment techniques indicated that the coefficients of variation of differences incurred from asking subjects to estimate the weight of food portions may be in the 50% range for foods and 20% for

nutrients. She indicated that the coefficient of differences in nutrient intake over one day from the 24-hour recall method when compared with observed intakes ranges from 4 to 400%. Moreover the errors are random and she concluded that unbiased retrospective estimates of diet are unable to fulfill the epidemiological purposes for which they were intended. A more serious potential source of error is the systematic bias due either to differences between different methods of dietary assessment or from the deliberate over- or under-reporting by the subjects themselves. Modern techniques of validating the results by the use of food markers enable the investigator to improve on the validity and reliability of the results but the subjects must remain free-living. However no matter how accurate the techniques become, the results so obtained still indicate only the intake at the time of investigation and not over the many previous years and without experimental proof cannot be used to indicate the likelihood of the diet having an effect on CHD or atherosclerosis.

Conceding short-term assessments may be accurate and repeatable, they remain of no consequence since individual diets vary qualitatively and quantitatively within wide limits during a whole life time. Attempts to correlate the dietary content of fat or any other constituent from one or two weeks with the incidence of CHD or even the severity of atherosclerosis which develops over a life time are unacceptable scientifically and provide no evidence for a cause and effect relationship. Such short-term dietary surveys do not take into account lifelong dietary habits or even the short-term detrimental effect of dietary constituents or deficiencies which could be significant and nonregressive. Some transient adverse dietary constituents seem to be cumulative and in technologically advanced countries with which CHD epidemiologists are primarily concerned, diets have become considerably more varied since the end of the Second World War. However to correlate short-term studies of individuals' diets with a disease process that develops throughout life would have to provide "black and white" evidence, rather than the soft, inconsistent correlations based on low quality dietary data that characterize the literature on the lipid hypothesis today. No experimentalist would accept data based on similar variation in animal diets.[10]

Every individual has a totally individualistic dietary history and metabolism and differs from others in so many other ways that there is need to consider the heterogeneous response to dietary fat and other constituents within the population. Epidemiologists have resorted to generalizations and compared average types of diet for populations and therefore conclusions using this methodology must be confirmed by hard biological and experimental evidence in individuals within the populations.

INDIVIDUAL DIETARY CONSTITUENTS

A. PROTEIN

Protein availability for consumption in the USA is said to have been constant from 1907 to 1972 although the ratio of animal to vegetable protein doubled and paralleled CHD mortality.[26,34] Dietary proteins influence plasma cholesterol and the development of lipid lesions in rabbits.[11,12] Several authors have reported a positive correlation between animal protein intake and CHD mortality rates[35,36] and Yerushalmy and Hilleboe[4] found the correlation with CHD to be stronger with animal protein than with fat although they considered the association to be of no etiological significance for it emphasized the nonspecificity of dietary fat and the inadequacy of the alleged causal relationship with fat. Blackburn and Gillum[37] however discredit any correlation between animal protein intake and CHD mortality rates because Anitschkow[1] found dietary lipid rather than protein produced arterial lipid deposits in rabbits which in itself is a fallacious correlation (Chapter 2).

B. CARBOHYDRATE

A causal role of carbohydrate intake (especially refined sugar) in atherogenesis has been invoked by several authors[38-41] as has the fact that decreased sugar tolerance and diabetes are associated with an enhanced incidence of CHD. Little et al[42] consider any link between sucrose and CHD mortality to be unproven. Yudkin[39] considers dietary sugar correlates better with CHD than dietary fat and both correlate with affluence. Kritchevsky[26] stated that in the USA from 1909 to 1972 carbohydrate available for consumption fell by 21% and the ratio of di-

etary starch to simple carbohydrates dropped from 2.15 to 0.89. Variations in dietary carbohydrate are known to influence serum cholesterol levels[43,44] depending on the type of carbohydrate. Simultaneous changes in other constituents and long-term adaptive changes have not been adequately studied. Sugars have a common metabolic pathway to fats and disturbances in carbohydrate metabolism can be associated with abnormal fat metabolism.[45] Refined sugar consumption correlates with affluence[39] and a high fiber diet correlates with the reverse as well as a lower CHD mortality rate. The repeated comparisons between populations of western and third world countries by CHD epidemiologists are not significant when the differences between these peoples are vastly more numerous than dietary factors, blood chemistry and CHD mortality rates. Their nutrition is often not satisfactory, the prevalence of indigenous diseases requires documentation as well as their longevity and accurate autopsy data on causes of death etc., are necessary.

The Working Group on Arteriosclerosis of the National Heart, Lung and Blood Institute (NHLBI)[8] found (i) a negative correlation between major sources of complex carbohydrate in the diet (grains, legumes, fruit and vegetables) and CHD mortality and (ii) a positive association between refined and processed sugars and CHD mortality. It was concluded from other clinical and animal studies that refined sugars are not closely related to serum cholesterol and lipoproteins or to atherogenesis except when inducing caloric imbalance and obesity.

The role of fiber in reducing serum cholesterol is controversial. Dietary fiber has been recommended to sustain good health by providing roughage to stimulate intestinal motility and because of the ecological negative correlation between national mortality rates and the dietary intake of unrefined carbohydrate. The food industry took up the recommendations with considerable enthusiasm and consumption of roughage has become one of the features of the so-called prudent diet. It is difficult to accept that relatively indigestible cellulose can be as beneficial as claimed by either stimulating peristalsis or acting as an inert absorbent for some constituent in the alimentary tract. If dietary fiber is really beneficial, the effect of nutrients associated with the fiber needs investigation. Morris et al[46] reported that men with a high fiber diet had a reduced incidence of clinical CHD. The effect of dietary fiber on serum cholesterol levels is controversial[47] but a slight reduction is claimed though within the range of individual variability. The substitution of serum cholesterol as a surrogate of severity of atherosclerosis is again an example of the invalid substitution game and any cause and effect relationship of dietary fiber to atherosclerosis and CHD is an assumed one. Since the mode of action of the increased roughage is unknown, the possible secondary quantitative and qualitative effects on the diet of the trial subjects are uncertain and no demonstrable effect on atherosclerosis has been documented. The validity of the hypothesis must be seriously questioned. Because both dietary surveys and CHD mortality rates are fallacious, any correlation with dietary carbohydrate as with protein must be considered unproven.

C. Dietary Fats

It is widely believed and sedulously promulgated that diets high in cholesterol and saturated animal fats and low in polyunsaturated fats tend to raise the plasma cholesterol levels by 10% to 20% in some individuals[48] and are therefore assumed to be atherogenic. In other words an effect on blood cholesterol levels is assumed to have a similar effect on the severity of atherosclerosis. This is a common but fallacious extrapolation that pervades CHD epidemiological studies of lipids ("substitution game")[9]. In many animal species, the feeding of large amounts of cholesterol results in severe hypercholesterolemia. This is particularly well seen in rabbits, chickens and even some primates. Some animals require thyroidectomy or thyroid suppression to facilitate the rise in plasma cholesterol concentrations. In humans only small rises in cholesterol concentration can be induced by dietary means. Rats can absorb large quantities of cholesterol yet are remarkably resistant to hypercholesterolemia. Some humans may be responders and others may not be just as in pigeons for there is considerable heterogeneity of response.

Preoccupation with lipids has occasioned a preponderance of dietary studies related to fat intake but evidence incriminating diets high in animal fat is essentially circumstantial or indirect. Short-term experimentation may elevate serum cholesterol levels in some individuals. Biological adaptation in the long-term may minimize the effect. More to the point, mild elevation of plasma cholesterol is not necessarily atherogenic and there is no scientific evidence that this is so in man. Evidence for the alleged role of dietary animal fat and cholesterol is primarily based on correlations of the *per capita* fat available for human consumption with CHD mortality rates for countries where vital statistics are available and incorrectly assumed to be sufficiently accurate for epidemiological use. Nevertheless the plausibility of the epidemiological evidence and the validity of estimates of the food consumed are in question and much contradictory evidence exists regarding the role of animal fats in atherogenesis.

In the USA, from 1909 to 1965, when the national mortality rates for CHD allegedly rose, there was a fall of 7% in the animal fat available for consumption and a rapid increase (181%) in vegetable polyunsaturated fat.[14,49-51] This does not suggest that the ingestion of animal fats is responsible for the allegedly increased national CHD mortality rate, nor does the dietary intake of polyunsaturated fats correlate with CHD mortality rates. Epidemiologists have ignored this evidence for an increasing intake of vegetable fats and oils. In the UK, Trenchard[52] reviewed fat consumption and claimed that on the available evidence and after reappraisal of past estimates, animal fat consumption had probably remained constant from 1909-1913 to 1975 except for wartime and shortage periods. This evidence is not strong but basically no weaker than other epidemiological evidence of its type. Besides, the estimated total dietary animal fat does not correlate with the severity of atherosclerosis at autopsy.[53]

Segall,[54] comparing milk consumption and the incidence of CHD for 43 countries, found that milk consumption gave the strongest correlation with total caloric intake, meat intake, fats, oils and proteins. Such correlations tend to negate causality because of their very nonspecificity. However, rather than raising serum cholesterol levels, milk has a hypocholesterolemic effect[55-57] as has yogurt.[58] In African pastoral tribes the high intake of calories and fat (mainly as milk) is associated with a lower serum cholesterol level and a low CHD mortality rate.[15,59]

Yudkin[60] found no correlation between CHD mortality rates and butter fat (from butter, milk and cheese) nor (positive or negative) between dietary vegetable fat and CHD mortality. Similarly in the USA, there was no correlation between the consumption of dairy products from 1910 to 1970 and the alleged epidemic rise of CHD during that time.[61,62] Despite such anomalies between national dietary intake of cholesterol or fat and CHD mortality rates and the doubtful validity of the data, the inconsistencies have been essentially ignored.

The effect of eggs on serum cholesterol levels is variable and often misrepresented but without the dire consequences so often alleged.[63-65] Much depends on other dietary constituents and food additives. Flynn et al[66] studied the effect of consuming two eggs daily for three months and the elimination of eggs for three months before or after eating eggs for a similar period of time. There was no significant increase in serum cholesterol after six months and no significant association of dietary cholesterol intake from eggs with either serum cholesterol or triglyceride. Similar studies for shorter intervals have revealed no significant difference in serum cholesterol levels between those who ate one egg per day and those on eggless diets[57] and even the Framingham study[67] found no relationship between egg consumption, blood cholesterol level and CHD mortality. Then there was the anecdotal report of an 88-year-old man accustomed to consuming 25 eggs per day yet having a normal blood cholesterol level.[68] Despite evidence from the above studies, lipid protagonists persist in advocating reduction in egg consumption and drinking skim milk rather than whole milk. It is important to realize that in the USA milk, eggs and beef provide up to 30% of the saturated fat and 57% of the cholesterol in the food available for human consumption and also 30% of the protein content. The committee on medical aspects of food policy admitted that the evidence for dietary intake of saturated fats leading to CHD "falls short of proof".[69] Extremes of fat intake in another study[70]

were accompanied by the same serum cholesterol levels, no difference in nutrient and caloric intake was found except for carbohydrate.

Many studies based on individuals have provided contradictory results but reviewers agree there is little or no association of fat consumption or dietary cholesterol with either serum cholesterol concentration, coronary atherosclerosis, or CHD at an individual level.[8,71-74] Nevertheless epidemiologists continue to make the invalid extrapolation from population studies to the individual, perpetuating the "ecologic fallacy".[75] Autopsy studies in large population groups have shown an association between fat intake and atherosclerosis but this has not been shown to be independent of other dietary and/or societal factors. Yet no correlation has been found between individual levels of fat intake and individual plasma cholesterol levels within those populations.[8,74] Despite the alleged strong evidence for the role of dietary fat in atherogenesis, serum cholesterol differences observed between individuals are largely unexplained by their diet[71] and Gordon et al[76] concluded "Investigations within populations, for example, seldom suggest any relation between the intake of dietary fats and blood lipid concentrations". Lack of correlation at the individual level[8] invalidates a causal relationship between the average blood cholesterol, dietary fat and CHD mortality rates in population studies. The CHD epidemiologists should by now acknowledge this fact because if it were true, it would be more readily demonstrable at an individual level than in population studies.

Differences in CHD mortality between males and females may be due to hormonal, genetic or behavioral differences. Caloric and percentage fat intakes of the sexes have been found to be almost identical[73] and do not explain differences in CHD incidence. Lack of correlation between dietary fat intake and CHD mortality rates of different races[73] do not suggest a causal relationship between dietary fat and CHD.

The effect of saturated and polyunsaturated fatty acids on serum cholesterol concentrations has been extensively studied and yet the mechanism of effect remains an enigma.[8] Polyunsaturated fats produce a decrease in serum cholesterol in some individuals especially when

institutionalized and tissue storage of cholesterol in others. In large amounts they can decrease serum LDL levels but again the effect of
biological adaptation in the long-term has not
been adequately studied. Long-term deleterious
effect of diets rich in polyunsaturated fatty acids remains unknown[77] but is potentially hazardous.[78] Reduction of these animal food nutrients and emphasizing vegetable food matter can
lead to imbalance or reduction in other nutrients. The tendency at present is for considerable and perhaps excessive emphasis on carbohydrate. It seems incongruous that man
synthesizes considerable quantities of saturated
fatty acids and cholesterol, yet exogenous animal fat is regarded as noxious.

Over the last few years there has been more
acknowledgment by lipid protagonists that diet
has relatively little effect (in free living individuals) on blood cholesterol levels which are
principally determined by genetics, but this too
has been knowledge available for many years.[79,80]
In a survey of 434 pairs of adults female twins,
genetics played a dominant role in determining
the serum levels of LDL cholesterol, HDL cholesterol and triglycerides as well as relative
weight. Genetic control of blood lipids was
thought a possible explanation for high levels
of these risk factors in some women despite
their adhering to current dietary recommendations.[81] To select certain features of a lifetime of
eating in subjects who develop clinical CHD
and retrospectively compare their diets with
those of individuals without clinical CHD is
pointless and so is comparing the average presumed diet of a Western citizen with that of a
third world inhabitant and then correlating the
difference in fat consumption and type of fat
believed to be consumed with the national differences in unreliable CHD mortality rates. Moreover severe atherosclerosis can occur in lower animal species on a vegetarian diet and despite
methodologic inadequacies there are many reports
either contradicting or inconsistent with the alleged correlation of animal or saturated fats with
CHD mortality rates during this century.

Lack of correlation has been reported between (i) serum lipids and CHD mortality rates
in certain groups or populations[73,82-85] or the
severity of atherosclerosis,[86-87] (ii) the diet and
CHD mortality rates[26,71,88,89] or the severity of

atherosclerosis in man[90] or lower animals[91,92] and
(iii) dietary fat and serum cholesterol levels.[93-96]

Brisson[97] indicated serious inconsistencies
between CHD mortality and dietary cholesterol,
only 36% of the variation in mortality could be
accounted for by dietary cholesterol and 64%
was due to other variables. In 11 of 20 countries there was a negative correlation and there
were instances in which for virtually the same
cholesterol intake CHD mortality could more
than double. Likewise correlation between CHD
mortality and the percentage of calories derived
from animal foods (eggs, meat, poultry, dairy
products) was again poor with considerable
variation for the same mortality or the same
dietary intake of animal foods.

In a study of commodity consumption in
England and Wales there were many correlations with CHD mortality but considerable
variability between the sexes and with time.[98]
The absence of sex differences in CHD mortality rates in some countries cannot be explained
on dietary grounds. Thom et al[99] compared
trends in total mortality and CHD mortality
for men and women 45 to 64 years of age in six
time periods during 1950 and 1978 for 26
countries. CHD epidemiologists usually place
considerable store on parallel trends, but these
results exhibit such gross divergence between
CHD mortality rates for men and women in
the involved countries that the results should
have led to doubts about the validity of the
lipid hypothesis. CHD mortality for males increased in most countries and that for women
decreased in all countries. Inconsistencies always indicate the need for caution in interpreting this type of study. However the multiplicity and variation in these correlations suggest
nonspecificity and noncausal relationships.

Undeveloped third world countries, with
which comparisons of diet and mean serum
cholesterol values are often made, do not have
CHD mortality rates available for consideration.[100] Much evidence about the infrequency
of CHD in such countries is semianecdotal or
experiential.[101,102] There is evidence that the
severity of atherosclerosis is less in the Africans
but many never reach hospital when sick or
dying[103] and detailed studies of their blood lipids is lacking. Isaacson[104] reported a substantial
increase in the incidence of myocardial infarc-

tion in the Bantu at autopsy between 1959 and 1976. Nevertheless environmental and lifestyle differences between Africans and the American population are numerous and more than the quality and quantity of dietary fat. No matter how plausible such epidemiological data may be, it does not prove a causal relationship.

The mean serum cholesterol level in India is lower than that in the USA and the low incidence of CHD thought to occur in India has been refuted.[105,106] Malhotra and Pathania[105] reported on 867 fatal cases of CHD from India and considered the frequency difficult to determine because of the lack of medical services, inadequacy of vital statistics and the remoteness of country villages. Many of the characteristics (age, sex distribution, family history, profession, association with diabetes and hypertension) are similar to those in the western world. Most were vegetarian with a relatively low dietary fat intake and differed in body build and way of life. The authors considered them no less prone to CHD than the omnivorous westerner and were skeptical of the alleged role of dietary fat in the etiology of CHD.

Good nutrition in affluent countries has long been regarded as encompassing a plentiful supply of meat, dairy products, fruit and vegetables. The less well-to-do eat proportionately less meat, milk and eggs and while fruit and vegetables may be more readily available, farinaceous foods are used as filling agents in most countries. Better nutrition is associated with greater body size, immunity and intelligence. Poor nutrition is associated with poor physical and mental development, apathy, susceptibility to infectious diseases and a shortened life span. Many Africans are said to have almost a subsistence diet with wide fluctuations in food supply. The significance of the respective blood cholesterol levels is uncertain and the optimal level in our own community is unknown.

From the foregoing the blood cholesterol level cannot be assumed to be determined by dietary fats. This is supported by evidence provided by the Masai who have low serum cholesterol and LDL levels compared to people in the USA despite (i) an average caloric intake of 3000 calories with 66% provided from animal fat (milk supplemented by blood and meat), (ii) an estimated average daily cholesterol intake from

0.6 to 2.0 gm and (iii) a low CHD incidence and low severity of atherosclerosis.[107,108] They live under primitive conditions with an unknown rate of parasitic infestations and infectious diseases. Shaper[109,110] reported other African tribes with an unusually high milk intake and yet the CHD prevalence appeared to be low with either low serum cholesterol levels or levels approximating those in western man. This African experience casts further doubt on the role of a high fat/cholesterol diet as being important in atherogenesis and suggests that other factors in the African lifestyle either protect or fail to enhance the rate of development of atherosclerosis.

Many dietary variables have been found to be significantly correlated with CHD mortality rates in numerous countries including dairy fats, but also animal protein, total protein, meat, refined carbohydrates with a negative correlation with cereals and vegetables. The multiplicity of such correlations indicates only their nonspecificity[111] and the need to determine which correlations, if any, are of biological and pathological significance rather than selecting fat because of a preconceived idea.

Kritchevsky[14] stated that attempts to correlate CHD with the diet provide anomalous data and no conclusive proof of a causal relationship between dietary fat or cholesterol and serum cholesterol or the severity of atherosclerosis. Those accepting such a relationship harbor a misplaced faith in (i) the authenticity of interpretations of evidence accruing from dietary-induced cholesterolosis of arteries in experimental animals[112,113] and of the alleged premature atherosclerosis in subjects with familial hypercholesterolemia (FH)[114,115] and (ii) the validity of CHD epidemiological methodology. Moreover they will be hard pressed to explain the experimental production of atherosclerosis in herbivorous animals by hemodynamic means under conditions analogous to those occurring in man.[116,117] At present it must be concluded that there is no substantial scientific evidence to warrant recommendations regarding the desirable intake of relative proportions of saturated/unsaturated fats.

CHOLESTEROL AND LIPOPROTEINS

Brown and Goldstein[118] in their Nobel Lecture called cholesterol "a Janus-faced molecule" stating, "The very property that makes it useful in cell membranes, namely its absolute insolubility in water, also makes it lethal". This unfortunate view of cholesterol by two very eminent biochemists denigrates the important role of cholesterol in human biology. Such a view could well apply to any metabolite when there is an interruption of its normal metabolic pathway. It results in tissue storage of the excessive accumulation of the metabolite with secondary consequences affecting other tissues. Their opinion is due to misrepresentation of the pathology of the vascular lesions of FH which are not purely atherosclerotic but fat storage phenomena (Chapter 2). If pathologists had been as nondiscerning in their appraisal of tumors as they have been in differentiating atherosclerosis from the vascular lesions of FH, it is possible we might still be at the stage of not knowing the difference between benign and malignant tumors.

Cholesterol is not a lipid but a lipidic steroid alcohol. It is the most abundant steroid in the animal kingdom and the only one that occurs in appreciable quantities throughout the body. Dietary cholesterol is of animal origin and plant steroids, except ergosterol (pro-vitamin D), are poorly absorbed by humans. The molecular structure of cholesterol is based on the four ring hydrocarbon perhydrocyclopentanophenanthrene and contains 27 carbon atoms, a single hydroxyl group and four methyl groups (Fig. 5.1). It is practically insoluble in water and therefore closely related physically and metabolically to lipids. In the body's aqueous milieu it is usually in complex associations with fatty acids and proteins.

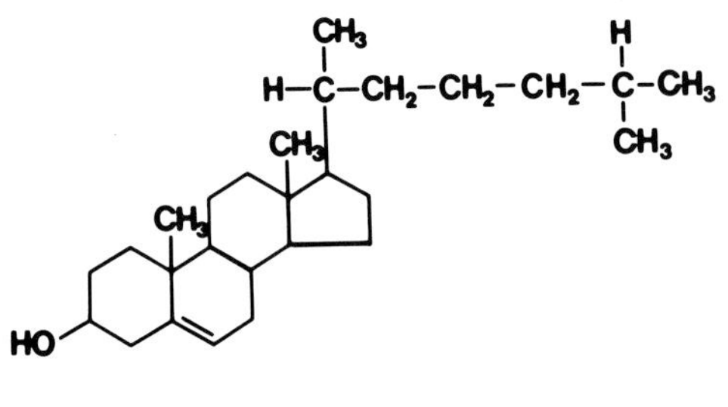

Fig. 5.1. Molecular structure of cholesterol.

Of the 140g or so of cholesterol in the body, less than 7% is present in the plasma.[119] Cholesterol, triglycerides and other lipids are transported in body fluids in association with protein as lipoproteins which are classified according to increasing density (Table 5.1). The lipoproteins consist of a core of hydrophobic lipids surrounded by a shell of polar lipids and apoproteins. Chylomicra are the largest of the lipoproteins and are about one-third to one-fourth protein. The remaining constituents include triglycerides, cholesterol, cholesterol esters and phospholipids. Chylomicra are formed in the intestinal mucosa following the ingestion of fat and for the most part the others are formed in the liver although small quantities of HDL are synthesized in the intestinal epithelium during postprandial absorption of dietary fat. The primary function of lipoproteins is the transport of lipid in the blood and tissue fluids in a soluble form.

The apolipoproteins are synthesized partly in the liver and partly in the intestinal mucosa. Their main function is to form macromolecular complexes with lipids and cholesterol, i.e., lipoproteins for transport in the blood and body fluids. Some apolipoproteins can inhibit or activate enzymes in the metabolism of lipid and some react with cell membrane markers.

The principal apolipoproteins (A-1, A-2, A-4, B-48, B-100, C-1, C-2, C-3, E) are synthesized and secreted by the liver and intestines. They solubilize highly hydrophobic lipids in this way and regulate the movement of particulate lipids into and out of specific target cells and tissues. The lipoprotein particles participating in the exogenous and endogenous cycles involving lipid metabolism all contain cholesterol (Table 5.1), though primarily the low-density lipoprotein (LDL) has been incriminated in atherogenesis.

LDL is the primary carrier of cholesterol and has a central hydrophobic core of about 1500 cholesterol ester molecules (mostly linoleate) surrounded by a shell of phospholipids and unesterified cholesterol with a single copy of the large apoprotein B-100.[120] Approximately 75% of serum cholesterol is in the LDL fraction. The role of LDL is to transport cholesterol to the tissues and to regulate cholesterol synthesis at these sites.

Cholesterol is a component of the plasma membranes of all higher animals and contributes to membrane fluidity. As such it is essential for the growth and viability of cells in higher organisms. In general, cells outside the liver and intestines obtain cholesterol from the plasma rather than synthesizing it de novo and consequently their primary source is LDL. The B-100 apoprotein binds to a specific receptor protein in coated caveolae or pits resulting in endocytosis of the LDL particles. The vesicles thus formed fuse with lysosomes in which protein is hydrolyzed to free amino acids, and cholesterol esters are hydrolyzed by lysosomal acid lipase, the LDL receptor returning to the plasma membrane to function as such again. Unesterified cholesterol is used for membrane synthesis or reesterified for intracellular storage (mainly as oleate and parmitoleate).[120] When there is sufficient intracellular cholesterol, no new LDL receptors are synthesized so that this negative feedback regulatory system within the cell reduces or stops further uptake.

At least 80% of the cholesterol required is synthesized in vivo, primarily in the liver and to a lesser extent in the intestinal epithelium. This is the major source of blood cholesterol but it is likely that all cells are able to manufacture it when necessary. All cholesterol required can be synthesized if necessary as occurs with people on strict vegetarian diets. When intestinal absorption of cholesterol diminishes, endogenous synthesis is increased and vice versa. The feedback regulatory system tends to maintain blood cholesterol at a relatively stable level and the bulk of exogenous cholesterol is recoverable as bile acids in the bile.[122] At least in normal subjects the plasma cholesterol concentration is not influenced significantly by variation in the dietary intake of cholesterol over a wide range (0 to 700 mg). Normal subjects without metabolic lipid disorders have the capacity to synthesize up to 2 gm daily from acetate.[122] A low plasma cholesterol level is found in the presence of severe chronic infection, including autoimmune deficiency syndrome, anemia, massive liver damage and usually also in malnutrition.

The principal functions of cholesterol include the following:

1. An essential and significant structural constituent of all plasma and intracellular membranes, it helps to limit permeability of the lipid bilayer to small water soluble molecules, to maintain the fluidity, flexibility and mechanical stability of the cell membrane.

2. Its importance to plasma membrane structure is reflected in cerebral tissue and myelination of nerve fibers since up to 17% of the dry weight of the brain is cholesterol. It is also a component of the membranes of intracellular organelles.

3. It is the precursor of the five groups of steroid hormones (progesterone, estrogens, male steroids, corticosteroids and mineral corticoids).

4. It is a precursor of vitamin D.

5. The most abundant use of cholesterol (as much as 80%) takes place in the liver to form

Table 5.1. Characteristics of major plasma lipoproteins

Plasma Lipoproteins	Major Core Lipids	Apolipoproteins	Size
Chylomicron	Dietary triglyceride	A-1, A-2, A-4, B-48	80-500 nm
Chylomicron remnants	Dietary cholesterol esters	B-48, C, E	
Very low density lipoprotein (VLDL)	Endogenous triglyceride (25% cholesterol)	B-100, C, E	30-80 nm
Intermediate density lipoprotein (IDL)	Endogenous cholesterol esters (45% cholesterol)	B-100, E	30 nm
Low density lipoprotein (LDL)	Endogenous cholesterol esters	B-100	15-25 nm
High density lipoprotein (HDL)	Endogenous cholesterol esters (less than 25% cholesterol)	A-1, A-2, (C and E are minor components)	5-12 nm

N.B. The apolipoprotein component of the lipoproteins varies considerably in the literature[48,120,121]

cholic acid which is conjugated with other substances to form bile salts. The large bulk of exogenous cholesterol is recoverable as bile salts in bile.[122] Bile salts emulsify dietary fat thereby facilitating their lipolysis and possibly activating pancreatic lipase. They also facilitate the absorption of lipid-soluble substances such as cholesterol, vitamin D and E and bilirubin. Together with phospholipids they maintain cholesterol in the bile in a soluble state, thus preventing it from precipitating out of solution in the gall bladder.

6. A large amount of cholesterol is present in sebaceous secretions that permeate the stratum corneum of the skin making the skin resistant to absorption of water-soluble substances and to the action of many chemical agents. It also helps to prevent water evaporation.[123]

The functional importance of cholesterol in cell membranes cannot be overemphasized. Mutant animal cells unable to synthesize cholesterol rapidly lyse and break down but the addition of cholesterol to the medium permits incorporation of cholesterol into the plasma membrane thus contributing to the survival of the cells.[124] All human cells require a constant supply of cholesterol which is provided from the diet or by biosynthesis in the liver. The cholesterol content of smooth muscle cells is higher than other striated muscle cells but the reason for this is obscure.[125]

Hemolysis of human erythrocytes occurs in subjects with cardiac valvular disease such as mitral stenosis[126,127] and also in association with a traumatic arteriovenous fistula with disappearance of the hemolysis following surgical closure of the shunt.[128] This micro-angiopathic anemia suggests that the plasma membrane fragility was induced by the vibrational stress of turbulent flow. Under less severe flow disturbances one might expect a much lower grade of hemolysis such as in the anemia of hypertension, sports, and marathon runners. These same hemodynamically induced vibrational stresses have been invoked as the reason for the augmented cellular turnover at arterial forks and for the vesiculogranular degeneration of smooth muscle cells in human atherosclerosis, human and experimental aneurysms and arteriovenous fistulas.[129] The degenerative changes are also the consequence of plasma membrane fragility, since

fragments of plasma membrane of variable length are found in the interstitial matrix in association with membrane bound vesicles which have a propensity for lipid accumulation and mineralization.[130,131] Lipid accumulation in atherosclerosis and in experimental models of atherosclerosis in herbivorous animals on a stock diet is merely an example of the well recognized nonspecific affinity of this cell debris for lipid and minerals.[132] It is pertinent therefore that a primary function of cholesterol is to maintain the fluidity and strength of the plasma membranes of cells and LDL is the principal carrier of LDL. Constituent molecules of cell membranes may be recycled and it is known that membranes repair themselves or their ends reunite if disrupted.

Phospholipids and cholesterol account for nearly 95% of the total lipid of the red cell membrane and the cholesterol in the erythrocyte membrane undergoes rapid exchange with the plasma. Half of the membrane cholesterol is replaced in a few hours and the rapid exchange rate depends on LDL supply of cholesterol.[133] Decrease in plasma LDL results in a decreased turnover of cholesterol in the membrane and an increase in cholesterol content in the red cell membrane with acanthocytosis and hemolysis. This cholesterol exchange implies that there may be some molecular alterations occurring that may be related to the membrane fragility. In any case the chemical composition of the plasma membranes would be of vital importance to the integrity of the cell which, if breached, could augment the vesiculogranular degeneration of smooth muscle cells and endothelium and the monocyte/macrophage population. Foam cell infiltration must interfere with the normal viscoelastic properties of the wall and would be unlikely to withstand the hemodynamic stresses to which the wall is continuously subjected.

The matrix vesicle population in the arterial wall is known to be increased by hypertension and also increases in the walls of aneurysms and arteriovenous fistulae in which atherosclerosis runs an accelerated course.[134,135] I believe the underlying mechanism is mechanical failure of vascular wall constituents due to the incessant pulsatile vibrational stresses rather than to shear stress as is so often alleged. The shear stress is alternating and therefore also vibrational and must be contributory. The basic evidence for simple shear stress is false and does not explain the acquired, all encompassing fragility of the entire wall. Alternating stresses are known to be peculiarly damaging in the production of poststenotic dilatations and dissecting aneurysms beyond valvular stenoses [129] and to red cells under similar stress.[126,127] There is evidence for molecular fragmentation of elastin under similar conditions.[136] It is also known that molecular fragmentation of long chain polymers occurs in highly disturbed flow. This, I contend, is the underlying mechanism of plasma membrane fragility in atherosclerosis.

It is not suggested that cholesterol is the principal molecule essential for cell membrane strength. Obviously phospholipid and the membrane proteins such as spectrin contribute to the mechanical strength. Plasma membrane abnormalities in ion transport have been reported in many cell types including lymphocytes, red blood cells and vascular smooth muscle cells in hypertension.[137] Whether or not these are independent or associated with hemodynamic stress is not known but physicochemical changes in the plasma membrane could well be manifested in many ways and possibly aggravated by abnormal or unusual constituents in the cell membranes.

Incorporation of fatty acids foreign to the body and chemically produced industrially in some substitute food products could be deleterious to cellular integrity and function and thus secondarily enhance the progression of atherosclerosis. The experimental evidence available is that cholesterol is one of the most important factors promoting cell membrane integrity and that a continual supply of cholesterol is vital to sustain the blood vessel wall physiologically. Therefore iatrogenic mechanisms interfering with the supply and turnover of this essential metabolite in normolipidemic subjects must be fraught with some hazard. Thus it is important that the evidence for reduction of dietary cholesterol is based on sound science not on the judgment of CHD epidemiologists and cardiologists who capriciously promote change in the human omnivorous diet knowing that conclusive evidence for their beliefs is not yet available.

Progressively as the lipid hypothesis developed and accumulated supporters, cholesterol became the dominant factor of atherosclerosis. For more than 30 years the public has been exposed to intense adverse publicity concerning the presumed role of cholesterol in heart disease. Since atherosclerosis is ubiquitous and occurs widely amongst lower animals, it is unlikely that an essential metabolite of every cell in humans and other vertebrates could cause such a widespread degenerative disease. The belief that it is noxious under physiological conditions is anathema to biological science. The epidemiology of CHD has centered on cholesterol and the epidemiology of cholesterol is essentially that of LDL or LDL cholesterol.

Pathologically, cholesterol accumulation is but one of many biochemical and morphological changes in the late stage lesions of atherosclerosis. Some regard it as the major chemical constituent or hallmark of the disease, a contention pathologically untenable as its presence does not explain the pathogenesis and complications of atherosclerosis. It is found in atherosclerosis, chronic inflammatory and degenerative disorders, cholesteatomas, old cerebral infarcts, cysts lined by squamous epithelium and at times in older degenerative regions of long-standing benign tumors. However its involvement in such disorders does not indicate a causative role nor make it pathogenic. It should be considered in a wider context with due regard for cholesterol's essential metabolic role in health. A case in point, hemosiderin in macrophages may persist in old areas of hemorrhage in hemophilia and in old healed splenic infarcts but it is not noxious except when its normal metabolic cycle is disturbed and the result is pathological accumulation of the metabolite with secondary complications ensuing.

Framingham Study reports have been inconsistent in evaluations of its significance. In 1957 no marked correlation was found between any dietary constituent and serum cholesterol.[138] Kannel and Gordon[139] reported serum cholesterol was not discriminatory between 54 and 61 years of age. In 1971 Kannel et al[140] considered the most useful lipid estimation in discriminating men likely to die of CHD was the total serum cholesterol level. In women over the age of 50 years in Framingham[140] the serum cholesterol had no predictive value and after 65 years was no longer regarded as a risk factor.[141] In 1982 Kannel and Gordon[142] declared that cholesterol was not a strong risk factor in the way hypertension was for stroke and for CHD no such strong risk factor existed. Now the serum cholesterol level is regarded as having no predictive value over 50 years of age in males or females.[143,144] Its lack of importance as a CHD risk factor can be fully appreciated on reference to Figures 1.1, 1.2 and Table 4.2, in which it is apparent that even at Framingham the value of a serum cholesterol as a so-called CHD risk factor is minimal since it is applicable to only a very small minority of deaths from CHD.

Epidemiological studies initially focused almost exclusively on total serum cholesterol and its relationship to CHD but most serum cholesterol is carried in the LDL fraction. It has been accepted that "much of what has been learned in the past about the ill effects of a high serum total cholesterol can be attributed to the associated levels of LDL or cholesterol carried in this lipoprotein fraction".[141] Others allege the epidemiology of serum cholesterol and LDL cholesterol is statistically equivalent[145] but Truswell[57] considers total blood cholesterol a better predictor of CHD than LDL cholesterol and less expensive to determine.

Cholesterol is mostly synthesized in vivo (at least 80%) with the utilization rate dependent on the rate of cellular turnover in the tissue concerned. Absorption of exogenous cholesterol in man is variable but low, increasing when large amounts are ingested and single large doses of cholesterol produce only transient, trivial changes in serum cholesterol.[146] It has been estimated from short-term studies that the relationship of dietary to serum cholesterol is linear with a daily consumption of cholesterol ranging from 0 to 600 mg. The estimated increase in serum cholesterol ranges from 3 to 12 mg per dL of plasma per 100 mg of dietary cholesterol consumed per 1,000 kilocalories.[74] More than 600 mg of dietary cholesterol per day produces little additional effect in most people.[8] These conclusions were derived essentially from short-term studies and not from free living individuals. Biological adaptation in the long-term may alter the end result though diet is believed to account for only 25% of the serum cholesterol and twin studies indicate a strong genetic influence on serum cholesterol.[79,81] A larger intake is offset by greater excretion and reduced synthesis although actual cholesterol absorption, it is thought, does not exceed 0.3 g per day. Taylor et al[147,148] consider the principal protection of humans from dietary cholesterol is their limited capacity for intestinal absorption. In carefully controlled metabolic ward studies of individuals, increased dietary cholesterol intake resulted in plasma cholesterol levels that rose in some, and fell or remained the same in others.[149] Plasma lipoproteins can be manipulated within limits by altering the ratio of one nutrient to another. Such studies have little relevance to real-life long-term situations where there is heterogeneous response of plasma lipids to similar diets because of variable dietary, environmental and individual differences that interact.

In the Tecumseh Study trained interviewers obtained details of food consumed during 24 hours prior to venepuncture and the subjects (both sexes) were classified into tertiles according to each serum cholesterol and triglyceride level. The mean daily consumption of each dietary component was virtually identical and the serum lipid values were unrelated to the quality, quantity or proportions of fat, carbohydrate or protein consumed during the 24 hour recall period.[96] Ahrens[150] considered that any one diet produces different results in different people and with a specific diet it is impossible to predict what proportion of the population will show a decline in plasma cholesterol levels or to what degree. Oliver[151] said dietary cholesterol contributes no more than 10% of the serum cholesterol and that within the average range of cholesterol intake (250 to 750 mg per diem) serum cholesterol would not change by more than 10 mg/dL. Kannel[152] considers that cholesterol intake above 400 mg per diem has no discernible effect on serum cholesterol. Keys and Anderson[153] contend that the cholesterol content of natural diets has no significant effect on serum cholesterol or atherogenesis in man.

A moderate cholesterol-lowering diet in the Lipid Research Clinical Coronary Primary Prevention Trial (LRCCPPT)[154,155] reduced the total serum cholesterol levels of 1903 middle-aged males with primary hypercholesterolemia by an average of only 14.3 mg/dL (4.9%) after seven years—an insignificant amount in view of (a) the methodological laboratory error involved, (b) the tendency to regression to the mean independently of any dietary manipulation[156] and (c) the tendency for the level to fall in males after 50 years of age independently of diet. If the dietary effect is so small in subjects with primary hypercholesterolemia, even less can be expected in normocholesterolemic subjects.

Barnes and Barnes[157] reported that a high fat diet even over 17 years did not produce hypercholesterolemia when thyroid function was adequate. The idea that diet has a direct long-term effect on plasma cholesterol levels remains to be proven[158] because the extent of long-term adaptation has yet to be determined. There appears to be a significant correlation between biological or blood relatives and total serum cholesterol and LDL cholesterol.[151] Correlations for spouses were not significant, suggesting the genetic influence is stronger on serum cholesterol and LDL cholesterol levels than can be explained environmentally. Oliver[151] considered the relationship of serum cholesterol to CHD to be weak since man is less sensitive to dietary cholesterol than other species like rabbits and chickens. Kannel[152] admitted that serum cholesterol is not the sole determinant and found difficulty in proving a causal relationship between cholesterol and CHD or atherosclerosis. He added that in free-living affluent populations no difference had been demonstrated in nutrient composition of the diet between those with and those without CHD, nor was there a correlation between diet and serum cholesterol values on an individual basis. Olson[62] essentially concurred with his views and so did McGill[74] and a Special Committee of the NIH.[8] The fact that the level of serum cholesterol that is a risk factor varies from country to country[159,160] detracts from its specificity and importance. Moreover there is no correlation between serum cholesterol and sudden cardiac death.[151,161]

Accordingly the relationship of serum cholesterol with the incidence of CHD has assumed undeserved importance in atherogenesis.[162] In reality it is weak and inconclusive even using the unreliable and fallacious dietary and CHD data as indicated earlier. Whether the increase in serum cholesterol is partly or wholly attributable to a corresponding increase in age, blood pressure or other age dependent risk factors is uncertain. The significance of the relationship to affluence and what has for years been regarded as a good, nutritious high protein diet is unknown but even within three distinct races, an increase was noted in serum cholesterol with affluence and its trappings.[163] The fact that in chronic diseases and anemia the blood cholesterol level is low suggests that the higher levels in technologically advanced countries may be associated with better nutrition, immunity and greater longevity. To attribute the greater severity of atherosclerosis or the higher incidence of the imprecise diagnosis of CHD to a high intake of dietary (animal) fat is an unproved assumption and should never have been accepted without more convincing evidence than is currently available.

In the past this concept of the role of animal fats depended on evidence from cholesterol-fed animal experiments and the pathology of FH, the lesions of which are lipid storage phenomena superimposed on atherosclerosis.[112-115] Neither can evidence from population studies of diets and mortality rates of CHD be used in support of the lipid hypothesis. The fact that atherosclerosis is not species-specific and occurs in lower animals including herbivores with low serum cholesterol values (even below 100 mg/dL)[116,117,164] indicates that at most hypercholesterolemia can only be an aggravating factor and not causal even if the epidemiological data were valid. Diet, blood lipids, atherosclerosis and the complications of the disease have not been plausibly integrated by the lipid hypothesis. Nor does it explain the prelipid phase of atherosclerosis, the mural connective tissue changes or the development of any complications of the disease (Chapter 2).

Several other problems require consideration in the evaluation of cholesterol levels.

(I) ACCURACY OF LABORATORY CHOLESTEROL ESTIMATIONS

Laboratory estimations of serum cholesterol have been notoriously inaccurate[165] with errors of 10 to 40%. The lack of standardization of laboratory techniques for cholesterol estimations can result in variations of 25% or more in the same laboratory.[166] In 1958 three sets of duplicate serum samples were submitted to five laboratories on different days: results were consistently higher in some laboratories than in others but the rank-order of the cholesterol estimations also varied.[167] Reproducibility of results from the one sample of blood was poor, the average deviation being ± 27 mg/dL. One sample varied from 180 to 312 mg/dL in different laboratories and another 311 to 529 mg/dL.

In any study there is no way of appraising the accuracy of or knowing which studies consistently contained the most reliable biochemical estimations. In recent years with greater emphasis on national quality control studies of laboratory results, a greater degree of accuracy and therefore comparability between laboratories and countries of similar technological advancement can be expected but the degree of accuracy of each laboratory must be determined for any particular study. Dawber[168] declared that difficulty in obtaining accurate, repeatable plasma cholesterol estimations plagued the Framingham Study and no doubt many other clinical and epidemiological studies also. Recently Blank et al[169] reported markedly different cholesterol values according to the techniques currently in use in the USA, indicating the need for individual laboratories to standardize their methodology and the possible lack of comparability when interpreting published values. This inaccuracy of serum cholesterol estimations throws doubt on the validity of older CHD studies and the overall quality of CHD epidemiological data. One has to wonder whether old Framingham Study data has been discarded.

Cholesterol measurements may be affected by many factors including whether the patient is sitting or standing when the blood is taken, how long the tourniquet is left on and even how the specimens were taken and stored. Roberts[170] indicated that the reading may be in error by 50 mg/dL. This variability was regarded as indicating that a single estimation was virtually meaningless. Lack of standardization of diet consumed in the period preceding the analysis influences serum cholesterol levels and triglycerides particularly by as much as 20% depending on fatty acid composition and the cholesterol content of the diet in the preceding 10 to 14 days.[166]

In 1990 it was stated that half of the US conventional clinical laboratories participating in proficiency testing surveys in 1985 and 1987 were unable to meet the current accuracy standards recommended by the Laboratory Standardization Panel. The commercial cholesterol testing systems that meet the most stringent analytic standards still misclassify a large proportion of individuals whose cholesterol value is close to critical decision levels.[171] The biological variability within one year can range from 3.9% to 12.4% and superimposed on this is the analytical variability of up to 5%. It is not surprising that current practice is to request multiple estimations which are also needed for other lipids.

(II) INDIVIDUAL VARIABILITY

Substantial intraindividual variation can occur within hours and appears to be relatively independent of the time of day or intervening meals.[17] Peterson et al[172] reported hourly variation in some young individuals whose mean cholesterol was somewhat higher than a control less-labile group. Variations from 40 to 80 mg/dL were observed during a control period. Even greater changes were associated with psychological stress. The extreme variability in the individual and between subjects nullifies the value of single serum cholesterol estimations.[162]

Within one year intraindividual variation has ranged from 3.9 to 10.9% for serum cholesterol, 12.9 to 40.8% for triglycerides and from 3.6 to 12.4% for HDL-cholesterol.[173] It was estimated that more than 60% of the variability was due to biological fluctuation and the remainder to analytical variation. Others have given the variation for cholesterol as 5 to 10% even when the diet is controlled in metabolic studies.[174]

Ten subjects on essentially similar diets and given a placebo treatment had serial cholesterol estimations from at least two months after suffering a myocardial infarction and monthly thereafter.[167] The fluctuations in results were wide in some subjects and negligible in others, the weighted average standard deviation being ± 30 mg/dL. In another study[175] over 12 years the standard deviation for all subjects was ± 43 mg/dL. Variability varied from person to person. Variability was greater with longer intervals between blood sampling. In a cohort of

177 male army personnel (aged 40 to 60 years) over a period of five years individual cholesterol levels fluctuated from 5% to 100% with a mean variation of approximately 25%. There was also variability of serum cholesterol levels in the same subjects over a period of 10 to 20 years without consistency in the direction of change: values increased significantly more than they fell and without relationship to health status.[162,176] Institutionalized or free-living subjects vary between 11.5 mg/dL to 24.4 mg/dL[17] and greater intraindividual variability occurs amongst subjects with serum cholesterol levels nearer the upper limit of the reference range.[177]

(III) NORMAL OR DISCRIMINATION VALUES FOR SERUM CHOLESTEROL

The term "normal values" is being discarded because of ambiguities and misconceptions regarding "normal" and healthy.[178] The discrimination values being adopted by clinical chemists represent the level of serum cholesterol which discriminates those subjects requiring further investigation because of the probability of a diseased state from those within the discrimination values who are in all likelihood "healthy". The term "normal values" refers to values determined statistically and is neither arbitrary nor infallible but should meet certain basic requirements.[178] The serum cholesterol range for adults in the USA has been given as 159 to 317 mg/dL with variation for age and sex.[179] The upper limit of the reference range has varied from 180 to 310[95,141,180-182] with the suggestion that individuals should endeavor to reduce their blood cholesterol level to below 180 mg/dL. This almost universal hyperlipidemia is unrealistic and unlike the experience with other diseases and laboratory data. Use of different arbitrary discrimination values for hypercholesterolemia by different authors in different countries will lead to further confusion and misrepresentation in the cholesterol controversy. Scott et al[183] consider there is a CHD risk for all levels of serum cholesterol and no discrimination value exists, implying in effect that cholesterol is noxious at all blood levels. Similar views have been expressed by others who advocate that entire populations should be on cholesterol lowering diets. Since CHD occurs at all blood cholesterol levels, rather than

reviewing the basis on which the hypothesis rests in detail, the upper discrimination value is being manipulated to make population serum lipid levels meet the criteria and opinions of CHD epidemiologists. In other words the conventional "normal values" do not indicate health as regards the likelihood of CHD or for that matter atherosclerosis. In reality no discrimination value for any biochemical parameter is applicable to the universal disease atherosclerosis. These are not logical grounds for altering the time honored conventional use of "normal" or discrimination values. Indeed laboratories are being advised not to distribute discrimination values for serum cholesterol.

The reference or discrimination values for serum cholesterol vary from country to country and the level determining "risk" in one area or country is not necessarily considered a risk factor elsewhere. Roberts[184] stated that whether or not hypercholesterolemia is a prerequisite for coronary atherosclerosis depends on the definition of hypercholesterolemia and suggests that the upper discrimination value should be 180 mg/dL rather than the 250 mg/dL often given. This loose usage of coronary atherosclerosis which is universal adds further to the existing confusion. Kannel et al[141] reported most laboratories used a reference range for adults from 180 to 310 mg/dL and Kritchevsky[26] gave 330 mg/dL for the upper value for adults 50 to 59 years of age. Therefore a better reason for changing it is needed than that currently provided by CHD epidemiologists.

If 180 mg/dL is taken as the discrimination value, 90% of Americans are hypercholesterolemic and using the NIH consensus development conference criteria, 49% of middle-aged British males can be regarded at moderate or severe risk requiring therapy to reduce their plasma cholesterol.[185] The situation would be worse if therapy was dependent on the views of Rifkind and Lenfant[186] who suggested that the physiological serum cholesterol level for adults might be 110 to 150 mg/dL, which would indicate an even higher prevalence of hypercholesterolemia and a greater national drug bill.

The discrimination values cannot under any circumstances be considered as an arbitrary value determined by preconceived ideas. Since hypertension usually indicates a shortened life span and hypotension indicates longevity with less chance of developing CHD, the analogous situation would be to arbitrarily declare the upper discrimination level for hypertension at 100 mm Hg systolic and 60 diastolic or even lower and to argue that most of the population is hypertensive and in need of drug therapy. The fallacy in the argument is that the biochemical or physiological parameter must be known to be related to the disease in question and rather than changing the discriminating blood cholesterol levels, the relevance of serum cholesterol levels to CHD (excluding the FH, type II hyperlipoproteinemia) should be questioned. The relationship to atherosclerosis is even more remote.

Hypercholesterolemia can be defined as a plasma cholesterol level above the 95th percentile, i.e., values above the range of 275 to 290 mg/dL for middle-aged Americans. The conflicting view expressed by lipid protagonists is that hypercholesterolemia indicates a plasma level associated with significantly increased CHD risk. Grundy et al[187] regard any value above 200 mg/dL as hypercholesterolemic. The NIH consensus development conference[188] considered levels of 240 mg/dL for middle-aged adults entailed moderately increased risk and indicated a high risk for levels above 260 mg/ dL. However in view of (i) the large diagnostic error for CHD (both false positives and false negatives), (ii) the problems associated with single cholesterol estimations (with individual diurnal, weekly, cyclical, seasonal and temporal

variability,[172,189,190] (iii) individual variation in serum cholesterol levels being greater than that of other blood constituents,[191] (iv) the failure to exclude or account for other variables (age, blood pressure, diabetes mellitus, body mass, nutrition status, the presence or absence of infections and FH), (v) the poor correlation of CHD with plasma cholesterol on an individual basis and (vi) the inappropriate use of CHD as a surrogate for atherosclerosis, the validity of "a significant increase in risk" must be questioned and CHD cannot be used as a marker to determine the upper discrimination value for serum cholesterol.

SERUM CHOLESTEROL AND AGE

In technologically advanced and affluent countries the serum cholesterol levels increase with age with the consumption of what has been traditionally regarded as a good nutritious diet. The mean cholesterol levels of umbilical cord blood in 1800 American neonates was 63.8 ± 18.7 mg/dL with no racial differences between black and white.[192] The upper arbitrary discrimination value for neonates was taken as 100mg/dL. Type II hyperlipoproteinemia was identified in the parents of a small number of those whose parents were available for study and the serum cholesterol level of an infant is independent of the maternal serum cholesterol level. The cholesterol level rises to 155 mg/dL at three months stabilizing at this level for the first four months of life.[193] For children from one to two years of age the mean cholesterol level has been reported as 159 mg/dL, 165 ± 25 mg/dL for two to six years and 170 ± 25 mg/dL for preadolescent and adolescents.[194] The serum cholesterol level need not rise with age,[176,195] but mean values in the USA tend to rise for males from adolescence through middle age with a curvilinear relationship. Thereafter the curve tends to flatten or actually decline somewhat after approximately 50 to 55 years of age[16,196,197] when CHD mortality is highest (Fig. 5.2). Female levels do not increase at the same rate but at about 50 years their level surpasses that of the males and may then flatten or decline somewhat[197] (Fig. 5.2). There is wide variation in each age group[199] and the lack of parallelism of male and female graphs lends no support for dietary factors as being primarily

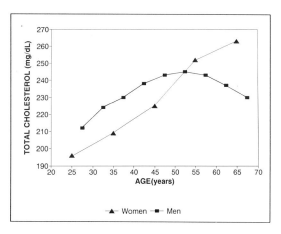

Fig. 5.2. Graph displaying the variation of serum cholesterol levels for both sexes without clinical CHD. (Adapted from data in Lawry et al.[198])

responsible for blood cholesterol levels. Moreover CHD mortality rates for males and females increase rapidly after 55 years of age and do not parallel the age-related serum cholesterol levels as would be expected if serum cholesterol was the determining factor (Fig. 1.1 and 1.2).

METABOLIC DISORDERS AND SERUM CHOLESTEROL LEVELS

Attention has already been drawn to the invalid inclusion of subjects suffering from FH in epidemiological studies involving CHD essentially because CHD is not pathognomonic of atherosclerosis and the pathogenesis of CHD in FH differs from that in atherosclerosis. It is likely therefore that subjects with FH and the few cases of familial defective apolipoprotein B-100 (FDB) can seriously affect CHD epidemiological studies and produce misleading and fallacious results. Quite obviously inclusion of FH with other diseases associated with CHD studies is contrary to modern medical science and also clinical practices.

Following the Second World War increasing note was made of the association of elevated serum cholesterol levels in groups of middle-aged men with clinical CHD[200] and it was shown by Lawry et al[198] that the younger the two groups (those with CHD and the clinically healthy) the greater was the difference in serum cholesterol. Kinsell[201] reported that in a study of subjects with CHD, there was an impressive correlation with elevated blood lipids in young adults but no relationship was found in coronary patients aged 60 years and older.

A meaningful correlation between high serum cholesterol levels and CHD was said to be demonstrated consistently only in certain subsets of patients, especially those with FH.[202] In 200 CHD patients the serum cholesterol levels were higher on an average than for control patients, but hypercholesterolemia was most noticeable in males less than 40 years of age.[203] A similar concentration of elevated serum cholesterol levels has been noted amongst the 40 to 49 year age group[204] and in those 21 to 30 years.[205] Oliver[206] found type II hyperlipoproteinemia was the commonest lipid disorder amongst women under 45 years with CHD and Rissanen[207] declared that familial hyperlipidemia and hypertension accounted for most of the

strong familial component of CHD in young adults. Schubert[193] indicated that FH could account for at least half the incidence of CHD in subjects under 65 without invoking other risk factors.

Consistently similar observations have been made indicating the high representation of FH amongst those with premature clinical CHD. Of 100 men with CHD, only 19 had serum lipids or the glucose tolerance test within normal limits[208] and Nikkilä and Aro[209] estimated that up to one-third of those with premature CHD had a familial trait of hyperlipidemia. In 83 persons with FH, the absolute amount of carbohydrate, fat, protein and cholesterol in the diet had no demonstrable effect on plasma cholesterol levels.[210]

If up to 20% of patients admitted to a coronary care unit had an abnormal lipid profile, they could substantially increase the mean plasma cholesterol level for the group as a whole.[211] Slack[212] also reported an undue tendency for subjects with heterozygous FH to manifest clinical CHD at a young age. Since heterozygotes have an incidence in the population of 0.02% and in a few countries the frequency is 0.5%, the prevalence of FH amongst subjects presenting with premature CHD clinically will be unduly high (Table 2.1). The more severe the FH, the higher will be the plasma cholesterol level for affected individuals. Since most clinical CHD studies and indeed most clinical trials involve male subjects under the age of 50 or 55 years the study group is a nonrepresentative minority because most CHD deaths occur after 60 years of age (Fig. 1.1 and 1.2). By virtue of this selection bias for young subjects, one would expect a biased over-representation of subjects with FH, because 50% of male heterozygotes with FH have CHD by the age of 50 years.[212,213] Not only should subjects with lipid dystrophies be excluded from CHD studies of normolipidemic subjects but the use of young subjects with the intention of seeking predisposing factors for premature CHD has inadvertently led to a selection bias for inclusion of FH. This is analogous to Berkson's bias, and inclusion of such patients with varying grades of the familial disorder can suggest a graded response for plasma cholesterol and CHD in population samples particularly in the young age group usually studied. This is particularly so since most deaths from CHD occur after the age of 60 years (Table 4.2) and serum cholesterol levels cease to be a "risk factor" for CHD after the age of 50 years.[143,144]

In 27 patients with severe angina pectoris who died during or after surgical procedures,[214] the serum lipoprotein pattern was unknown in 22 patients. Of these six had type II, one had type III and one had type IV hyperlipoproteinemia. This is an unduly high incidence of hyperlipidemia, especially of type II even though the numbers are small. Since FH leads to stenoses of the coronary arteries and their ostia,[114,115] the mean cholesterol levels of a study group (due to the bias resulting from the unduly high representation of FH) will be higher than in an unaffected group matched for age and sex. Such bias could have affected many epidemiological studies in the past. All patients with hyperlipoproteinemia affecting the coronary arteries should be treated as separate entities.

Carlson[215] reported a lipid or carbohydrate metabolic disorder in 81% of subjects with clinical cardiovascular disease, indicating the nonspecificity of metabolic aggravation of atherosclerosis per se or of the effects of its complications. Yet there was no correlation between the serum cholesterol in 1700 surgically treated patients with PVD or aneurysms, nor was there correlation between the serum cholesterol level and the nature and extent of the atherosclerotic lesions.[214] This indicates the need to carefully study the incidence of metabolic disorders in the base population to avoid selection bias.

Plasma cholesterol levels of 280 mg/dL for both sexes at ages under 25 years, and 320 mg/dL for men and 330 mg/dL for women over 44 years were considered suitable values from which to discriminate between normalcy or health and FH by Epstein et al.[181] There is some overlap in the highest quintile since some heterozygotes for FH have values lower than the majority of those similarly affected.

In a comparison of plasma cholesterol levels of men 30 to 62 years of age in the Framingham study with those of 68 men with FH displaying xanthomatosis there was little overlap in cholesterol levels.[168] Most subjects with FH had distinctly higher cholesterol levels suggesting that only very high levels are indicative of an underlying disease but some mild cases no doubt exist or may represent a separate disease entity.

It would be wrong to regard atherosclerosis as a disorder of lipid metabolism because of the ubiquity of the disease in man, the widespread distribution in the animal kingdom and reproduction of the disease in lower animals and in man without dietary manipulation.[116,117] It would seem that a characteristic of populations of more affluent countries is to have on average a higher plasma cholesterol level than those from less developed areas. When comparisons are made with third world populations including African tribesmen it is well to remember that the variables in the populations are multiple, one is diet and another is the state of nutrition and health. Differences in body mass, longevity, indigenous diseases, immune state, lifestyle and socio-economic stresses must be considered. The basic mechanisms responsible for blood cholesterol levels remain unknown but both cholesterol and LDL levels are primarily determined by genetics. Higher cholesterol levels in the affluent populations may be indicative of better nutrition, health, immunity and longevity rather than the severity of atherosclerosis or the risk of CHD. The possibility that blood cholesterol levels may be influenced by severe ulcerative atherosclerosis has not been excluded[132] and the most desirable blood level has yet to be determined but it cannot be ascertained by the use of inappropriate epidemiological methodology. Currently there is no scientific reason for altering the conventional statistical methods of determining the cholesterol discrimination values.

Other genetic metabolic disorders that either aggravate atherosclerosis or directly induce CHD by virtue of storage of metabolites including FDB should be excluded from both epidemiological and pathological investigations. Results from investigations involving a mixture of diseases are not applicable to the individual diseases and can give false results. There could well be other yet to be discovered metabolic diseases that will warrant consideration in the same light. An analogous situation would be seen in the use of aortic aneurysms as a surrogate of atherosclerosis. In such studies all nonatherosclerotic diseases would be treated separately according to the specific diseases responsible for the aneurysms but to include genetically determined connective tissue diseases with a propensity for aneurysms would be unwise but analogous to including FH in studies of CHD.

THE RELATIONSHIP OF PLASMA CHOLESTEROL TO CHD

In view of (i) the misrepresentation of the vascular pathology of FH and dietary-induced hypercholesterolemia in lower animals, (ii) the invalid inclusion of FH in epidemiological studies of CHD, (iii) the fallacious and unscientific nature of monocausal national mortality rates for CHD, (iv) the substantial, indeterminate and fluctuating diagnostic error for CHD clinically and (v) the use of a nonrepresentative minority of subjects with CHD by virtue of selection by age, any conclusions regarding the relationship of plasma cholesterol to CHD are precluded.

Reference to Figure 5.2 showing the age changes in serum cholesterol levels in the population should be contrasted with the mortality from CHD in the USA and UK (Fig. 1.1 and 1.2). When the CHD mortality is increasing exponentially the blood cholesterol level in the males declines and the mortality for females does not parallel their blood cholesterol levels. To confine CHD studies for the most part to those under 55 and then to extrapolate to the entire population is conjecture and not science.

The Working Group on Arteriosclerosis of the National Institutes of Health (NIH)[7,8] in 1981 concluded that in epidemiological studies of large national or regional population groups there was generally (but not invariably) a correlation between dietary cholesterol and both the concentration of serum cholesterol and the morbidity and mortality rates for CHD but conceded it "has not been possible to show an unequivocal association between the ingestion of dietary cholesterol and either the concentration of serum cholesterol or the incidence and prevalence of atherosclerotic disease through surveys of individuals within population groups." The current hypothesis of a positive correlation between blood cholesterol levels and CHD incidence is invalidated by this absence of a correlation at the individual level. The NIH Working Group acknowledged individual and daily variation in the concentration of serum

cholesterol levels amongst individuals on the same diet and admitted to substantial error in dietary assessments. The probability is that the associations reveal only characteristics of the population under study. The NIH Working Group on Arteriosclerosis[7,8] concluded that high-order intercorrelations among the dietary carbohydrate variables, along with dietary calories, total fat, saturated fats, cholesterol, proteins, and animal proteins, make it difficult to determine whether these suggested associations reflect a causal relation. Their very nonspecificity suggests otherwise.[4]

McGill's conclusions[74] were basically the same viz: (i) comparison of CHD among nations and large population groups with dietary cholesterol and egg consumption produced a weak or absent relationship when other interrelated variables were taken into account and (ii) the associations could not be considered evidence for a causal relationship. Kannel[152] in 1974 said that the serum cholesterol level was not the sole determinant of CHD and admitted finding difficulty in proving a causal relationship between cholesterol and CHD or atherosclerosis. He added that in free-living affluent populations there was no demonstrable difference in nutrient composition of the diet between those with and those without CHD and no correlation was found between the diet and serum cholesterol values on an individual basis. Eventually similar views were expressed by Olson[62] and the fact that the serum cholesterol level that has been regarded as a risk factor in the past varied from country to country detracts from its specificity and importance. Moreover there is no correlation between serum cholesterol levels and sudden death.[151,161] In 1988 in the Framingham Study the serum cholesterol level was most strongly related to CHD in men under 65 years, was less so with PVD and the relationship was weakest with atherothrombotic brain infarction in males and possibly significantly inversely related in women.[216] Such are the inconsistencies in the lipid hypothesis which displays overall weakness and not strength, yet the supporters still fail to review their stance.

The association demonstrated between CHD mortality rates and the sale of radio and television sets in England and Wales[60] usually meets with derision but the lesson to be learnt is that statistical correlations and parallel graphs, no matter how plausible they may seem or how conveniently consistent they may appear to be, do not establish a cause and effect relationship. It must not be assumed and requires proof by nonepidemiological means. Similar correlations have been demonstrated with protein, fat and carbohydrate intake, the educational standards, national per capita income, energy consumption, automobiles, socio-economic stress, radios, television and telephones.[111] Under the circumstances no importance can be attributed to the association which appears to be with national affluence and all that is entailed thereby. To continue to invoke the validity of the population correlation between dietary fat, serum cholesterol levels and CHD mortality in the absence of validity at the individual level within those populations is perpetuating an ecological fallacy and relying on fallacious vital statistics.

SERUM CHOLESTEROL LEVELS AND ATHEROSCLEROSIS

It has been alleged that virtually everyone accepts an association between cholesterol levels and atherosclerosis[217] and that a causal association between dietary fat, hypercholesterolemia and CHD is proven beyond all reasonable doubt.[218] Gotto[219] has alleged that every epidemiological study on hyperlipidemia has found that an elevation of serum cholesterol is a predictor of coronary artery disease (CAD). This carefully worded ambiguous statement encompasses subjects predominantly with FH but does not specify atherosclerosis. Since CAD is used synonymously in the literature with CHD and atherosclerosis and in western countries most epidemiological studies are conducted on middle aged men (under 55 years) when serum cholesterol levels, the incidence of CHD and the severity of atherosclerosis all increase with age, Gotto's statement is misleading. Moreover in this particular age group it has been demonstrated that blood cholesterol levels, body bulk or obesity and the incidence of diabetes mellitus and hypertension are each age and genetically dependent and have some inexplicable interrelationship but both CHD and atherosclerosis are also age dependent. Under such circumstances it is most unlikely that even sophisti-

cated statistics could separate the independent effect of blood cholesterol on the incidence of CHD.[220] Its effect on atherosclerosis, determined by the methodology used by CHD epidemiologists, would be even more unlikely if that is possible. Again these results are still confounded by the inclusion and selection bias for FH by virtue of the age group used. Dock[221] alleged that cholesterol is the cause of atherosclerosis just as the tubercle bacillus is the cause of tuberculosis and Roberts[222] now alleges there is only one risk factor, viz, a serum cholesterol level greater than 150mg/dL or more specifically an elevated serum LDL-cholesterol level.

The above statements are scientifically untenable. It is misrepresentation to classify cholesterol or LDL as noxious humoral agents. Animal fat and cholesterol are not the only dietary constituents that can affect blood cholesterol levels and the primary determinant of the cholesterol level in health within a population is probably genetic. The accumulation of fat and cholesterol in the vessel wall is ubiquitous in humans, commencing in infancy when blood levels are at their lowest and continuing after 50 to 55 years when blood levels are leveling off or declining. Lipid accumulates in the vessel walls at low levels in humans and in herbivores preferentially at sites of augmented hemodynamic stress. The false relationship of serum cholesterol levels to atherosclerosis that has been promulgated has been greatly influenced by the alleged support provided by FH and cholesterol overfed animals. In a number of autopsy studies in which an attempt has been made to correlate the dietary intake of animal fat, blood cholesterol levels and atherosclerosis severity the correlation coefficients have been zero or weak and probably not of biological significance.[223] Scrimshaw and Guzmán[30] reported a near zero correlation between atherosclerosis and animal fat intake (0.07) and blood cholesterol levels and animal fat intake (0.07) in 31,000 autopsies from 15 different countries (International Atherosclerosis Project). The relationship between raised lesions and animal fat consumption was actually negative (-0.17)[223] As Smith[223] has documented, these results have unfortunately been repeatedly misrepresented in the literature by the lipid protagonists. The blood cholesterol levels were not measured on the same subjects and whilst attempts were made to standardize the assessment of severity by the use of pictorial standards, inevitably in such a massive undertaking standards of performance would vary. It is inappropriate however to claim a causal relationship between dietary intake of fat and atherosclerosis on weak ecological correlations especially since the results are confounded by the inclusion of subjects with familial hypercholesterolemia. Correlations in pathology are no more causal than they are in epidemiology.

In the Honolulu Heart Program the correlation coefficient between total cholesterol and atherosclerosis severity was low and even lower and not significant for the correlation with LDL, with an almost zero correlation for HDL (-0.09).[224] In the most recent report from the Pathological Determinants of Atherosclerosis in the Youth Research Group, Wissler[225] declared that the serum lipoprotein cholesterol concentrations were strongly "additive" as important determinants of the early stages of atherosclerosis in adolescents and young adult males who were victims of violent deaths. The assessment methods were dependent on the percentage area of involvement using lipid-stained gross specimens which is a poor technique for assessing atherosclerosis severity because the emphasis is on the lipid ("athero") and it ignores the sclerotic element which has limited permeability to lipid stains. Nevertheless in the more detailed report[226] although total cholesterol levels were performed they did not report either correlation coefficients for total cholesterol, LDL or LDL cholesterol suggesting that no correlations were found. They reported only combined VLDL + LDL cholesterol values (0.24 and 0.16) for the total area involved and for raised lesions of the right coronary artery respectively. The values for the abdominal and thoracic aortas were equally unimpressive. The values for HDL cholesterol for the area involved of thoracic and abdominal segments of the aorta were 0.15 and 0.14 respectively and for raised lesions and the right coronary were all close to zero (varying from 0.01 to 0.06). Since subjects with FH or FDB were not specifically excluded from these studies the results support the conclusion that there is no pathological support for a biologically significant or causal relationship between serum cholesterol levels and atherosclerosis (excluding all subjects with lipid dystrophies). It is curious that now Wissler[225] is alleging that the lipid accumulation in the arterial wall is the result of intimal binding or trapping of combined LDL and VLDL associated with the metabolic failure of intimal cells to digest and excrete the excessive amounts of these cholesterol-containing lipoproteins associated with hyperliproteinemia. This is an example of assumed causality and ignores the fact that lipid can accumulate in blood vessel walls at very low blood cholesterol levels that could not remotely be regarded as hyperliproteinemia.[116,117]

In any case it is difficult to reconcile a primary causative role for serum cholesterol in view of the many inconsistencies with the pathological and experimental evidence (Chapter 2). Yet a low plasma cholesterol level does not indicate freedom from atherosclerosis or from the likelihood of developing CHD. The many inconsistencies and contradictions in the relationship of serum cholesterol to CHD and atherosclerosis have been indicated and are extensively documented by Smith[223] but rather than reviewing the premises on which the lipid hypothesis rests, epidemiologists have ignored them or rationalized by invoking a multicausal etiology, methodological differences or unknown risk factors.

Though an elevated serum cholesterol level is not causal, the possibility that it may aggravate atherosclerosis cannot be denied. In hypercholesterolemic rabbits, trauma localizes lipid deposition at least temporarily. In experimental hemodynamically induced atherosclerosis in the veins of arteriovenous shunts and in venous pouch aneurysms of rabbits, superimposing dietary induced atherosclerosis leads to preferential lipid deposition in those vessels, more so than in the afferent artery of the arteriovenous shunt or the traumatized control artery. The affected vessel walls, as explained (Chapter 2), manifest pronounced foam cell infiltration rather than accelerating the pathogenesis of atherosclerosis and there appears to be no propensity for lipid deposition in the atrophic lesions of atherosclerosis. In humans hypercholsterolemia (such as FH, FDB and hypercholsterolemia type III) superimposes fat storage on the conventional proliferative lesions of atherosclerosis. A high fat diet in untreated diabetes results in xanthomatous infiltration similar to FH (Chapter 2) and in a limited study intimal proliferation of some arterial forks in FH did not exhibit a propensity for lipid deposition as occurs readily in the rabbit.[115] At present there is no evidence that FH aggravates the effects of naturally occurring atherosclerosis or enhances the advanced proliferative lesions of bypass grafts and the veins of therapeutic arteriovenous fistulas. Though significant reduction of serum cholesterol levels might reduce the lipid storage in the affected vessel wall of subjects with FH thereby giving the impression angiographically that regression of the vascular pathological lesions was occurring, at present there is no convincing evidence that a cholesterol-lowering diet has significant effect on lipid depletion from atherosclerotic arteries in normolipidemic humans.

COMMENTARY ON CHOLESTEROL

Cholesterol could one day be recognized as the most important steroid in human biology. Cholesterol is no more noxious than oxygen, calcium or hemosiderin. To refer to good cholesterol (HDL) and bad cholesterol (LDL) is unscientific. Use of such terminology to lead the public into accepting a contentious and unproven hypothesis is reprehensible. Promulgation of such concepts in the public arena when there is intense public interest in food and health has led to confusion and an undeserved phobia of cholesterol and in the long-term leads medicine into disrepute.

CHD is most prevalent in the more prosperous, better-fed and long-living communities. Yet, within those communities it is most prevalent in the lowest socio-economic group. The western diet had led to an increase in height and weight and a much reduced infant mortality.[211] Rising affluence is associated with increased longevity and greater resistance to infectious diseases. Caution is needed before instituting alterations to the human diet and it is inadvisable to institute changes on the basis of a controversial and unproven hypothesis. There is evidence that even moderate dietary-induced hypocholesterolemia in young children is potentially hazardous to brain and body development and may endanger the cholesterol

degradative mechanism.[211] What the serum cholesterol level should be for optimal physiological function at any age is unknown.

It must be concluded that in inherited metabolic disorders in man and several lower species, the grossly elevated blood cholesterol or LDL levels may induce metabolic storage phenomena in the blood vessels, cardiac valves and extravascular tissues but in normolipidemic subjects there is no scientific evidence that cholesterol or LDL is noxious at all blood levels nor that they cause atherosclerosis. In effect there should be no cholesterol controversy.

HIGH-DENSITY LIPOPROTEIN (HDL)

High-density lipoprotein (HDL) contains only 20 to 25% of the cholesterol in the plasma, and problems with inaccuracies in its measurement are greater than with total plasma cholesterol the intraindividual variability over time having been shown to vary[173] by as much as 12.4%. It contains the highest protein concentration (approximately 50%) and has been divided into three subfractions based on ultracentrifugal behavior. HDL_1 the least dense, is a minor component and HDL_3 is the form in which HDL is released from the liver following synthesis. HDL_2 results from an increase in cholesterol ester content due to the transfer of fatty acid (mainly linoleic acid) from lecithin to free cholesterol by the enzyme activity of lecithin-cholesterol acyl transferase (LCAT) in the plasma. The free cholesterol is partly derived from HDL_3 and partly from other plasma sources. HDL is thought to be concerned with the removal of cholesterol from the body by mobilizing cholesterol from the tissues and transferring it to the liver where it is partly converted to bile acids and salts and also contributes apoprotein C and cholesterol esters to the synthesis of VLDL.

In the plasma it tends to have an inverse relationship to plasma LDL levels. When HDL is high, the LDL level is low and vice versa. As a consequence it has been alleged that an elevated HDL level is beneficial and actively retards the progression of atherosclerosis by efficiently removing cholesterol from the blood and thus reducing its deposition in the arterial wall.[227] A low serum level is regarded as deleterious and atherogenic with the subjects assumed to be at enhanced risk of developing CHD. This hypothesis suffers from the basic defects of the lipid hypothesis and is essentially dependent on circumstantial evidence using LDL blood levels as a substitute for the severity of atherosclerosis a maneuver called the "substitution game".

This is not to deny the importance of HDL in the removal and transport of unwanted cholesterol for excretion but there is no direct evidence that high blood levels directly impede atherogenesis. The hypothesis presupposes that lipid accumulation is the crucial pathological change in atherogenesis when it is only one of many, although from the commercials and documentaries consequent upon the anti-cholesterol campaign, this is the impression presented to the public. It is currently commercially advantageous to do so.

The purpose and effects of high and low blood levels of HDL are unknown. Kannel et al[141] considered HDL the single most powerful predictor of risk over the age of 50 years yet in British men HDL does not appear to be a significant risk factor.[228] Whilst total serum cholesterol and LDL usually vary inversely with that of HDL, there are exceptions[229] and Oliver[151] considered there was no correlation within a given community between HDL cholesterol and total serum cholesterol or LDL. In one dietary study in North Karelia (Finland)[230] the three values diminished whilst the middle aged men were on the diet with reversal of the effect when the participants returned to their original diets. In underdeveloped communities low serum cholesterol and HDL are compatible with a low incidence of CHD.[151]

Holme et al[231] reported that in 129 autopsies the HDL/cholesterol ratio correlated with raised coronary artery lesions but the absolute value for blood HDL had a weak association whereas blood pressure and blood cholesterol had stronger associations. In an angiographic study of coronary arteries, men with high coronary artery scores tended to have low plasma HDL especially HDL_2 cholesterol which did not correlate with the size of the lesions or the number of complete and partial stenoses.[232] Nor was there any correlation with plasma apolipoproteins A-1, A-2 and E. However the numbers in these two series were small.

Kannel et al[141] consider the value of the HDL level is mostly in those over 50 years of age with the importance in younger subjects yet to be determined. In Tangier disease where there is little HDL in the blood, premature severe CHD might be expected to be prevalent but this is not so.[233,234] These subjects frequently survive to middle-age without obvious large vessel disease or obvious lipid storage in the vessels. The blood LDL level is also low and the relative absence of HDL suggests only a circumstantial association of low serum HDL. Other mechanisms seem to be responsible for the premature development of severe atherosclerosis.

Until more is known of HDL in cholesterol metabolism, in the absence of finite evidence of a role in atherosclerosis and in view of inconsistencies in the relationship of HDL to CHD[235] and the inability to extrapolate from CHD to atherosclerosis, no scientific conclusion can be reached regarding its role in atherogenesis.

LIPOPROTEIN (A) [LP(A)]

Lipoprotein (a) [Lp(a)] refers to a family of lipoprotein particles that are closely related to or variants of LDL. They are highly polymorphic with considerable variation in molecular weight and LDL and Lp(a) are similar in lipid composition. The protein moiety of apolipoprotein-B100 in Lp(a) is linked by disulphide bonds to one or two molecules of the glycoprotein apolipoprotein (a) [apo(a)] that has extensive homology with the fibrinolytic zymogen plasminogen. The latter contains a domain homologous to the family of serine proteinases. The amino terminal contains a series of five disulphide-stabilized loop-like structures called kringles. The apo(a) subunit contains up to 37 copies of a kringle homologous to kringle-4 of plasminogen, a single copy of a kringle homologous to kringle-5 of plasminogen, and a region homologous to the catalytic domain at the carboxyl terminal of plasminogen.[236] This similarity suggests that apo(a) may be involved in fibrinolysis and that elevated blood levels may suppress normal fibrinolytic activity and thus enhance thrombosis. The apo(a) subunit however cannot be activated by tissue plasminogen activator a urokinase due to the replacement of arginine by serine (site 560 in plasminogen).[237]

Lp(a) appears to be synthesized in the liver,

secreted directly into the blood and catabolized by the LDL-receptor pathway. Plasma levels are under strong genetic control. Chemical treatment can remove apo(a), leaving a particle that looks and behaves like LDL.

Whilst it is ubiquitous in humans, except possibly for those with abetalipoproteinemia, plasma levels of lp(a) vary widely among individuals in the order of thousand-fold despite relatively little intraindividual variation. African Americans tend to have higher blood levels and there is a high degree of inheritance with a Mendelian mode of transmission. Plasma Lp(a) levels appear unrelated to those of other lipoproteins and apolipoproteins.[237] The various isoforms of Lp(a) complicate the evidence currently available.

Diet appears to have no effect on the levels of Lp(a) and this is true for hypolipidemic drugs such as cholestyramine. Its physiological role in lipid metabolism is unknown but it has been linked with atherogenesis predominantly epidemiologically.

Currently it appears that Lp(a) competes with plasminogen for various vascular binding sites and inhibits plasmin generation by several plasminogen activators in vitro but it is unknown whether it has any effect on the fibrinolytic system in vivo. It has been thought that high plasma levels of Lp(a) suppress the fibrinolytic system and secondarily facilitate enlargement of the mural thrombus which might then become occlusive but without any direct effect on atherogenesis or the development of the intimal tear.

The blood level of Lp(a) is low in those with liver disease and alcoholics but is within the normal range in the one subject with abetalipoproteinemia so far examined.[238]

Elevated plasma levels occur in diabetes mellitus and chronic renal disease but any alleged effect on atherogenesis would need to be carefully investigated by virtue of the independent metabolic defects in diabetics and the frequency of hypertension in both disorders. Even so any independent role of Lp(a) in the disorders would be one of aggravation rather than cause in its strictly logical sense.

Since Lp(a) binds with endothelial cells, it has been suggested that Lp(a) may help promote healing by providing a source of cholesterol for endothelial cell membrane synthesis in vascular injuries.[239] Be this as it may, until the physiological roles of these lipoprotein particles (and the isoforms) are established it is inappropriate to speculate about a possible role in healing or atherosclerosis.

It has been suggested that almost one-quarter of heart attacks in men younger than 60 years occurs in those who have inherited high blood levels of Lp(a) and that most of the genetic component of CHD not attributable to other risk factors, rests with levels of Lp(a).[239] Lp(a) is currently regarded as atherogenic and its relationship to CHD is based predominantly on epidemiological evidence.[240] It has been suggested that it may promote atherogenesis by preventing the normal uptake of apo B_{100}-containing particles by the LDL (apo B,C) receptor. Its plasma concentration is considered to correlate well with clinical CHD and angiographically documented CHD, cerebrovascular atherosclerosis and saphenous vein graft stenosis. The limitations of these techniques notwithstanding, a cause and effect relationship cannot be assumed between Lp(a) blood levels and atherosclerosis.[241]

Lp(a) has been demonstrated in atherosclerotic plaques immunohistochemically in the human aorta and in coronary venous bypass grafts but the nature of its involvement is unknown. It may be an innocent bystander or be incorporated into the wall with other plasma constituents by virtue of the increased endothelial permeability or mural disruption. In subjects with elevated plasma LDL levels the cardiovascular risk of elevated Lp(a) concentration is thought to be significantly increased.

Lp(a) plasma levels are greatly increased in heterozygotes with FH but this may be due to deficiency of or defective LDL receptors which normally catabolize Lp(a). As with LDL, lipid storage may occur within the vessel wall if there is an interruption in the normal metabolic pathway with diminished catabolism and increased blood levels as a consequence.

In dietary-induced hypercholesterolemia in transgenic mice expressing high levels of apo(a), the development of lipid-staining lesions in the aorta was accentuated and the lesions also contained apo(a).[242] Transgenic mice on a normal diet apparently did not exhibit lipid deposition. The apo(a) increased the blood cholesterol levels but had no effect on HDL.

Most of the evidence that serum Lp(a) is related to CHD is based on case control studies with myocardial infarction rather than prospective studies.[238] There are however difficulties with blood level measurements and the skewed distribution in the general population creates the problem of which estimates of the mean to use and many studies have compared the proportion of people above and below some arbitrary Lp(a) level. This is a major problem in view of the extraordinarily wide range of blood levels and the optimum level is unknown.

A study of blood Lp(a) levels in 103 untreated hypercholesterolemic normotensive middle-aged males showed a correlation with carotid but not with aortic or femoral plaques.[243] This cannot be regarded as evidence although it was concluded that early atherosclerosis was influenced by serum Lp(a). The numbers were too few and the assumed causality typical of many clinical studies in this field.

Armstrong et al[244] found that the risk associated with Lp(a) was dependent on the prevailing serum LDL cholesterol level. Mbetu and Durrington[238] considered Lp(a) to be less discriminating than apo B or A-1 but such studies suffer from the defects in the epidemiological methodology as explained in Chapters 3 and 4, and also assume a causal relationship without ever demonstrating the direct effect of Lp(a) on atherogenesis.

The risk associated with Lp(a) appears greatest in subjects with FH, since elevation of LDL and Lp(a) both occur secondarily to either defective or a deficiency of LDL receptors. According to Mbetu & Durrington[238] the risk in FH is greater than for polygenic hypercholesterolemia for a given blood LDL level and this may be because Lp(a) is also elevated in FH or high Lp(a) blood levels may potentiate the effect of FH on the vessel wall at least in some heterozygotes[237] as it augments lipid deposition in the dietary-induced hypercholesterolemic monkey and transgenic mice[242] expressing human apo(a). Mbetu and Durrington[238] believe elevated blood levels of Lp(a) have an independent risk for CHD and as explained above this may not be due to its effect on atherosclerosis but to enhancing the development of the mural thrombus secondary to intimal disruption. There is no evidence as yet that elevated Lp(a) is associated with its increased deposition in the vessel wall. Nevertheless, abnormal blood levels may aggravate the atherogenesis independently of other factors.

In our present state of knowledge it must be concluded that Lp(a) cannot cause atherosclerosis which occurs at all blood levels of Lp(a) and also in lower animals that do not have Lp(a) at all in their blood. Nor does Lp(a) explain the initiation and pathogenesis of the disease nor its topography and complications. Its function is unknown and yet blood levels believed to be elevated have been incriminated as atherogenic without a cause and effect relationship being demonstrated. Blood levels in African Americans are higher than those of white Americans yet without increased CHD.[245] Whether its presence in atherosclerosis or in assumed high blood levels has a direct effect on the pathogenesis of atherosclerosis is unknown. The potentiating effect of apo(a) in hypercholesterolemic transgenic mice[242] has no direct bearing on atherogenesis. In abnormalities of Lp(a) metabolism an effect on atherosclerosis may occur but it is not causal.

LIPOPROTEIN X

Lipoprotein X is observed only in subjects with obstructive jaundice and in those with a deficiency of the plasma enzyme lecithin-cholesterol acyl transferase (LCAT).[246] Apo F and Apo G are believed to be minor immunologically distinct apolipoprotein components of HDL.[247]

TRIGLYCERIDES

There has been much controversy over the effect blood triglycerides have on atherosclerosis and CHD. The blood triglyceride level exhibits a diurnal variation of up to 30% indicating the need for repeated estimations but also raises doubt about the reliability of any relationship to CHD. Although triglycerides and cholesterol are closely associated through mutual lipoprotein carriers, the evidence incriminating plasma triglycerides as an independent "risk factor" is surprisingly weak. In clinical practice hypertriglyceridemia is mostly secondary to a variety of disorders such as obesity, alcoholism, certain drugs, diabetes mellitus, chronic renal disease, liver disease occasionally metabolic and endocrine disorders. Some of these are also associated with severe atherosclerosis or secondarily due to the associated hypertension. Certainly there is little support for treating or attempting to reduce plasma triglyceride levels although obviously the primary disorders with which this finding is associated require attention.

Brunzell et al[248] reported CHD in adults with familial hypertriglyceridemia under the age of 40 to 50 years. In subjects with familial hypertriglyceridemia in whom the blood level is grossly elevated, lipid storage in the arterial wall may be augmented. This does not relate to atherogenesis although theoretically lipid storage may have a propensity for atherosclerosis just as dietary-induced hypercholesterolemia has a propensity for lipid deposition in hemodynamically induced atherosclerosis in the rabbit.[249,250] At present the histological features of blood vessels from such patients are unknown and it is generally acknowledged that there is no benefit to be derived in reducing elevated blood triglyceride levels.

APOLIPOPROTEIN E

In humans, the structural gene locus for plasma apolipoprotein E (apo E) is polymorphic, there being three common alleles with three major apo E isoforms in the plasma (apo E4, apo E3 and apo E2). Apo E is important in modulating the metabolism of apo B-containing lipoproteins linked with atherosclerosis[251] and therefore affects the LDL levels in the blood but apo E2 is alleged to be protective. Involvement of these apolipoproteins in CHD epidemiology is open to the basic criticisms of using CHD as a surrogate without direct incrimination in atherogenesis or demonstrated affect on the severity of atherosclerosis. Obviously it cannot be denied that the various isoforms of the apolipoproteins each may have a varying effect on atherogenesis, probably with the effects modified by many other blood constituents. However the important conclusion that must be reached in our present limited state of knowledge, is that the various apo E phenotypes are not causal in atherosclerosis though they may play important roles in the pathogenesis. Some mutants are associated with several dyslipidemic individuals but such disorders are distinct from atherosclerosis.

LDL (OXIDATIVE MODIFICATION)

Spontaneous autoxidation products of cholesterol have been considered to aggravate the vascular effects of cholesterol overfeeding of rabbits and angiotoxicity of oxygenated sterols has been considered to play a possible role in atherogenesis.[252] Many investigators have been quick to incriminate them in atherogenesis. Oxygenated sterols have also been implicated as inhibitors of cholesterol biosynthesis and as regulators of sterol metabolism.[252] Not all oxygenated sterols are angiotoxic. Purified cholesterol has been shown to have no cytotoxicity and minimal inhibition of cholesterol biosynthesis.[253]

There has been progressive interest in the possible effects of oxidized LDL of which modifications are immunogenic and as a consequence autoantibodies to such products have been found in the serum and atheromatous tissue.[254]

When the cell cholesterol level is increased, the activity of LDL receptors is decreased and this has led to the belief that some other mechanism accounts for the cholesterol and lipid accumulation in the cells of the blood vessel wall such as monocytes. Recent evidence[255,256] has fostered the belief that oxygenated modification of LDL may lead to its unregulated uptake by macrophages through a specific receptor in the acetyl LDL or scavenger receptor.[255] This concept is based on the belief that intimal retention by phagocytosis in the intima of LDL with its incorporated cholesterol percolating through the vessel wall plays a primary role in atherogenesis and the progressive accumulation of cell debris with its known affinity for lipid not only precedes lipid accumulation but has been completely ignored by lipid protagonists. Witztum[257] believes that oxidative modification of LDL in the vessel wall may be responsible for the chemotaxis of monocytes and may be a prerequisite for LDL uptake and accumulation of cellular cholesteryl ester in the intima. Intervention studies in the LDL receptor deficient Watanabe hereditary hypercholesterolemic (WHHL) rabbit, using probucol as an antioxidant, have reduced the lipid uptake and development of the foam cell lesion. Rather than having an effect on atherosclerosis, these experiments only reveal effects on macrophagic uptake of modified LDL in a lipid storage disease. The assumption in this hypothesis is that foam cells are deleterious whereas the correct approach is to seek the basic reason for their presence in atherosclerosis. A more plausible explanation is that monocytes enter the intima to phagocytose the cell debris (matrix vesicles) which has an affinity for lipid. Since the matrix vesicles progressively accumulate in abundance there seems to be little value in inhibiting their phagocytosis which in effect equates with inhibiting or at least delaying attempts at clearance of the cell debris.

For the most part the mechanisms involved in the study of oxygenated sterols are dependent on tissue culture rather than in vivo and in view of the essential role of LDL for all cells, it is unlikely that such an uncontrolled mechanism would occur only in vivo in arteries at specific sites and not in other tissues as well. Allegations have been made that oxidation modification of LDL may play a significant role in progression of coronary atherosclerosis in a limited number of middle aged males[254,258] but the incidence of FH in the cohorts is unknown and associations do not prove causality. The possibility remains that LDL modification may be the consequence of the atherosclerotic process or that it occurs in the abundant matrix vesicles and cell debris in atherosclerosis. The half life and effective concentration of these oxidation products are unknown and to suggest that they play a dominant pathogenic role in atherogenesis is speculative and overlooks the protective role of the immune system and also the antioxidant defense system[259] involving thiols, carotenoids, tocopherols and vitamin C. It remains to be proven that the sterol oxidation products play a significant and specific role in atherogenesis for their presence is suspected in other tissues and in blood vessels throughout the body.

Intermediate Density Lipoproteins (IDL)

After a meal chylomicra are released from the gut and very low density lipoproteins (VLDL) from the liver. In the process of lipolysis of chylomicra and VLDL, so-called remnant lipoproteins or intermediate density lipoproteins (IDL) are formed due to inadequate lipolysis or abnormalities in the metabolism of remnant lipoproteins. Epidemiological studies have provided some indication that blood IDL levels are high in hypercholesterolemia and also in CHD subjects[260] but such studies suffer from the same deficiencies as using serum cholesterol, LDL and CHD as surrogates of atherosclerosis. It is most unlikely that IDL is involved in the etiology of atherosclerosis as Slyper[260] has assumed on the fallacious epidemiological methodology.

DIETARY FATTY ACIDS

Fatty acids in the diet are ingested mostly in the form of triglycerides which are partially hydrolyzed by pancreatic lipase. The resulting fatty acids and 2-monoglycerides are absorbed by the intestinal epithelium where they are resynthesized into triglycerides. Fatty acids in phospholipids or cholesteryl esters traverse a similar pathway and are used for lipid synthesis by the mucosal cells, and incorporated into chylomicrons which are very rich in triglycerides. Many of these triglycerides are hydrolyzed by circulating lipoprotein lipase and released fatty acids pass into the tissues to be used directly as a source of energy or stored as triglycerides.

Medium-chain fatty acids from dietary triglycerides are released into the portal blood and are transported as free fatty acids to the liver where they are oxidized as a source of energy or used to synthesize palmitic acid which is the principal saturated fatty acid in humans. Fatty acids can also be synthesized from glucose. These saturated fatty acids can be desaturated to form monounsaturated fatty acids which have been regarded as "neutral" in their effect on plasma cholesterol in dietary experiments. Thus it was concluded that they are less harmful than saturated fatty acids. This is another example of the substitution of serum cholesterol for atherosclerosis with the implicit assumption that monounsaturated fatty acids would have a similar effect.

Polyunsaturated fatty acids are derived from the diet and cannot be synthesized by humans but after absorption they can be elongated or desaturated by the tissues as required. The two main types of polyunsaturated fatty acids are the N-6 class including linoleic acid derived primarily from plant oils (corn, safflower, soybean and sunflower oil) and the second class, N-3 fatty acids, includes linolenic acid derived from plants and the long-chain fatty acids primarily from fish oils. The two classes cannot be connected one to the other and both are essential dietary components. Fatty acids serve as a source of energy and have many specialized functions according to cell and tissue type. In the liver they are used to produce the lipoprotein VLDL to transport fatty acids in the form of triglyceride for storage in adipose tissue.

Ingested fatty acids, saturated and unsaturated, are absorbed and incorporated into the body's fat depots, which can be sampled to determine the nature of the food intake. There appears to be some preference for saturated fatty acids even though some unsaturated fatty acids are essential and cannot be synthesized by the body. Humans are able to synthesize saturated fatty acids when fed a fat-free meal and saturated fatty acids are preferred in the absorption of dietary fat, deposition of adipose fat and anabolism of endogenous triglycerides. Moreover triglycerides of chylomicra are more saturated than those consumed if dietary fat is highly unsaturated. In view of this preferential usage it is unlikely that saturated fats are detrimental.

In the evolutionary process there has been a progressive decline in the number of fatty acids in depot fat culminating in predominance of oleic, palmitic, linoleic and stearic acids in higher land animals. Other trends have been towards mixed glycerides, i.e., containing two or three different fatty acids per molecule, a higher degree of saturation and the main acids being (monounsaturated) oleic and (saturated) palmitic acids.[261] Phylogenetic influences seem to be the most important determinant of the fatty acid composition of adipose tissue in the various species and there appears to be active regulation of the triglyceride composition in the tissue itself.[261] There is no significant difference in sampling site or with age and sex. The fatty acids usually comprise more than 90% of the total mixture given by Jeanrenaud[261] as follows: myristic (2.4%), palmitic (24.6%), palmitoleic (5.6%), stearic (6.0%), oleic (49.9%) and linoleic (9.5%) but the fatty acid composition tends to reflect to some degree the dietary intake particularly if weight gain is rapid. Weight reduction is not associated with any

discrimination for loss or retention of fatty acid types.[262]

TRANS FATTY ACIDS

Margarines and shortenings are the products of modern technology based on chemical and physicochemical reactions which modify the chemical composition of the parent fats and oils. This introduces into the human diet fatty acids not found in naturally occurring untreated vegetable oils. These new fatty acids have the same carbon-chain length and the same number of double bonds as the natural compounds. They are positional isomers when the double bonds are at different locations on the fatty acid chain and geometrical isomers when the molecule has the *trans* configuration around the double bonds.[97]

The physical and chemical properties of shortenings and margarines largely depend on the degree of hydrogenation of the vegetable oils which are high in unsaturated fatty acids. Partial hydrogenation reduces the degree of unsaturation of vegetable oils and gives them physical and chemical properties more acceptable to the food industry and for baking in particular. Thus the three major unsaturated fatty acids (linoleic, linolenic and oleic acids) are drastically changed with the production of many new chemical isomers, the properties of which are still unknown but potentially hazardous in the long-term such that the oblivious general public is participating in an uncontrolled long-term experiment.

The digestion, absorption, transport and catabolism of fatty acids containing *trans* unsaturation differ little from the *cis* counterparts, but because of differences in molecular shape and some physicochemical properties, it has been suggested they should be treated in much the same manner as saturated fatty acids.[263] The hypercholesterolemic effect is variable but even when positive it is apparently of shorter duration. The effect on blood cholesterol or LDL is not of paramount importance but the direct or indirect effect on atherogenesis is unknown. The effect of possible changes on cellular metabolism and cell membrane function is also unknown and the possibility remains that the *trans* fatty acids may have a much more indirect metabolic effect that could hinder the resilience of the arterial wall and its reparative capacity.

The nature and quantity of these *trans* isomers are unpredictable and again unknown. The high content of *trans* isomers in margarine, shortening and salad oils produced commercially and consumed in our diets is of concern. Whereas polyunsaturated fatty acids consumed by cattle are biohydrogenated, thereby increasing the degree of saturation, milk, butterfat and meat as a result contain hydrogenated saturated fatty acids and monounsaturated fatty acids. The low *trans* fatty acid content of butterfat and ruminant body fat has been recognized for some time. The suggestion is that they are probably more natural foods for humans than artificially manufactured *trans* fatty acids, the physiological or pathological effects of which in the long-term cannot be deduced.

Up to 12 g *per capita* of *trans* fatty acids are consumed in the USA per day[264] and the level may be as high as 27.6 g. Of this 95.2% comes from partially hydrogenated vegetable oils and only 4.8% from animal fat.[97,265] There is also a considerable intake when prepackaged crispy and tasty tidbits are consumed. Unfortunately these *trans* fatty acids are often included in the category of saturated fatty acids for the purposes of nutrition statistics, and nutrition labeling and mislabeling is frequent.[265] There is evidence that *trans* fatty acids are metabolized much more slowly and less effectively than the *cis* isomers. In experimental animals, the fetus contains very little *trans* fatty acid either due to the placental barrier or preferential use but the *trans* isomers are transferred to the milk. The concentrations of *trans* isomers are always lower in the brain than in other organs. Their possible effects on the human physiology are unknown but they could affect plasma membrane fragility and physiology and cell function throughout the body. The preference for *cis* isomers in natural synthesis of fatty acids and of the brain suggests that the *trans* fatty acids may be detrimental but suggested links have been made between both cancer and hypercholesterolemia.[97] The evidence is that *trans* fatty acids elevate serum LDL levels and lower HDL cholesterol[266] and yet current dietary recommendations frequently advocate the use of margarine rather than butter.

It is well-established that certain polyunsaturated fatty acids (linoleic and linolenic acids) are essential and cannot be synthesized in the body. Deficiency of these acids is associated with the well authenticated essential fatty acid deficiency syndrome and inadequate intake has been suggested as an aggravating factor in atherogenesis[267] which cannot explain the characteristic features of the pathology of the disease. It has never been adequately investigated as a possible aggravating factor. Whether or not essential fatty acid deficiency interferes with cholesterol transport is also unknown. Deficiency increases capillary fragility and whether this applies to larger blood vessels is not known but change in plasma membrane properties may result in increased matrix vesicle production. It is a serious matter that some margarines contain up to 23% of the total fatty acid in the *trans* configuration of these essential fatty acids which do not act as essential fatty acids and cannot treat essential fatty acid deficiency. Evidence suggests they may have an aggravating effect. The term physiologically active polyunsaturated fatty acids has been introduced.

The C18 fatty acids are necessary for the synthesis of prostaglandins, thromboxanes and leukatrienes, but the effect the *trans* isomers of these essential fatty acids have on the health of the population is unknown, unmonitored and uninvestigated. Inclusion of the *trans* fatty acid content on food labels and distinction between the *trans* fatty acids and *cis* fatty acids in all food statistics are both warranted. Increased research into the effect of *trans* isomers on the body is imperative and urgent.

More than one-third of brain fatty acids, mainly arachidonic and cervonic acids, are synthesized from dietary essential linoleic and linolenic acids. It is thought they play an important role in cell membrane function and the turnover of brain membranes is slow. It is therefore important to ascertain if the *trans* isomers of these essential fatty acids significantly alter brain function by their presence apart from effecting a diminished prostaglandin production.[268]

The increase in total cancer mortality in the USA correlated with the increase in vegetable fat intake and more specifically with the increased dietary availability of *trans* fatty acids.[265] There appears to be some interference with the immune response. Enig[269] has indicated the following list of reported observations on the effect of *trans* fatty acids by various research groups:

(i) Elevation of serum cholesterol levels by 20 to 30%.

(ii) The immune response is affected by the lowering of the efficiency of B cell response and increasing the proliferation of T cells.

(iii) The amount of cream is lowered in milk from lactating females in various species including humans, thus reducing the overall quality of the milk but also increasing the *trans* fatty acid content of the milk for infant consumption.

(iv) Decrease in insulin binding with a possible deleterious effect on diabetes.

(v) Inhibiting membrane related enzyme function such as delta-6-desaturase with decreased conversion of linoleic acid to arachidonic acid.

(vi) Alteration in activities of enzymes concerned with metabolism of chemical carcinogens and pharmaceutical drugs.

(vii) Alteration in physiological properties of biological membranes including membrane transport and membrane fluidity.

(viii) Alteration in size and number of adipose cells with alteration of lipid adipose fat and tissue.

(ix) Interaction with fish oil omega-3 fatty acids.

(x) Interaction with essential fatty acid deficiency.

The possible serious deleterious effects on subjects with FH is of concern and *trans* fatty acids would mitigate the very effect modern drugs are being used to produce in those with particularly high serum cholesterol and LDL levels.

It must be concluded that the emphasis on the use of polyunsaturated fatty acids and vegetable oil products is more harmful than the consumption of saturated fatty acids, the ill effects of which have not been demonstrated, only incriminated by indirect evidence from ecological studies typified by poor methodology and fallacious vital statistics and dietary data.

In a recent workshop on the role of these various dietary fatty acids in atherogenesis and thrombogenesis,[270] it was concluded that no prothrombotic effect of saturated dietary fatty acids had been established although N-3 fatty acids were believed to be antithrombotic.

N-3 POLYUNSATURATED FATTY ACIDS (FISH OILS)

The interest in the possible role of fish oils in preventing atherosclerosis derives from the epidemiological evidence of the Greenland Inuit. The low incidence of CHD in the Inuit with relatively high blood cholesterol levels was correlated with their high intake of fish oil. Analysis of the population revealed that it was small and young with relatively few (11%) being between 45 to 74 years and sustained a particularly high mortality from accidents (58%).[271] It was not surprising that there were few deaths from CHD. Once again it is not CHD but atherosclerosis that is the principal concern and there was no reliable data on its comparative severity. The alleged benefit had been attributed to N-3 polyunsaturated fatty acids in fish or whale meat, about 400 to 500 g of which is consumed per head per day and the N-3 fatty acids, particularly eicosapentaenoic acid, were incorporated into the phospholipids of their platelet surface membranes resulting in prolonged bleeding time and decreased in vitro platelet aggregation.[272] Subsequent studies have demonstrated only moderate effect on platelet function and this is associated with large individual variations in the experimental data.[273] The weakness of other correlations that have been attempted to support the view derive from the unreliability of national CHD mortality rates and the low quality of dietary data.

The overall effects of N-3 polyunsaturated fatty acids lie in the structural similarity of eicosapentaenoic and docosahexaenoic acids, which are incorporated into plasma membranes, with arachidonic acid and this affects the platelet behavior and function and impairs monocytic chemotaxis, decreases synthesis of interleukin-1 and tumor necrosis factor, platelet-activating factor and toxic oxygen-derived free radicals.[272] It is postulated that these activities may participate in various stages of atherogenesis as well as exerting a variable effect on blood lipids, but to demonstrate these various individual properties or reactions in vitro is quite different from demonstrating such activities in vivo when biological and cellular activities have many checks and balances and are usually the result of a finely-tuned balance of many pharmacodynamic reactions. The proof of such a train of events is difficult, the ultimate proof being dependent on animal experimental studies.

The administration of N-3 polyunsaturated fatty acids to experimental animals with dietary-induced hypercholesterolemia has resulted in reduced lipid deposition as determined by planimetric estimations of the intimal surface involvement.[272] Such experimental studies in the guise of investigating the effect of the N-3 fatty acids on atherosclerosis have in reality more applicability to lipid storage diseases such as FH or type III hyperlipoproteinemia. They are not applicable to atherosclerosis.

In studies of the effect of N-3 fatty acids on restenosis following angioplasty in humans, the results are in conflict. In one study there was limitation of restenosis in single vessel coronary artery disease but no difference in multivessel disease. Such studies are not applicable to atherosclerosis because of the artificial disruption of the wall and the complications of superimposed thrombosis and repair. The anticipated benefit to be derived from these N-3 fatty acids has not been forthcoming although it is thought that small increases in dietary fish might prevent secondary mortality after myocardial infarction and might reduce CHD mortality.[272] Again we are faced with the lack of consideration of the diagnostic error and the use of the wrong endpoint. It is therefore not possible to accept a thesis of any benefit or harm from the ingestion of N-3 polyunsaturated fatty acids for healthy normolipidemic subjects. To recommend administration of concentrated fish oils would be unwise in our current state of knowledge, although such a viewpoint is too conservative for some.

GENETICS OF ATHEROSCLEROSIS

When genetics of atherosclerosis is discussed FH is usually introduced but since this is a lipid storage disorder, its mode of inheritance is peculiar to FH. Likewise other metabolic disorders are not pertinent to atherosclerosis itself. It has been reiterated that CHD tends to run in families and it may probably run in every

family but family histories without confirmation are not reliable. What is needed is documentation of the assessed severity of atherosclerosis at a specific age and this is not possible.

Searching for genetic defects in subjects with clinical CHD and using nonCHD subjects as controls will lead to grossly misleading data. It is an unscientific approach to atherogenesis because it is based on three misconceptions, (i) that CHD is a synonym of atherosclerosis, (ii) that CHD is a specific disease, and (iii) that atherosclerosis is essentially a metabolic disorder of lipids.[274] At best such investigators might stumble on a genetic defect that aggravates atherosclerosis but much time and energy will be wasted.

The use of molecular genetics and transgenic mice can be of considerable interest and value in studying metabolic lipid storage disorders but has no direct applicability to atherogenesis.

If atherosclerosis is due to mechanical failure of the vessel wall as contended,[129] then it is certainly likely that genetics will be important just as it is in timbers etc., and connective tissue disorders will have an aggravating effect on atherogenesis as with hypertension and diabetes mellitus. Whilst these may be genetically determined, it is likely that ubiquitous atherosclerosis can only be discussed in terms of the genetics of diseases that have an aggravating effect on its pathogenesis.

If it were possible to determine genetic defects and mutations that aggravate atherosclerosis and bring about early development of the complications of atherosclerosis, molecular genetics might one day be able to intervene to avoid premature mortality. However this concept presupposes that the severity of atherosclerosis can be assessed accurately and that the pathogenesis of the disease is well understood.

CONCLUSIONS

Dietary fat intake explains only a small proportion of the variance in plasma lipid in free living normolipidemic subjects and there is considerable heterogeneity of response. It is not possible to determine the effect of a life-long diet on the pathogenesis or severity of atherosclerosis. Dietary assessments are unreliable and do not represent the diet in the long-term for it must be remembered that atherosclerosis has a long silent developmental or incubation stage of some 50 years and more.

Ecological correlations between dietary fat and national mortality statistics are nonspecific and indicate only that affluent societies are long-lived and no causal relationship can be assumed and no direct effect on atherosclerosis has been demonstrated. This is further reinforced by the invalid epidemiological methodology and fallacious data.

Cholesterol has been maligned but some metabolic disorders of lipids exhibit nonspecific lipid storage phenomena. Nonlipid metabolic disorders demonstrate some similarities to the pathology of FH.

On the balance of evidence and taking into account deficiencies and weaknesses in the epidemiological methodology, dietary lipids and cholesterol do not cause atherosclerosis. The presence of lipid and cholesterol in the vascular lesions is only one of the manifestations of atherosclerosis and does not appear to be the initiating factor. The possibility that lipid storage in the vessel wall in a normolipidemic subject aggravates atherosclerosis has not been demonstrated but lipid storage as in FH can be superimposed on atherosclerosis. These views are strongly supported by experimental production of atherosclerosis by hemodynamic means in herbivores on a stock diet under conditions analogous to those occurring in humans.

It can only be concluded that the detrimental role of serum cholesterol, LDL levels and dietary saturated fats has been seriously misrepresented and that reduction in the dietary intake of animal foodstuffs with replacement by substitute or modified natural foods is unwarranted.

References

1. Anitschkow N. Experimental arteriosclerosis in animals. In: Cowdry EV, Ed. Arteriosclerosis. New York: MacMillan Co, 1933: 271-322.

2. Hueper WC. Arteriosclerosis. Arch Pathol 1944; 38:162-81,245-85,350-64. 1945; 39:51-65,117-31,187-216.

3. Keys A. Atherosclerosis: A problem in newer public health. J Mt Sinai Hosp 1953; 20:118-139.

4. Yerushalmy J, Hilleboe HE. Fat in the diet and mortality from heart disease, NY State J Med 1957; 57:2343-53.

5. Vastesaeger MM. The contribution of comparative atherosclerosis to the understanding of human atherosclerosis. J Atheroscler Res 1968; 8:377-80.

6. Roberts WC. We think we are one, we act as if we are one, but we are not one. Am J Cardiol 1990; 66:896.

7. Report of the Working Group on Arteriosclerosis of the National Heart, Lung, and Blood Institute. Arteriosclerosis Vol 1. US Dept Health Human Serv. NIH Pub, No81-2034. 1981.

8. Report of the Working Group on Arteriosclerosis of the National Heart Lung, and Blood Institute. Arteriosclerosis Vol 2. US Dept Health Human Serv. NIH Pub, No 82-2035. 1981.

9. Yerushalmy J, Palmer CE. On the methodology of investigations of etiologic factors in chronic diseases. J Chr Dis 1959; 10:27-40.

10. Stehbens WE. Diet and atherogenesis. Nutr Rev 1989; 47:1-12.

11. Epstein FH. Epidemiology of coronary heart disease. In: Jones AM, ed. Modern Trends in Cardiology. vol 1. London: Butterworths, 1960: 155-71.

12. Carroll KK. Hypercholesterolemia and atherosclerosis: Effects of dietary protein, Fed Proc 1982; 41:2792-6.

13. Carroll KK, Hamilton RMG. Effects of dietary protein and carbohydrate on plasma cholesterol levels in relation to atherosclerosis. J Food Sc 1975; 40:18-23.

14. Kritchevsky D. Diet and atherosclerosis. Am J Pathol 1976; 84:615-32.

15. Lowenstein FW. Epidemiologic investigations in relation to diet in groups who show little atherosclerosis and are almost free of coronary ischemic heart disease. Am J Clin Nutr 1964; 15:175-86.

16. Stamler J. Population studies. In: Levy RI, Rifkind BM, Dennis BH et al, Nutrition, Lipids, and Coronary Heart Disease. Vol Nutrition in Health and Disease. New York: Raven Press, 1979. 25-88.

17. Keys A. Dietary survey methods. In: Levy RI, Rifkind BM Dennis BH et al, Nutrition, Lipids and Coronary Heart Disease. New York: Raven Press, 1979. 1-23.

18. Arroll B, Beaglehole R, Jackson R et al. The Auckland diet: Results from a seven day food diary. NZ Med 1991; 5:1-3.

19. Lilienfeld AM, Graham S. Validity of determining circumcision status by questionnaires as related to epidemiological studies of cancer of the cervix. J Nat Cancer Inst 1958; 21:713-20.

20. Baumgarten M, Siemiatychi J, Gibbs GW. Validity of work histories obtained by interview for epidemiologic purposes. Am J Epidemiol 1983; 118:583-91.

21. Petitti DB, Friedman GD, Kahn W. Accuracy of information on smoking habits provided on self-administered research questionnaires. Am J Publ Health 1981; 71:308-11.

22. Mann JM. A prospective study of response error in food history questionnaires: Implications for foodborne outbreak investigation. Am J Publ Health 1981; 71:1362-6.

23. Groover ME, Boone L, Houk PC et al. Problems in the quantitation of dietary surveys. JAMA 1967; 201:86-8.

24. Eagles JA, Whiting MC, Olsen RE. Dietary appraisal. Problems in processing dietary data. Am J Clin Nutr 1966; 19:1-9.

25. Gardner MJ, Heady JA. Some effects of within—person variability in epidemiological studies. J Chr Dis 1973; 26:781-95.

26. Kritchevsky D. Dietary Interactions. In: Levy RI, Rifkind BM, Dennis BH et al, eds. Nutrition, Lipids and Coronary Heart Disease. New York: Raven Press, 1979: 229-46.

27. Beaton GH, Milner J, Corey P et al. Sources of variance in 24-hour dietary recall data: Implications for nutrition study design and interpretation. Am J Clin Nutr 1979; 32:2546-59.

28. Chappell GM. Long-term individual dietary surveys. Brit J Nutr 1955; 9:323-39.

29. Block G. A review of validations of dietary assessment methods. Am J Epidemiol 1982; 115:492-505.

30. Scrimshaw NS, Guzmán MA. Diet and atherosclerosis. Lab Invest 1968; 18:623-8.

31. Rhoads GG. Reliability of diet measures as chronic disease risk factors. Am J Clin Nutr 1987; 45:1073-9.

32. Bingham SA. The dietary assessment of individuals; methods, accuracy, new techniques and recommendations. Nutr Abstracts Rev (Series A) 1987; 57:706-42.

33. Bingham SA. Limitations of the various methods for collecting dietary intake data. Ann Nutr Metab !991; 35:117-27.

34. Kritchevsky D. Experimental atherosclerosis in primates and other species. NY Acad Sc 1969; 162:80-8.

35. Annand JC. Atherosclerosis-the case against protein-continued. J Coll Gen Pract 1961; 4:567-96.

36. Annand JC. Hypothesis: Heated milk protein and thrombosis. J Atheroscler Res 1967; 7:797-801.

37. Blackburn H, Gillum RF. Heart disease. In: Last, JM ed. Maxcy-Rosenau Public Health and Preventive Medicine. 11th Ed. New York: Appleton-Century-Crofts, 1980: 1116-201.

38. Judkin J. Dietary fat and dietary sugar in relation to ischaemic heart-disease and diabetes. Lancet 1964; 2:4-5.

39. Yudkin J. Evolutionary and historical changes in dietary carbohydrates. Am J Clin Nutr 1967; 20:108-15.

40. Yudkin J, Roddy J. Levels of dietary sucrose in patients with occlusive atherosclerotic disease. Lancet 1964; 2:6-8.

41. Lopez A, Hodges RE, Krehl WA. Some interesting relationships between dietary carbohydrates and serum cholesterol. Am J Clin Nutr 1966; 18:149-53.

42. Little JA, McGuire V, Derkson A. Available carbohydrates. In: Levy RI, Rifkind BM, Dennis BH et al, eds. Nutrition Lipids, and Coronary Heart Disease. New York: Raven Press, 1979. 119-48.

43. Hodges RE, Krehl WA. The role of carbohydrate in lipid metabolism. Am J Clin Nutr 1965; 17:334-46.

44. Groen JJ, Balogh M, Yaron E et al. Effect of interchanging bread and sucrose as main source of carbohydrate in a low fat diet on the serum cholesterol levels of healthy volunteer subjects. Am J Clin Nutr 1976; 19:46-58.

45. Masironi R. Dietary factors and coronary heart disease. Bull WHO 1970:42:103-14.

46. Morris JN, Marr JW, Clayton DG. Diet and heart: A postscript. Br Heart J 1977; 2:1307-14.

47. Stewart FM, Neutze JM, Newsome-White R. The addition of oatbran to a low-fat diet has no effect on lipid values in hypercholesterolaemic subjects. NZ Med J 1992; 105:398-400.

48. Robbins SL, Cotran RS, Kumar V. Pathologic Basis of Disease. 3rd Ed. Philadelphia: WB Saunders, 1984: 506-18.

49. Risek RL, Friend B, Page L. Fat in today's food supply—level of use and sources. J Am Chem-

ists' Soc 1974; 51:244-50.

50. Enig MG, Munn RJ, Keeney M. Dietary fat and cancer trends-a critique. Fed Proc 1978; 37:2215-20.

51. Klurfeld DM, Kritchevsky D. The western diet: An examination of its relationship to chronic disease. J Am Coll Nutr 1986; 5:477-85.

52. Trenchard Viscount, Fat consumption assumptions and the long-term trends, Meat Trades J 1977; Sept 29:4-5.

53. McGill HC, Arias-Stella J, Carbonell LM et al. General findings of the International Atherosclerosis Project. Lab Invest 1968; 18:498-502.

54. Segall JJ. Is milk a coronary health hazard? Br J Prevent Soc Med 1977; 31:81-5.

55. Mann GV. Hypocholesterolaemic effect of milk. Lancet 1977; 2:556.

56. Marks J, Howard AN. Hypocholesterolaemic effect of milk. Lancet 1977; 2:763.

57. Truswell AS. Diet and plasma lipids—a reappraisal. Am J Clin Nutr 1978; 31:977-89.

58. Mann GV. A factor in yogurt which lowers cholesterolemia in man. Atherosclerosis 1977; 26:335-40.

59. Lapiccirella V, Lapiccirella R, Abboni F et al. Enquête clinique, biologique et cardiographique parmi les tribes nomades de la Somalie qui se nourrissent seulement de lait. Bull WHO 1962; 27:681-97.

60. Yudkin J. Diet and coronary thrombosis. Hypothesis and fact. Lancet 1957; 2:155-62.

61. Kahn HA. Change in serum cholesterol associated with changes in the United States civilian diet, 1909-1965. Am J Clin Nutr 1970; 23:879-82.

62. Olson RE. Is there an optimun diet for the prevention of coronary heart disease? In: Levy RI, Rifkind BM, Dennis BH et al, eds. Nutrition, Lipids and Coronary Heart Disease. New York: Raven Press, 1979: 349-64.

63. McNair AL. Eggs and cholesterol. Lancet 1984; 1:1127

64. Ahrens EH. Eggs and cholesterol. Lancet 1984; 1:1127-8.

65. Bronsgeest-Schoute DC, Hermus RJJ, Dallinga-Thie GM et al. Dependence of the effects of dietary cholesterol and experimental conditions on serum lipids in man. III The effect on serum cholesterol of removal of eggs from the diet of free-living habitually egg-eating people. Am J Clin Nutr 1979; 32:2193-7.

66. Flynn MA, Nolph GB, Flynn TC et al. Effect of dietary egg on human serum cholesterol and triglycerides. Am J Clin Nutr 1979; 32:1051-7.

67. Dawber JR, Nickerson RJ, Brand FN et al. Eggs, serum cholesterol, and coronary heart disease. Am J Clin Nutr 1982; 36:617-25.

68. Kern F. Normal plasma cholesterol in an 88-year-old man who eats 25 eggs a day: Mechanisms of adaptation. N Engl J Med 1991; 324:896-9.

69. Marmot MG. Epidemiology and the art of the soluble. Lancet 1986; 1:897-900.

70. Browe JH, Morlley DM, Logrillo VM et al. Diet and heart disease in the cardiovascular health center. J Am Diet Assoc 1967; 50:376-84.

71. Meade TW, Chakrabarti R. Arterial-disease research: Observation or intervention? Lancet 1972; 2:913-6.

72. Kuller LH. Epidemiology of coronary heart disease. In: Perkins EG, Visek WJ, eds. Dietary Fats and Health. Am Oil Chemists' Soc Campaign, 1983: 466-75.

73. Friedman M, Rosenman RH. Comparison of fat intake of American men and women. Possible relationship to incidence of clinical coronary artery disease. Circulation 1957; 16:339-47.

74. McGill H. The relationship of dietary cholesterol to serum cholesterol concentration and to atherosclerosis in man. Am J Clin Nutr 1979; 32:2664-702.

75. Feinstein AR. Clinical Epidemiology, The Architecture of Clinical Research. Philadelphia: WB Saunders, 1985.

76. Gordon T, Fisher M, Rifkind BM. Some difficulties inherent in the interpretation of dietary data from free-living populations. Am J Clin Nutr 1984; 39:152-6.

77. Oliver MF. Prevention of coronary heart disease-propaganda, promises, problems and prospects. Circulation 1986; 73:1-9.

78. Kaunitz H. Repair function of cholesterol versus the lipid theory of arteriosclerosis. Chemistry & Industry 1977; 17th Sept:761-3.

79.. Pikkarainen J, Takkunen J, Kulonen E. Serum cholesterol in Finnish twins. Am J Human Genet 1966; 18:115-26.

80. Oliver MF. Serum cholesterol—the knave of hearts and the joker. Lancet 1981; 2:1090-5.

81. Austin MA, King M-C, Bawol et al. Risk factors for coronary heart disease in adult female twins. Genetic heritability and shared environmental

influences. Am J Epidemiol 1987; 125:308-18.

82. Toor M, Katchalsky A, Agmon J et al. Serum-lipids and atherosclerosis among Yemenite immigrants in Israel. Lancet 1957; 1270-3.

83. Groen JJ, Tijong KB, Koster M et al. The influence of nutrition and ways of life on blood cholesterol and the prevalence of hypertension and coronary heart disease among Trappist and Benedictine monks. Am J Clin Nutr 1962; 10:456-70.

84. Paterson JC, Armstrong R, Armstrong EC. Serum lipid levels and the severity of coronary and cerebral atherosclerosis in adequately nourished men, 60 to 69 years of age. Circulation 1963; 27:229-36.

85. McMichael J. Prevention of coronary heart disease. Lancet 1976; 2:569.

86. Mathur KS, Patney NL, Kumar V et al. Serum cholesterol and atherosclerosis in man. Circulation 1961; 23:847-52.

87. Holman RL, McGill HC, Strong JP et al. Filtration versus local formation of lipids in pathogenesis of atherosclerosis. JAMA 1959; 170:416-20.

88. Schlierf G, Arab L. Associations between coronary heart disease and nutrient intake with particular reference to European data. In: Fidge NH, Nestel PJ, eds. Atherosclerosis VII. Amsterdam: Excerpta Med. 1986: 667-70.

89. Shaper AG. Cardiovascular mortality in Great Britain. Br Med Bull 1984; 40:366-73.

90. Schroeder HA. Degenerative cardiovascular disease in the Orient. 1. Atherosclerosis. J Chr Dis 1958; 8:287-333.

91. Vastesaegar MM, Dalcourt R. The natural history of atherosclerosis Circulation 1962; 26:841-54.

92. Detweiler DK, Ratcliffe HL, Luginbühl H. The significance of naturally occurring coronary and cerebral arterial disease in animals. Ann N Y Acad Sc 1968; 149:868-81.

93. Mann GV, Muñoz JA, Scrimshaw NS. The serum lipoprotein and cholesterol concentrations of central and north Americans with different dietary habits. Am J Med 1955; 19:25-32.

94. Mann GV. A short history of the diet/heart hypothesis. In: Mann GV, ed. Coronary Heart Disease. London: Janus Paul Co, 1993. 1-17.

95. Morris JN, Marr JW, Heady JA et al. Diet and plasma cholesterol in 99 bank men. Br Med J 1963; 1:571-6.

96. Nichols AB, Ravenscroft C, Lamphiear DE et al. Daily nutritional intake and serum lipid levels. The Tecumseh Study. Am J Clin Nutr 1976; 29:1384-92.

97. Brisson GJ. Lipids in Human Nutrition. Englewood: Jack K Burgess Inc, 1981.

98. Armstrong BK, Mann JI, Adelstein AM et al. Commodity consumption and ischemic heart disease mortality, with special reference to dietary practices. J Chr Dis 1975; 28:455-69.

99. Thom TJ, Epstein FH, Feldman JJ et al. Trends in total mortality and mortality from heart disease in 26 countries from 1950 to 1978. Int J Epidemiol 1985; 14:510-20.

100. Anonymous. The inequality of death. Assessing socioeconomic influences on mortality. WHO Chron 1980; 34:9-15.

101. Becker BJP. Cardiovascular disease in the Bantu and coloured races of South Africa. Sth Afr J Med Sc 1946; 11:97-105.

102. Higginson J, Pepler WJ. Fat intake, serum cholesterol concentration, and atherosclerosis in the South African Bantu. Part II. Atherosclerosis and coronary artery disease. J Clin Invest 1954; 33:1366-71.

103. Laurie W, Woods JD. Atherosclerosis and its cerebral complications in the South African Bantu. Lancet 1958; 1:231-2.

104. Isaacson C. The changing pattern of heart disease in South African blacks. S A Med J 1977; 52:793-98.

105. Malhotra RP, Pathania NS. Some aetological aspects of coronary heart disease. An Indian point of view based on a study of 867 cases seen during 1948-55. Br Med J 1958; 2:528-31.

106. Sarvotham SG, Berry JN. Prevalence of coronary heart disease in an urban population in Northern India. Circulation 1968; 37:939-53.

107. Ho K-J, Biss K, Mikkelson B et al. The Masai of East Africa: Some unique biological characteristics. Arch Pathol 1971; 91:387-410.

108. Mann GV, Spoerry A, Gray M et al. Atherosclerosis in the Masai. Am J Epidemiol 1972; 95:26-37.

109. Shaper AG. Cardiovascular studies inn the Samburu tribe of Northern Kenya. Am Heart J 1962; 63:437-42.

110. Shaper AG, Jones KW, Jones M et al. Serum lipids in three nomadic tribes of Northern Kenya. Am J Clin Nutr 1963; 13:135-46.

111. Stehbens WE. The controversial role of dietary cholesterol and hypercholesterolemia in the eti-

ology of atherosclerosis. Pathology 1989; 21:213-221.

112. Stehbens WE. An appraisal of cholesterol-feeding in experimental atherogenesis. Progr Cardiovasc Dis 1986; 29:107-28.

113. Stehbens WE. Vascular complications in experimental atherosclerosis. Progr Cardiovasc Dis 1986; 29:221-37.

114. Stehbens WE, Wierzbicki E. The relationship of hypercholesterolemia to atherosclerosis with particular emphasis on familial hypercholesterolemia, diabetes mellitus, obstructive jaundice, myxedema and the nephrotic syndrome. Progr Cardiovasc Dis 1988; 30:289-306.

115. Stehbens WE, Martin M. The vascular pathology of familial hypercholesterolemia. Pathology 1991; 23:54-61.

116. Stehbens WE. The lipid hypothesis and the role of hemodynamics in atherogenesis. Progr Cardiovasc Dis 1990; 33:119-36.

117. Stehbens WE. Experimental induction of atherosclerosis associated with femoral arteriovenous fistulae in rabbits on a stock diet. Atherosclerosis 1992; 95:127-35.

118. Brown MS, Goldstein JL. A receptor-mediated pathway for cholesterol homeostasis. Science 1986; 232:34-47.

119. Sodhi HS, Kudchodkar BJ, Mason DT. Clinical methods in study of cholesterol metabolism. Monograph on Atherosclerosis. 9: Basel: Karger, 1979.

120. Stryer L. Biochemistry 3rd Ed. New York: WH Freeman & Co, 1988.

121. Lewis B. The hyperlipidaemias. Clinical and laboratory practice. Oxford: Blackwell Scient Publ, 1976.

122. Latner AL. Cantarow and Trumper. Clinical Biochemistry. 7th Ed. Philadelphia: WB Saunders, 1975.

123. Guyton AC. Textbook of Medical Physiology. 8th Ed. Philadelphia: WB Saunders, 1991: 754-64.

124. Alberts B, Bray D, Lewis J et al. Molecular Biology of the Cell. 2nd Ed. New York: Garland Publ Inc, 1989: 275-340.

125. Goudie RB. Molecular and cellular pathology of tissue damage. In: Anderson JR, ed. Muir's Textbook of Pathology. 12th Ed. London: Edward Arnold. 1985: 3-8.

126. Ziperovich S, Paley HW. Severe mechanical hemolytic anemia due to valvular heart disease

without prosthesis. Ann Int Med 1966; 65: 342-6.

127. Westring DW. Aortic valve disease and hemolytic anemia. Ann Int Med 1966; 65:203-9.

128. Chamberlain JK, O'Brien JF, Christ LM et al. Intravascular hemolysis with traumatic arteriovenous fistula. NY State J Med 1974; 74: 686-8.

129. Stehbens WE. Hemodynamics and the Blood Vessel Wall, Springfield: CC Thomas, 1979.

130. Rogers KM, Stehbens WE. The morphology of matrix vesicles produced in experimental arterial aneurysms in rabbits. Pathology 1986; 18:64-71.

131. Stehbens WE. Cerebral atherosclerosis. Arch Pathol 1975; 99:582-91.

132. Stehbens WE. The role of lipid in the pathogenesis of atherosclerosis. Lancet 1975; 1:724-7.

133. Chien S. Red cell membrane and hemolysis. In: Hwang NHC, Norman NA, eds. Cardiovascular Flow Dynamics and Measurements. Baltimore: Univ Park Press, 1975. 757-97.

134. Stehbens WE. The ultrastructure of the anastomosed vein of experimental arteriovenous fistulae in sheep. Am J Pathol 1974; 76:377-400.

135. Stehbens WE. The ultrastructure of experimental aneurysms in rabbits. Pathology 1985; 17:87-95.

136. Davis PF, Ryan PA, Manning JN et al. Isolation and characterization of salt-soluble cross-linked elastin from vascular tissue. Angiology 1984; 35:38-44.

137. Rinaldi G, Bohr D. Plasma membrane and its abnormalities in hypertension. Am J Med Sc 1988; 295:389-95.

138. Kagan A, Dawber TR, Kannel WB et al. The Framingham Study: A prospective study of coronary heart disease. Fed Proc 1957; 21(4 part II):52-7.

139. Kannel WB, Gordon T. The Framingham Study. An Epidemiological Investigation of Cardiovascular Disease. Washington: Sect 23 US Gov Print Office, 1969.

140. Kannel WB, Castelli WP, Gordon T et al. Serum cholesterol, lipoproteins, and the risk of coronary heart disease. Ann Int Med 1971; 74:1-12.

141. Kannel WB, Castelli WP, Gordon T. Cholesterol in the prediction of atherosclerotic disease. Ann Int Med 1979; 90:85-91.

142. Kannel WB, Gordon T. The search for an

optimun serum cholesterol. Lancet 1982; 2:374-5.

143. Gordon T, Castelli WP, Hjortland MC et al. Predicting coronary heart disease in middle-aged and older persons. The Framingham Study. JAMA 1977; 238:497-9.

144. Anderson KM, Castelli WP, Levy D. Cholesterol and mortality. 30 years of follow-up from the Framingham Study. JAMA 1987; 257:2176-80.

145. Hopkins PN, Williams RR. Identification and relative weight of cardiovascular risk factors. Cardiol Clin 1986; 4:3-31.

146. Keys A, Mickelson O, Miller EvO et al. The concentration of cholesterol in the blood serum of normal man and its relation to age. J Clin Invest 1950; 29:1347-53.

147. Taylor CB, Ho K-J. A review of human cholesterol metabolism. Arch Pathol 1967; 84:3-14.

148. Taylor CB, Mikkelson B, Anderson JA et al. Human cholesterol metabolism. Med Times 1967; 95:489-501.

149. Samuel P, McNamara DJ, Shapiro J. The role of diet in the etiology and treatment of atherosclerosis. Ann Rev Med 1983; 34:179-94.

150. Ahrens EH. Dietary fat and coronary heart disease: Unfinished business. Lancet 1979; 2:1345-48.

151. Oliver MF. Diet and coronary heart disease. Br Med Bull 1981; 37:49-58.

152. Kannel WB. The role of cholesterol in coronary atherogenesis Med Clin N Am 1974; 58:363-79.

153. Keys A, Anderson JT. The relationship of the diet to the development of atherosclerosis in man. In: Symposium on Atherosclerosis. Washington: Nat Acad Sc Publ 338 Nat Res Council, 1955: 181-97.

154. Lipid Research Clinics Program. The Lipid Research Clinics Coronary Primary Prevention Trial Results. 1. Reduction in incidence of coronary heart disease. JAMA 1984; 251:351-64.

155. Lipid Research Clinics Program. The Lipid Research Clinics Coronary Primary Prevention Trial Results. II The relationship of reduction in incidence of coronary heart disease to cholesterol lowering. JAMA 1984; 251:365-74.

156. Ederer F. Serum cholesterol changes: Effects of diet and regression toward the mean. J Chr Dis 1972; 25:277-89.

157. Barnes BO, Barnes RW. Physiology and clinical management of atherosclerosis and coronary heart disease. Fed Proc 1957; 16:7.

158. Grundy SM. Cholesterol and coronary heart disease. A new era. JAMA 1986; 256:2849-58.

159. Epstein FH. The epidemiology of coronary heart disease. J Chr Dis 1965; 18:735-74.

160. Walker ARP. Studies bearing on coronary heart disease in South African populations. S A Med J 1973; 47:85-90.

161. Werkö L. Diet, lipids and heart attacks. Acta Med Scand 1970; 206:435-9.

162. McMichael J. Fats and arterial disease. Am Heart J 1979; 98:409-12.

163. Bronte-Stewart B, Keys A, Brock JF et al. Serum-cholesterol, diet, and coronary-heart disease. Lancet 1955; 2:1103-7.

164. Stout C, Bohorquez F. Aortic atherosclerosis in hoofed animals. J Atheroscler Res 1969; 9:73-80.

165. Levy RI. Changing perspectives in the prevention of coronary heart disease. Am J Cardiol 1986; 57:17G-26G.

166. Vergroesen AJ, Gottenbos JT. The role of fats in human nutrition: An introduction. In: Vergroesen AJ, ed. The Role of Fats in Human Nutrition. London: Academic Press, 1975. 1-41.

167. Rivin AV, Yoshino J, Shickman M et al. Serum cholesterol measurement-hazards in clinical interpretation. JAMA 1958; 166:2108-11.

168. Dawber TR. The Framingham Study. The Epidemiology of Atherosclerotic Disease. Cambidge: Harvard Univ Press, 1980.

169. Blank DW, Hoeg JM, Kroll MH et al. The method of determination must be considered in interpreting blood cholesterol levels. JAMA 1986; 256:2867-70.

170. Roberts L. Measuring cholesterol is as tricky as lowering it. Science 1987; 238:482-3.

171. Belsey R, Baer Dm. Cardiac risk classification based on lipid screening. JAMA 1990; 263:1250-2.

172. Peterien JE, Wilcox AA, Haley MI et al. Hourly variation in total serum cholesterol. Circulation 1960; 22:247-53.

173. Demacher PNM, Schade RWB, Jansen RTP et al. Intra-individual variation of serum cholesterol, triglycerides and high density lipoprotein cholesterol in normal humans. Atherosclerosis 1982; 45:259-66.

174. Hegstad DM, Nicolosi RJ. Individual variation in serum cholesterol levels. Proc Nat Acad Sc 1987; 84:6259-61.

175. Groover ME, Jernigan JA, Martin CD. Variations in serum lipid concentration and clinical coronary disease. Am J Med Sc 1960; 239: 133-9.

176. Man EB, Peters JP. Variations of serum lipids with age. J Lab Clin Med 1953; 41:738-44.

177. Keys A, Fidanza F. Serum cholesterol and relative body weight of coronary patients in different populations, Circulation 1960; 22:1091-106.

178. Sunderman FW. Current concepts of "normal values", "reference values", and "discrimination values" in clinical chemistry. Clin Chem 1975; 21:1873-7.

179. Reed AH, Cannon DC, Wilkelman JW et al. Estimation of normal ranges from a controlled sample survey. I Sex- and age-related influence on the SMA 12/60 screening group of tests. Clin Chem 1972; 18:57-66.

180. Aranow WS, Starling L, Etienne F et al. Risk factors for coronary heart disease in persons older than 62 years in a long-term health care facility. Am J Cardiol 1986; 57:518-20.

181. Epstein FH, Bloch WD, Hand et al. Familial hypercholesterolemia, xanthomatosis aand coronary heart disease. Am J Med 1959; 26:39-53.

182. Editorial. Prevention of coronary heart disease. Lancet 1987; 1:601-2.

183. Scott RS, Lintott CJ, Bremer J et al. Hyperlipidaemia and the prevention of coronary heart disease. NZ Med J 1987; 100:717-9.

184. Roberts WC. Fat versus fatigue: Comments on causes of atherosclerosis. Cardiovasc Med 1977; 2:593-5.

185. Shaper AG, Pocock SJ. British blood cholesterol values and the American consensus. Br Med J 1985; 291:480-1.

186. Rifkind BM, Lenfant C. Cholesterol lowering and the reduction of coronary heart disease risk. JAMA 1986; 256:2872-3.

187. Grundy SM, Vega GL, Bilheimer DW. Causes and treatment of hypercholesterolemia. Atheroscler Res 1986; 15:13-39.

188. National Institutes of Health Consensus Development Conference. Lowering blood cholesterol to prevent heart disease. JAMA 1985; 253: 2080-6.

189. Gordon H. The regulation of the human serum-cholesterol level. Postgrad Med J 1959; 35:1 86-96.

190. Paul O, Lepper MH, Phelan WH et al. A longitudinal study of coronary heart disease. Circulation 1963; 28: 20-31.

191. Hurxthal LM, Balodimos MC, Kealey OJ. The predictive value of blood cholesterol for coronary artery disease. Geriatrics 1965; 20:438-58.

192. Glueck CJ, Heckman F, Schoenfeld M et al. Neonatal familial type II hypolipoproteinemia: Cord blood cholesterol in 1800 births. Metabolism 1971; 20:597-608.

193. Schubert WK. Fat nutrition and diet in childhood. Am J Cardiol 1973; 31:581-7.

194. Drash A. Atherosclerosis, cholesterol, and the pediatrician. J Pediatrics 1972; 80:693-6.

195. Sperry WM, Webb M. The effect of increasing age on serum cholesterol concentration. J Biol Chem 1950; 187:107-10.

196. Gertler MM, Garn SM, Bland EF. Age, serum cholesterol and coronary artery disease. Circulation 1950; 11:517-522.

197. Lewis A, Olmsted F, Page IH et al. Serum lipid levels in normal persons. Findings of a cooperative study of lipoproteins and atherosclerosis. Circulation 1957; 16:227-45.

198. Lawry EY, Mann GV, Peterson A et al. Cholesterol and beta lipoproteins in the serums of Americans. Am J Med 1957; 22:605-23.

199. Schilling FJ, Christakis GJ, Bennett NJ et al. Studies of serum cholesterol in 4,244 men and women: An epidemiological and pathogenetic interpretation. Am J Pub Health 1964; 54: 461-76.

200. Stamler J. Lectures on Preventive Cardiology. New York: Grune & Stratton, 1967: 47.

201. Kinsell LW. Relationship of dietary fats to atherosclerosis. In: Holman RT, Lundberg WO, Malkin T, eds. Progress in Chemistry of Fats to Atherosclerosis. Vol 6 Oxford: Pergamon Press, 1963: 137-70.

202. Kuo PT. Diet-drug treatment of hyperlipidemia in coronary artery disease. A rational and beneficial approach. Chest 1983; 83:165-6.

203. Oliver MF, Boyd GS. The plasma lipids in coronary artery disease. Br Heart J 1953; 15:387-92.

204. Biörck G, Blomqvist G, Sievers J. Cholesterol values in patients with myocardial infarction and in a normal control group. Acta Med Scand 1957; 156:494-7.

205. Underwood DA, Proudfit WL, Lim J et al. Symptomatic coronary artery disease in patients aged 21 to 30 years. Am J Cardiol 1985; 55:631-4.

206. Oliver MF. Ischemic heart disease in young women. Br Heart J 1974; 4:253-9.

207. Rissanen AM. Familial occurrence of coronary heart disease: Effect of age at diagnosis. Am J Cardiol 1979; 44:60-6.

208. Carlson LA, Wahlberg F. Serum lipids, intravenous glucose tolerance and their relationship studied in ischaemic cardiovascular disease. Acta Med Scand 1966; 180:307-14.

209. Nikkilä EA, Aro A. Family study of serum lipids and lipoproteins in coronary heart-disease. Lancet 1973; 1:954-9.

210. Wilkinson CF, Blecha E, Reimer A. Is there a relation between diet and blood cholesterol. Arch Int Med 1950; 85:389-97.

211. Corday E, Corday SR. Prevention of heart disease by control of risk factors: The time has come to face the facts. Am J Cardiol 1975; 35:330-3.

212. Slack J. Inheritance of familial hypercholesterolemia. Atherosclerosis Rev 1979; 5:35-66.

213. Motulsky AG. Genetic aspects of familial hypercholesterolemia and its diagnosis. Arteriosclerosis 1989; 9 Suppl 1:1-9.

214. Garrett HE, Horning EC, Creech BG et al. Serum cholesterol values in patients treated surgically for atherosclerosis. JAMA 1964; 189:655-9.

215. Carlson LA. Serum lipids and atherosclerotic diseases. In: Carlson LA, Pernow B, eds. Metabolic Risk Factors in Ischemic Cardiovascular Disease. New York: Raven Press, 1982: 1-16.

216. Kannel WB. Cholesterol and risk of coronary heart disease and mortality in men. Clin Chem 1988; 34:B53-9.

217. Lifshitz F, Moses N. Growth failure. A complication of dietary treatment of hypercholesterolemia. Am J Dis Child 1989; 143:537-42.

218. Gotto AM, LaRosa JC, Hunninghake D et al. The Cholesterol Facts. A joint statement by the American Heart Association and the National Heart, Lung and Blood Institute. Circulation 1990; 81:1721-33.

219. Gotto AM. Rationale of treatment. Am J Med 1991; 91 Suppl 1B:31S-6S.

220. Stehbens WE. The epidemiological relationship of hypercholesterolemia, hypertension, diabetes mellitus and obesity to coronary heart disease. J Clin Epidemiol 1990; 43:733-41.

221. Dock W. Atherosclerosis. Why do we pretend the pathogenesis is mysterious? Circulation 1974; 50:647-9.

222. Roberts WC. Atherosclerotic risk factors—are there 10 or is there only one? Am J Cardiol 1989; 64:552-4.

223. Smith RL. Diet, Blood Cholesterol and Coronary Heart Disease: A Critical Review of the Literature. Vol 2. Santa Monica: Vector Enterprises Inc, 1991.

224. Reed DM, Strong JP, Resch J et al. Serum lipids and lipoproteins as predictors of atherosclerosis. An autopsy study. Arteriosclerosis 1989; 9:560-4.

225. Wissler RW. Update on the pathogenesis of atherosclerosis. Am J Med 1991; 91 Suppl 1B:3S-9S.

226. Pathological Determinants of Atherosclerosis in Youth (P Day) Research Group. Relationship of atherosclerosis in young men to serum lipoprotein cholesterol concentrations and smoking. JAMA 1990; 264:3018-24.

227. Rosenfeld K. Lipoprotein analysis. Early methods in the diagnosis of atherosclerosis. Arch Pathol Lab Med 1989; 113:1101-10.

228. Editorial HDL and ischaemic heart disease in Britain. Lancet 1986; 1:481-2.

229. Miller GT, Miller NE. Plasma-high-density-lipoprotein concentration and development of ischaemic heart-disease. Lancet 1975; 1:16-9.

230. Ehnholm C, Huttunen JK, Pietinen P et al. Effect of diet on serum lipoproteins in a population with a high risk of coronary heart disease. NEJM 1982; 307:850-5.

231. Holme I, Enger SC, Helgeland A et al. Risk factors and raised atherosclerotic lesions in coronary and cerebral arteries. Arteriosclerosis 1981; 1:250-6.

232. Miller NE, Hammett F, Saltissi S et al. Relation of angiographically defined coronary artery disease to plasma lipoprotein subfractions and apoliproteins Br Med J 1981; 282:1741-4.

233. Brunzell JD, Miller NE. Atherosclerosis in inherited and acquired disorders of plasma lipoprotein metabolism. In: Miller NE, Lewis B, eds. Lipoproteins, Atherosclerosis and Coronary Heart Disease. Amsterdam: Elsevier/North Holland Biomed Press, 1981: 73-88.

234. Herbert PN, Assmann G, Gotto AM et al. Familial lipoprotein deficiency: Abetalipoproteinemia, hypobetaliproteimemia and Tangier disease. In: Stanbury JB, Wyngaarden JB, Fredrickson DS et al, The Metabolic Basis of Inherited Disease. 5th ed. New York: McGraw-Hill, 1983: 589-621.

235. Schlierf G, Arab L, Oster P. Influence of diet on

high density lipoprotein. Am J Cardiol 1983; 52:17B-9B.

236. Edelberg J, Pizzo SV. Why is lipoprotein (a) relevant to thrombosis? Am J Clin Nutr 1992; 56:791S-2S.

237. Scanu AM. Lipoprotein (a). A genetic risk factor for premature coronary heart disease. JAMA 1992; 267:3326-9.

238. Mbetu AD, Durrington PM. Lipoprotein (a): Structure, properties and possible involvement in thrombogenesis and atherogenesis. Atherosclerosis 1990; 85:1-14.

239. Lawn RM. Lipoprotein (a) in heart disease.Scient Am 1992; June:26-32.

240. Scanu AM. Lipopoprotein (a). A potential bridge between the fields of atherosclerosis and thrombosis. Arch Pathol Lab Med 1988; 112:1045-7.

241. Rader DJ, Brewer HB. Lipoprotein (a). Clinical approach to a unique atherogenic lipoprotein JAMA 1992; 267:1109-12.

242. Lawn RM, Wade DP, Hammer RE et al. Atherogenesis in transgenic mice expressing human apoliprotein (a). Nature 1992; 360:670-2.

243. Cambillau M, Simon A, Amar J et al. Serum Lp(a) as a discriminant marker of early atherosclerotic plaque at three extraordinary sites in hypercholesterolemic men. Arteriosclerosis 1992; 12:1346-52.

244. Armstrong VW, Cremer P, Eberle E et al. The association between serum Lp(a) concentrations and angiographically assessed coronary atherosclerosis. Dependence on serum LDL levels. Atherosclerosis 1986; 62:249-57.

245. Scott J. Lipoprotein (a) Thrombotic and atherogenic. Br Med J 1991; 303:663-4.

246. Gowenlock AH, McMurray JR, McLauchlan DM et al. eds, Varley's Practical Clinical Biochemistry. Boca Raton: CRC Press Inc, 1988.

247. Devlin TM, ed. Textbook of Biochemistry with Clinical Correlations. 2nd ed. New York, John Wiley & Sons, 1986: 98.

248. Brunzell JD, Schrott HG, Motulsky AG et al. Myocardial infarction in the familial forms of hypertriglyceridemia. Metabolism 1976; 25:313-20.

249. Stehbens WE. Experimental arteriovenous fistulae in normal and cholesterol-fed rabbits. Pathology 1973; 5:311-24.

250. Stehbens WE. Predilection of experimental arterial aneurysms for dietary-induced lipid deposition. Pathology 1981; 13:735-47.

251. Davignon J, Gregg RE, Sing CF. Apoliprotein E polymorphism and atherosclerosis. Arteriosclerosis 1988; 8:1-21.

252. Imai H, Werthessen NT, Subramanyam V et al. Angiotoxicity of oxygenated sterols and possible precursors. Science 1980; 207:651-3.

253. Peng S-K, Tham P, Taylor CB et al. Cytotoxicity of oxidation derivatives of cholesterol on cultured aortic smooth muscle cells and their effect on cholesterol biosynthesis. Am J Clin Nutr 1979; 32:1033-42.

254. Salonen JT, Ylä-herttuala S, Yamamoto R et al. Autoantibody against oxidized LDL and progression of carotid atherosclerosis. Lancet 1992; 339:883-6.

255. Steinberg D, Parthasarathy S, Carew TE et al. Beyond cholesterol. Modifications of low-density lipoprotein that increase its atherogenicity. N Engl J Med 1989; 320: 915-24.

256. Hoff HF, O'Neil J, Chisholm GM et al. Modicifation of low density lipoprotein with 4-hydroxynonenal induces uptake by macrophages. Arteriosclerosis 1989; 9: 538-49.

257. Witztum JL. Role of oxidized low density lipoprotein in atherogenesis. Br Heart J 1993; 69 Suppl:S12-8.

258. Regnström J, Nilsson J, Tornvall P et al. Susceptibility to low-density lipoprotein oxidation and coronary atherosclerosis in man. Lancet 1992; 339:1183-6.

259. DiMascio P, Murphy ME, Sies H. Antioxidant defense systems: The role of carotenoids, tocopherols, and thiols. Am J Clin Nutr 1991; 53:194S-205S.

260. Slyper AH. A fresh look at the atherogenic remnant hypothesis. Lancet 1992; 340:289-91.

261. Jeanrenaud B. Lipid components of adipose tissue In: Renold AE, Cahill GF, eds. Adipose Tissue, Section 5 in Handbook of Physiology. Washington: Am Physiol Soc, 1965: 169-76.

262. Hirsch J. Fatty acid patterns in human adipose tissue. In: Renold AE, Cahill GF, eds. Adipose Tissue, Section 5 in Handbook of Physiology. Washington: Am Physiol Soc, 1965: 181-9.

263. Gurr MI. Dietary lipids and coronary heart disease: old evidence, new perspective. Prog Lipid Res 1992; 31:195-243.

264. Holub BJ. Cholesterol-free foods: Where's the *trans*? Can Med Assoc J 1991; 144:330.

265. Enig MG. Status Report. *Trans* Fatty Acid Research Lipids Biochemistry Group. University of Maryland, 1987.

266. Mensinck RP, Katan MB. Effect of dietary *trans* fatty acids on high-density and low-density lipoprotein cholesterol levels in healthy subjects. N Engl J Med 1990; 323:439-445.

267. Sinclair HM. Deficiency of essential fatty acids and atherosclerosis. Lancet 1956; 1:381-3.

268. Kinsella JE, Bruckner G, Mai J et al. Metabolism of *trans* fatty acids with emphasis on the effects of *trans*, *trans*-octdecadienate on lipid composition, essential fatty acid, and prostaglandins: An overview. Am J Clin Nutr 1981; 34:2307-18.

269. Enig MG. Health and physiological effects of dietary *trans* fatty acids: A summary report from the University of Maryland Lipids Research Group. University of Maryland, 1988.

270. Hoak JC, Spector AA. Overview. Am J Clin Cutr 1992; 56:783S-4S.

271. Cliff WJ. Coronary heart disease: Animal fat on trial. Pathology 1987; 19:325-8.

272. Israel DH, Gorlin R. Fish oil in the prevention of atherosclerosis. J Am Coll Cardiol 1992; 19:174-85.

273. Nordøy A, Goodnight SH. Dietary lipids and thrombosis. Relationships to atherosclerosis. Arteriosclerosis 1990; 10:149-63.

274. Page IH, Stamler J. Diet and coronary heart disease. Med Concepts Cardiovasc Dis 1968; 37:119-23.

CHAPTER 6

RISK FACTORS, PREDICTION, CLINICAL TRIALS AND REGRESSION OF ATHEROSCLEROSIS

I t has been shown how the epidemiology of atherosclerosis is in reality the epidemiology of coronary heart disease (CHD) and reasons given why CHD and risk factors are inappropriate terms as currently used. Risk factors are essentially statistical associations with the incidence of CHD and no cause and effect relationship can be assumed. However CHD risk factors are equated with the causes of atherosclerosis. Other defects in the methodology have been mentioned and further deficiencies will be indicated.

RISK FACTORS

There are now in excess of 270 acknowledged CHD risk factors[1] and although most can have little or no bearing on the cause of atherosclerosis, some of the so-called major factors need to be discussed with due regard to the methodology and our present knowledge of the pathology of atherosclerosis.

For more than 30 years epidemiological studies have focused on the role of risk factors in the development of CHD and by extrapolation of atherosclerosis. It has been proposed that risk factors meet specific criteria before their acceptance as such but no risk factor meets all criteria and the "major" risk factors together do not explain the variance in incidence within or between populations.[2] All risk factors lose their predictive value in the elderly[1] and serum cholesterol, diabetes mellitus and psychosocial stress are not significant in unrecognized myocardial infarcts.[3] To account for inconsistencies in various studies and the variation in the level of the risk factors effective in different populations epidemiologists, rather than reviewing the premises on which their hypothesis rests as logic demands, have postulated the existence of as yet undiscovered risk factors.[2] Such rationalization reveals the will-o'-the-wisp nature of risk factor involvement whereby CHD is allegedly due to a variable mix of risk factors in any one individual—thus precluding verification or disproof of the contributory or causal role of any one factor.

Each observation should be reliable and accurate but the degree of disagreement between interviewers in determining the presence or absence of clinical symptoms (angina pectoris[4] intermittent claudication[5]), signs (blood pressure,[6] ankle pulses[7,8]), and electrocardiographic evidence of infarction or ischemia is of such magnitude that possibilities of error in determining risk factors cannot be regarded as inconsequential. The CHD epidemiologists use incidence of the risk factor in the respective populations or alternatively the average value according to the parameter assessed. The correct measurement should incorporate grade and duration of the desired parameter for comparison with the severity of atherosclerosis. Until it is possible to measure the severity of atherosclerosis during life, it is unlikely that the effect of aggravating diseases or the effect of therapy will be measured satisfactorily. Reliance on mean values for a population is an inherent weakness for there is no guarantee that within the group there is a correlation between the grade of risk factor and the grade of outcome. Dividing the population into quintiles does not overcome this ecological fallacy.

Sex

It is widely accepted that males develop severe coronary atherosclerosis at an earlier age than women possibly due to their greater physical activity, body size, mean heart size and heart weight. Consequently their coronary arteries have a larger diameter than those of females[9] and the larger the caliber the more severe atherosclerosis is likely to be. The difference in severity may be in part an independent expression of genetic or hormonal differences between the sexes and variation in physical activity.

McGill and Stern[10] declared it was not possible to extract a single unifying hypothesis to explain the sex difference in CHD and the effects of sex hormones on risk factors and disease. Serum lipid levels do not parallel the sex differences in incidence of CHD, nor do androgens or estrogens explain these discrepancies. Differences in established risk factors are not sufficiently great to explain the sex differences in the incidence of CHD or the severity of atherosclerosis. They concluded that factors other than conventional risk factors must be responsible and no consistent sex differences in experimental (cholesterol-induced) "atherosclerosis" have emerged from countless animal experiments.

Age

Atherosclerosis cannot be a function of the aging process since the severity of atherosclerosis varies from vascular bed to vascular bed. Certain vessels remain relatively unscathed, e.g. veins, and yet when they are subjected to augmented stress levels (coronary venous bypass grafts, arteriovenous shunts), atherosclerosis develops at an accelerated rate (Chapter 2). This indicates the importance of local hemodynamics and demonstrates that age is merely a time factor.

There is individual variability but in general the severity of atherosclerosis increases with age. Both age specific mortality rates and absolute mortality of CHD increase with age but most deaths from CHD and cerebrovascular disease (CVD) occur after 65 years (Fig. 1.1 and 1.2, Table 4.2). Most clinical studies have involved subjects under 55 years of age. As a consequence information on risk factors is relevant only to a young nonrepresentative minority who die of CHD. For example in the Report of the Inter-Society Commission for Heart Disease Resources,[11] a comparison was made of national CHD mortality rates and yet only male subjects aged 45 to 54 years were considered.

Hypercholesterolemia

Hypercholesterolemia is the dominant risk factor linked to excessive intake of dietary animal or saturated fats on the one hand and CHD on the other. Implicit in this concept is that hypercholesterolemia induces fat and cholesterol accumulation in the vessel wall, the hallmark of atherosclerosis.[12] The fallacies of these concepts and the reasons for not accepting such hypotheses have been indicated in earlier chapters together with reasons for not altering the conventional statistical method of determining discrimination values. However other aspects of this possible relationship should be considered.

Overall the total serum cholesterol is said to have a weak relationship with CHD[13] and none with sudden cardiac death or unrecognized infarcts.[3] In Framingham[14] the risk varies at any level of cholesterol according to the presence of other contributing risk factors, thus implying partial dependency on other risk factors. Serum cholesterol levels in affluent countries in which CHD is prevalent increase with age at least to the age of 55 years when the concentration levels off and declines slightly in the male (Fig. 5.2). In the age group usually considered in clinical studies (20 to 55 years), this elevation with age appears to be true.[12,15] In the Pooling Project[16] the risk of CHD increased with age for each quintile of serum cholesterol. It is therefore possible that the increase in CHD with serum cholesterol in clinical studies[17] may be due to age though inclusion of subjects with familial hypercholesterolemia (FH) would contribute to this relationship. Keys and Fidanze[18] found that subjects with CHD had higher body weight than control subjects.

Mathur et al[19] compared serum cholesterol levels with the severity of aortic, coronary and cerebral atherosclerosis in a series of medicolegal autopsies in which death was not sudden and no organic disease was evident at necropsy. A statistically significant association between serum cholesterol level and age was found and also between the severity of atherosclerosis and age but statistical analyses failed to reveal a correlation between the serum cholesterol level and the severity of atherosclerosis when age was taken into account. A similar lack of correlation between serum cholesterol and the severity of atherosclerosis or low correlation coefficients has been reported by others.[20-23]

HYPERTENSION

In a population sample, blood pressure (systolic, diastolic and pulse) increased with age[24] more so in some individuals than in others. The aggravating effect of hypertension on atherosclerosis is established on pathological grounds and increased systolic, pulse and diastolic pressures have all been incriminated as risk factors for CHD and particularly for CHD. Hypertension has been regarded as a stronger factor than serum cholesterol[17] and a progressively increasing risk of CHD with increasing systolic and diastolic pressures and age has been reported.[25] Since hypertension affects the vessel wall over time the correct correlation to be sought should be the severity and duration of the hypertension with the severity of atherosclerosis. However using the current epidemiological methods there is a positive association between hypertension and elevated serum cholesterol levels,[26] diabetes mellitus and body weight or obesity[27] and serum cholesterol levels tend to fall following some forms of antihypertensive therapy.[28]

BODY BUILD AND OBESITY

Methods of determining obesity lack precision and appropriate criteria and the pathological relationship to atherosclerosis is not clear. Body weight according to age and height is an unsatisfactory criterion because it fails to differentiate between obesity per se and muscle mass or body build. Carrying excess fat (ballast-effect) increases the cardiac workload and secondarily the coronary artery workload. Muscle bulk and a large body build will also contribute to cardiac and coronary arterial workload and blood vessels in skeletal musculature are larger in caliber and require more blood. Theoretically both muscle bulk and obesity could contribute to coronary atherosclerosis by affecting hemodynamic parameters in this way.

An increased risk of CHD for high relative weight for men in their forties has been reported[16] and also a correlation between (i) CHD and obesity, (ii) high blood pressure and obesity, (iii) serum cholesterol levels and obesity and (iv) body build with serum cholesterol and CHD.[26] Weight increase occurs with age[29] and a hereditary factor is believed to affect each of the above relationships.

In Framingham weight gain after the young adult years was reported to convey an increased risk of CHD.[30] This stepwise increase in CHD with increasing weight has been demonstrated by others. Body weight is also associated with other risk factors, e.g., hypertension, hypercholesterolemia, low levels of HDL cholesterol, smoking, hypertriglyceridemia and elevated plasma glucose levels.[27,31,32] Roberts[33] considered obesity, smoking and blood pressure were all interrelated. In all age-sex groups, blood pressure correlates with the average weight and by 65 years of age 40 to 45% of the population is hypertensive.[34]

DIABETES MELLITUS

On pathological grounds diabetes mellitus is recognized as an aggravating factor of atherosclerosis. It is not surprising that a disorder affecting carbohydrate and lipid metabolism of every cell in the body enhances bacterial and mycotic infections and aggravates atherosclerosis. However diabetics also have a tendency to hypercholesterolemia which is not as profound as in preinsulin days when lipid storage in blood vessels and extravascular tissues was frequent in those on a therapeutic high fat diet.

There may be incipient diabetes amongst any clinical group although not all abnormal glucose tolerance tests are due to diabetes. An association between CHD and diabetes mellitus and diminished glucose tolerance without frank diabetes has been recognized.[26] There is also a tendency for glucose tolerance to worsen with age. Both hypertension and diabetes mellitus are age dependent and aggravate the severity of atherosclerosis, thereby enhancing the chance of developing CVD, CHD or peripheral vascular disease (PVD) clinically. An integral relationship exists between abnormalities of insulin and glucose metabolism and the etiology and clinical course of hypertension[35] and several antihypertensive drugs adversely affect glucose, insulin and lipid metabolism.

GENETIC FACTORS AND SMOKING

A familial tendency to the complications of severe atherosclerosis has been long recognized clinically and basic biochemical metabolic pathways are no doubt genetically determined. These in turn will affect the response of vascular connective tissue to mechanical stresses in atherogenesis and other biochemical pathways. Genetic factors appear to determine blood cholesterol, blood pressure, blood sugar levels,[26] body build and possibly obesity. Familial hypercholesterolemia (FH) and hereditary connective tissue disorders either complicate or aggravate respectively the effects of atherosclerosis and no doubt subclinical phenotypes or variants of these disorders exist.

After studying twins Lundman[36] concluded from post-exercise electrocardiography that smoking probably had little or no effect on CHD and that a significant genetic component was evident. Monozygotic twin studies have revealed a strong hereditary impact and the possibility that CHD in smokers may be largely due to constitutional differences between smokers and nonsmokers rather than to smoking per se. Smokers and nonsmokers tend to be "self-selected" groups.

The role of smoking in CHD and atherosclerosis, if any, is obscure. There is no evidence that smoking has an effect on the severity of atherosclerosis, although if such a relationship exists it may be due to interference with amino acid cross-linking of elastin, thereby reducing its tensile strength.[37] The association is between smoking and CHD with all the deficiencies in such epidemiological methodology. Nevertheless there is the possibility that pharmacological agents absorbed by smokers may affect cardiac irritability in patients with moderate to severe coronary atherosclerosis thereby precipitating sudden fatal dysrhythmias. There is no conclusive evidence of a deleterious effect on atherosclerosis and smoking is not a risk factor for CVD.[38] Furthermore no controlled trial has specifically tested the effect of smoking on CHD.

Factors that appear to have a familial tendency are always a problem because of difficulty in differentiating between inherited genetic factors and inherited environment. Inherited psychosocial stresses and personality type appear to be important[39-41] in atherogenesis with hemodynamic responses to these stresses secondarily influencing disease development.

AGE DEPENDENCE

It has been shown previously that in the young age group (under 40 to 55 years) usually investigated a bias will result due to an unduly high representation of FH in clinical studies because heterozygotes have a high incidence of CHD before the age of 50 especially in males (Table 2.1). This has resulted in the oft repeated observation that hypercholesterolemia is particularly frequent in the young age group and is more common than in older subjects with CHD. It has also been suggested and seems to be so that those with CHD in the young age group could well constitute a separate entity.

In this young age group usually studied the blood cholesterol levels in males increase with age as do hypertension, diabetes mellitus and obesity. These four risk factors are genetically dependent and in some way inextricably interrelated one with another. It is also accepted on pathological grounds that hypertension and diabetes mellitus aggravate atherosclerosis and that atherosclerosis and CHD are also age dependent and probably genetically dependent. Under the circumstances it is highly unlikely that it is possible to determine the independent relationship of serum cholesterol levels to CHD and certainly not to atherosclerosis.[42] The age dependence of all these variables has been overlooked and providing numbers are sufficient, by dividing a study population into quintiles and again using averages, it is inevitable that the age relationship will become manifest. Their importance as risk factors could therefore be exaggerated without their having such a profound effect on the majority of CHD deaths over 80% of which occur after 65 years of age.

It has been estimated that to differentiate the causal effect of three independent variables a population of upwards of 8000 is required,[33] but more would be required to differentiate the role of the above four risk factors if it is at all possible. Multivariate statistical analyses were introduced to differentiate between the effects of multiple risk factors but the mutual interrelationship of the above four risk factors, their genetic and age dependence and the bias due to inclusion of FH would all have to be taken into account irrespective of other methodological fallacies. These are the conditions which Cochrane[43] would consider to be beyond the power of elaborate analyses to overcome. Statistics cannot launder this type of data and the selection bias by virtue of the age group used introduces bias with the FH element and precludes determination of the role of the blood cholesterol level in CHD and also in atherosclerosis.

PREDICTIVE VALUE OF RISK FACTORS

The reader is reminded of some basic facts. It has been shown why risk factors for CHD are irrelevant to the etiology of atherosclerosis and why both risk factors and CHD are inappropriate terms for the purposes for which they are used. Risk factors are essentially statistical associations with the incidence of CHD and no causal relationship can be assumed either with CHD or atherosclerosis. Despite this, risk factor is used synonymously with cause and CHD is equated with atherosclerosis, so that in studies of regression or prevention, it is risk factor modification that is instituted and the endpoint sought is usually CHD.

Risk factors for CHD were originally sought in attempts to determine the environmental factors responsible for the alleged epidemic of CHD and in the hope that risk factor modification might relieve the epidemic. However these factors have lost their actuarial significance and instead have become deeply entrenched in modern medicine to the extent that pathology is expected to explain such risk factors, as if a causal relationship had been demonstrated. Seeking so-called "risk factors" for CHD is basically illogical. Factors related to the initiation of atherosclerosis should be sought rather than those related to one of the nonpathognomonic complications of end-stage atherosclerosis, unless a different aim is instituted, that of seeking aggravating factors. Kannel[44] considered the assessment of risk factors inefficient and possibly misleading and I concur with his conclusions. In view of the fallacious nature and questionable validity of much of the contradictory data pertaining to risk factors because of diagnostic errors, misuse of the term and the inapplicability to atherosclerosis, reevaluation of current usage of the concept of "risk factors" as applied to atherosclerosis and CHD and also of past data in the same vein is essential. The usage and indeed misusage indicate the need for the term "risk factor" to be abandoned and such factors, if of any biological significance, should be designated according to their true role in the pathogenesis of atherosclerosis.[45] One aim of epidemiology is to reduce the morbidity and mortality of CHD and this is dependent on the ability to identify persons likely to develop CHD. Inherent in this risk factor concept is that there is a high predictive value of risk factors. It has become increasingly apparent that the predictive capacity is low. This weakness has been circumvented by the staunch defense of the population-wide strategy in the treatment of high blood cholesterol levels rather than initially treating only those with hypercholesterolemia. It has been indicated that prediction is no more precise than offering a one in six chance of a hitherto healthy man developing CHD within five years if he is at high risk. Prediction within a high risk group usually produces more incorrect forecasts than correct ones.[46] Smith[23] contends one can guess with greater accuracy than can be predicted by cholesterol levels. From pathology alone certain characteristics (middle and old age, male sex, hypertension, diabetes mellitus) are associated with a particular propensity for individuals to develop severe atherosclerosis and CHD, CVD and PVD. From mortality rates for the USA, almost half the population will die of CHD or CVD and as middle age advances the likelihood increases. Just from this information, it can be predicted that any male 55 to 65 years of age has a 50% chance of developing severe but nonfatal atherosclerosis with the likelihood being even greater in the presence of hypertension or diabetes mellitus.

Most emphasis has been on serum cholesterol estimation though the associated predictive value is controversial and many authors are unaware of the serious misrepresentation of the arterial pathology of FH which probably also includes familial defective apolipoprotein B-100 (FDB). These particular subjects are likely to die prematurely even if they are heterozygotes and a high proportion will have manifested clinical CHD by the age of 50 years (Table 2.1). Their CHD and deaths cannot be attributed to atherosclerosis and can be predicted more accurately but these subjects should be dealt with in special categories rather than in studies of atherosclerosis.

Prediction in normolipidemic subjects is much more difficult. Even without excluding lipid dystrophies, epidemiologists have demonstrated little ability to predict the clinical future of any one patient[47,48] or to indicate which subjects are likely to benefit from a blood cholesterol-lowering regime.[49] Kannel[44] stated that the major identified risk factors, even taken together, do not appear to explain entirely the variance in incidence either within or between these populations.

CHD risk factors do not have the same "significance of noxiousness" in different populations and risk factors fail to explain the variable CHD incidence in various ethnic groups.[50] Oliver,[5] after reviewing the "singularly disappointing" results of clinical intervention trials, attributed the major problem in CHD prevention to the low sensitivity and specificity of identifying individuals at risk. Moreover he doubted a graded relationship between CHD and serum cholesterol and Rose[48] believed the

great overlap in serum cholesterol levels between the Framingham male subjects (aged 30 to 62 years) who did or did not have CHD explains the poor predictive value in either sex over 50 years of age. Reference to Table 4.2 and Figures 1.1 and 1.2 reveals how few CHD victims of either sex are under 50 years of age. It is not surprising therefore that prediction is poor if extrapolations are made from the small nonrepresentative minority to the population at large. This minority will contain an unduly high proportion of FH subjects. Blood cholesterol alone is a poor predictor of British middle-aged males developing CHD in the next few years. It is less than in the USA, even though UK men have higher blood cholesterol levels on average than men in the USA.[53] Oliver[54] estimated that only one in seven (14.3%) coronary deaths in the UK between the ages of 45 and 54 years is associated with pronounced hypercholesterolemia though 35% of all deaths in this age group are due to CHD. Even so this indicates a disproportionately high incidence of hypercholesterolemia since FH has an incidence of only 0.2% and FDB 0.14% in the community, suggesting bias in the population because of the age selected.

In an editorial in 1977 it was stated, "If we take 100 men with the three major risk markers (smoking, hypertension, and raised serum cholesterol), only eight develop clinical manifestations of CHD over the next 10 years, while 92 do not; conversely, most previously fit patients who developed CHD while under observation in the Seattle "heart-watch" program had no conventional risk factors on entry. We must therefore realize that risk factors cannot be causal and that they have very poor predictive value".[55]

Jenkins[56] declared that most patients with CHD do not have blood cholesterol levels above 250 mg/dL, only a fraction are hypertensive and fewer are diabetic, whereas the simultaneous occurrence of two or three risk factors predicts only a small minority of CHD cases. Meade and Chakrabarti[46] concluded that the major risk factors predicted only one chance in six of a healthy man developing CHD within five years, and one in three or four of developing CHD within 10 years. Whyte[49] estimated that if 100 men who are nonsmokers with normal blood pressure and electrocardiograms lower their plasma cholesterol from 310 to 260 mg/

dL starting at 35 years of age, six could potentially benefit by avoiding a coronary incident, 94 would be likely to follow the regimen without apparent benefit, and eight of those would have an attack within 20 years despite adherence to the regimen. The potential benefit is less for women and for those who start the regimen at an older age.

Heller et al[57] reported that of middle-aged men in the top 15% of risk, only 7% of those initially free of CHD and 22% of those initially with CHD would actually develop myocardial infarction in the subsequent five years. Oliver[51] asserts that there is a significantly greater risk of CHD only in men whose serum cholesterol is in the top quintile of distribution and even so the actual risk there ranges from 7-17% which means that about 80% of these people would have to be treated unnecessarily. He estimated that two-thirds of healthy males (40 to 55 years old) with serum cholesterol values and blood pressure above the 80th percentile (excluding FH) will remain fit over the subsequent 25 years. From the Pooling Project[16] only 15% of those in the top quintile of blood cholesterol levels between the ages of 40 to 59 will develop CHD over the next 8.6 years and over a 25-year span only one-third of such high risk men (aged 40 to 64 years) will develop CHD. In some studies the risk was even lower.[58]

Taylor et al[59] calculated from existing data derived from clinical trials that persons aged 20 to 60 years at low risk will gain three days to three months of life respectively from a lifelong cholesterol reduction program. For those at high risk a gain of 18 days to 12 months can be expected assuming that cholesterol reduction is effective and safe in reducing the risk of CHD. However the safety of long-term reduction in serum cholesterol is presently unknown.

It is not solely serum cholesterol which is of low predictive value and risk factors alone or together cannot account for more than 25% of the "explanation" for raised lesions in the coronary arteries at autopsy[60] nor for more than a fraction of the striking age trend in the incidence of atherosclerosis.[61] Currently such aspects as chance, the inaccuracies of measurement and diagnosis and the weak and interrelated associations make appraisal of individual risk weak, inaccurate and misassessed.[46,48]

Kannel[44] considered risk factors could be used to identify "vulnerable segments of almost any population" but apparently not individuals within the population. Again the risk factors were regarded as atherogenic even though the correlations were with clinical CHD (Fig. 2.2). The realization that risk factors apply more to the population or parts thereof than to the individual has eventually resulted in the classification of CHD as a mass disease. Rose[48] said the commonest cause of death in a western man with the lowest levels of coronary risk factors was by far CHD and that everyone is a high-risk individual because it is a uniquely mass disease. However Kannel[44] contends that "evidence incriminating diet within free-living general populations continues to be elusive".

Rose[48] declared that it was almost impossible to demonstrate any relation between an individual's diet and his serum cholesterol and yet easy to show a strong association between population mean values for saturated fat intake and the serum cholesterol level and CHD incidence. Though he was convinced that dietary fat determined the CHD incidence, he acknowledged that it was nigh impossible to identify high-risk individuals. Now Marmot[62] suggests that the determinants for individual risks of disease may differ from the determinants of population risks! This assertion inevitably led to the concept that "risk characteristics for CVD are mass phenomena, and therefore require mass preventative approaches".[63]

Such convoluted reasoning is surely another example of the ecological fallacy. The belief is that because the application of the ecological correlation of dietary fat and serum cholesterol with CHD mortality does not accurately predict the development of CHD in the individual, prevention must be applied to the entire population rather than to those at greatest risk. Despite the strong negative association in the individuals within the "sick populations" Rose,[48] like others, fails to consider the possibility that the ecological correlations may be invalid and their lack of applicability at the individual level certainly suggests this is the case. The new dictum has it that each individual is expected to comply with the edicts of the lipid protagonists despite their acceptance that the changes in lifestyle may have no or minimal effect on most individuals.[64] This line of reasoning cannot be reconciled with the pathology of atherosclerosis. Alteration of my serum cholesterol level will not affect my neighbors' blood cholesterol levels or that of those in distant cities. If determinants or risk factors for CHD for the population differ from those in the individual,[63] then lipid propoganists must not only define the nature of these determinants but explain them in pathological and epidemiological terms. The only disorder which I can conceive of which would affect a population whereby the activities of one individual can affect or "infect" neighbors and populations at a distance is irrationality. Is it also supposed to follow that if the population or mass dietary strategy fails to reduce CHD mortality, those who failed to reduce their blood cholesterol levels by the required amount will be held responsible for the specified number of deaths?

According to Tunstall-Pedoe[65] data on risk factors have in the past been misrepresented, abused or presented in such a way as to enhance their apparent importance. It has been the presence or absence of the risk factor rather than the level, grade and duration of "exposure" that was considered. Fluctuating blood cholesterol levels, labile blood pressures and subclinical glucose intolerance compound the difficulties. In a review of factors relevant to low prevalence of CHD in population groups throughout the world, no consistent pattern for any of the currently popular "risk factors" or combinations of them has been found.[66] No one has yet established a convincing fit of trends for any risk factor with cardiovascular mortality trends.[51]

In view of the poor scientific basis of knowledge of "risk factors" for CVD, their poor predictive power and numerous inconsistencies, and the assumed causality associated with use of the term, cessation of the use of this risk concept is desirable. Preferable would be the use of such terms as aggravating, conditional or predisposing factors etc., which provide a more accurate indication of their specific roles in atherogenesis. Mensuration and mathematical analysis of the effect of natural phenomena (such as risk factors) are fraught with great difficulty and unless performed accurately and precisely, results are worthless and misleading. To admit weaknesses and then to allege strengths and

value of some of the data derived from investigations based on the methodology used by CHD epidemiologists is wishful thinking and the results never validate the methodology. To ignore even minor weaknesses only serves to perpetuate error and misrepresentation and the errors are far from minor.

CLINICAL TRIALS

The alleged epidemic and its supposed decline in many western countries led to the belief that CHD can be prevented. This belief was supposedly supported by observations on cholesterol-overfeeding of susceptible animals. It was stated that the lipid content of their vascular lesions could regress after the return of these animals to a normal stock diet.[67,68] Considerable fibrosis and some calcification resulted—a finding confirmed by others with Armstrong et al[69] reporting greater but unconfirmed success with Rhesus monkeys. However, in regression studies of atherosclerosis the criteria by which regression of the process is said to be judged must be specified, the one obvious prerequisite being that the lesion is indeed atherosclerotic. It has been shown that the experimental dietary-induced lesions represent fat-storage lesions and not atherosclerosis (Chapter 2). Likewise the xanthomatous lesions of FH (and probably FDB) are not atherosclerotic although combined lesions may coexist and some trials have a mixture of dyslipidemic and normolipidemic subjects. This subject mix invalidates the results since the object of the trials is to test the thesis that atherosclerosis can be reversed. Reduction in dietary fat and of serum cholesterol levels in such subjects may reduce the lipid content of arterial lesions, as can occur with skin xanthomata[70] and thereby may enlarge the lumen but whether or not lipid depletion of atherosclerosis in normolipemic subjects is possible and beneficial is unknown. Furthermore lipid depletion from atherosclerotic vessels is not necessarily indicative of regression of atherosclerosis. Though continuous depletion of lipid from the vessel wall is likely, the rate of depletion must at some time be slowed and possibly retarded given the evidence of impaired phagocytic activity in atherosclerosis.

In a number of clinical trials only dyslipidemic subjects have been used and this is acceptable since these unfortunate subjects obviously require treatment. Of concern is that two subjects with FH under probucol therapy[71] to lower their blood cholesterol levels had a diminution in visible xanthomatous infiltrations with the appearance of nonmacrophage lipid storage in nontraditional sites for xanthoma. The effect of the therapy on the vascular lesions was not known. In any event the vascular changes that occur in dyslipidemic subjects are not relevant to atherosclerosis.

Regression of atherosclerosis implies reversal of the pathogenesis. Many who speak of regression seem to be unfamiliar with its pathology for atherosclerosis appears to be inexorably and insidiously progressive although the rate may be slow. To the pathologist familiar with the gross architectural disruption of the vessel wall in atherosclerosis, it is difficult to conceive of significant regression or reversal of the degenerative changes characteristic of the disease. Some resorption of lipid and minerals, lysis and organization of mural thrombus and repair of ulcers or intimal tears might occur but regeneration, reversal and reorganization of the cellular and noncellular connective tissues are likely to be limited. Even a simple tear in the internal elastic lamina is not repaired or restored to its original appearance and there is no evidence that intimal proliferation at the ostia of branches ever disappears.

In biological repair of most tissues, excessive proliferation occurs initially and precedes a phase of regression to a more normal appearance with minimal scarring. This sequence is also seen with minimal arterial injuries in which the initial intimal thickening diminishes and condenses to form a thinner scar[72] with enlargement of the lumen though minimal. Dissection of the internal elastic lamina of a cerebral artery in an infant was not followed by restoration of the elastic lamina even after many years.[73] Destructive lesions of arteries, whether traumatic or inflammatory, are followed by healing and scarring and possibly some calcification but there is no evidence of any attempt to restore the artery to its original architecture. Since all neonates have intimal thickenings in the aorta and at branchings of distributing arteries which are considered early changes of atherosclerosis and compensatory in nature due to elastolysis and

medial thinning, inhibition of muscle proliferation is unlikely to be beneficial. There is no evidence that it can regress. Development of intimal proliferation in the rat aorta[74] similar to that in the human neonate,[75] occurs with aging and in hypertension and is diminished by hypotensive therapy.[74] Whilst this supports the concept that the proliferation is of hemodynamic origin it is unlikely that hypocholesterolemic therapy will do likewise because the blood cholesterol levels in the fetus are at their lowest levels likely to be attained during life. Freshly developed immature repair tissue could be even more susceptible to the stresses that caused the tear than neighboring mature intact tissue. There is also evidence that the acquired fragility that characterizes atherosclerosis is cumulative and not progressive as seen in the poststenotic dilatation, in the aneurysm on the afferent arteries of arteriovenous fistulas and in the vascular changes of vibrating tool disease.

Enlargement of the lumen or smoothing the contours of the luminal silhouette in response to augmented flow-induced stresses initiated by surface irregularities may be functionally beneficial but angiographic evidence of an enlarged lumen or a slightly improved average longevity of a group is not an infallible indicator of regression of atherosclerosis. Until it is possible to assess the severity of atherosclerosis in vivo, it will be difficult to determine the efficacy of therapy. Variation of the rate of progression is a possibility which will require pathological evidence (macroscopic, histological, ultrastructural and biochemical) from spontaneous or experimentally induced true atherosclerosis in lower animals. However there is no agreement on what parameter is the best criterion for progression or regression of the disease. In general, morphology is a crude means of assessing the functional state of tissues. Assessment of the physicochemical state or tensile strength of the vessel wall is the parameter requiring accurate assessment. This cannot be performed satisfactorily at present during life and the condition of one vessel probably has limited bearing on that of other vessels.

It has been widely held that the relationship between plasma cholesterol and CHD is continuous, graded and without a threshold.[76,79] Kannel et al[78] said, "atheromas are encountered throughout the range of lipids" and that virtually everyone in the U.S.A. appears to have sufficient circulating lipid to produce atheroma. The concept that lowering blood cholesterol causes regression of atherosclerosis is a contradiction of this no-threshold concept.[79] Repair no doubt can occur at all blood cholesterol levels, and lipid protagonists consider CHD and progression also occur at all blood cholesterol levels. It is therefore difficult to accept that a reduction of blood cholesterol will induce regression, particularly since atherosclerosis commences early in life and progresses when blood cholesterol levels are at their lowest. Moreover in clinical trials it is alleged that regression can occur at almost any cholesterol level (136 to 270 mg/dL) encompassing about 90% of all cholesterol levels in the human race[79] despite the absence of a discrimination level below which atherosclerosis does not progress. It is inconceivable that serum cholesterol levels can play such an important causative role in the progression of atherosclerosis over the range of blood cholesterol levels at which it also induces regression. In view of the inadequacy of the angiographic evidence that true regression occurs and because of the pathological evidence of the inability of the vessel wall to regenerate and for pathological changes to regress as distinct from repair, it is most likely that atherosclerosis cannot regress.

How reduction of blood cholesterol levels could achieve regression has never been explained but implicit in the concept is that cholesterol must be the dominant factor in initiating the disease and inducing the gamut of degenerative changes in the cellular and noncellular constituents of the vessel wall in atherogenesis. In contradiction to this hypothesis is the basic and incontrovertible fact that cholesterol-feeding in animals and homozygous FH does not reproduce atherosclerosis, its pathogenesis or complications.

Roussouw et al[80] alleged that reduction of the blood cholesterol level by 10% can be expected to reduce the rate of nonfatal reinfarction by 19% and of fatal myocardial infarction by 12%. More clear cut evidence of the benefit of lowering serum cholesterol levels is said to be found in secondary prevention studies[80,81] even though the alarmingly high death rate from noncoronary events tended to balance this. Less concern was expressed for noncoronary deaths but the total death rate is not subject to diagnostic error. In the light of the foregoing they have to explain the mechanism of the alleged prevention of myocardial infarction in pathological terms.

Many clinical trials have been instigated in the anticipation that reduction of dietary intake of animal saturated fat and cholesterol would result in regression of atherosclerosis and so prevent CHD or the recurrence of an acute clinical episode in end-stage disease or alternatively produce beneficial changes in the arteries studied angiographically. These trials have evoked criticisms, whilst other authors consider the lipid hypothesis is proven beyond all reasonable doubt. Though it is not possible here to review in detail all clinical trials, the purpose is to appraise the methodology and the results of some recent trials. Weaknesses and deficiencies in the epidemiological approach (already discussed) are applicable to these clinical trials viz.

(i) Misuse of the term CHD as a marker or endpoint of severe atherosclerosis rather than grading the severity of atherosclerosis.

(ii) Failure to exclude nonatherosclerotic causes of CHD particularly dyslipidemias, e.g., FH, FDB, type III hyperlipoproteinemia.

(iii) The diagnostic error in CHD is unquantifiable but greater than differences in incidence of CHD between the groups—an aspect not allowed for in any of the statistical analyses.

(iv) The extreme variability in individual life styles, environment and dietary and culinary habits over a life time would be unacceptable in animal experimentation where dietary or pharmacological effects are assessed over a comparatively short time span under rigidly controlled conditions usually in only small numbers of subjects.

(v) The mean reduction in cholesterol is often less than the methodological error of the possible analyses.

(vi) Implausibility of the basic hypothesis due to misrepresentation of the pathology of the cholesterol-fed animal and of FH (Chapter 2).

(vii) Extrapolation from CHD to atherosclerosis is invalid.

(viii) Inappropriate choice of study subjects on the basis of sex, age and selection bias for inclusion of FH.

Reviewers, even including lipid protagonists, consider that most primary and secondary clinical prevention trials prior to 1984 are inclusive or that they fail to satisfactorily support the hypothesis that a reduction in blood cholesterol lowers the CHD mortality rate. The factors responsible include design flaws, inadequate cholesterol reduction, unsatisfactory statistical analysis or inconclusive results.[25,51,82-86] Pooling of results from multiple center trials can mask a significant finding (positive or negative) because of variation in quality of the investigation and the diagnostic error pertaining in different centers. Moreover the use of "person-years of experience"[16] under surveillance can also dilute significant findings by the incorporation of too many short-term studies.

Some trials have been considered either suggestive or even promising[85,87-89] but nevertheless inconclusive. A 1972 *Lancet* editorial[90] declared the results of primary or secondary prevention trials of CHD had been particularly disappointing. In 1974 Kannel[91] contended there was no confirmed efficacy of lowering blood lipids. Werkö[83] in 1976 analyzed three epidemiological investigations indicating inadequacies and differences between the trial subjects and the populations, inconsistencies in reporting data, and lack of information on therapy administered to subjects who were overweight or hypertensive. Despite allegations of the importance of cholesterol in CHD, hypertension and smoking were more important than hyperlipidemia in the development of CHD. Olson[92] reviewed 11 large scale dietary trials of the lipid hypothesis in various countries over two to ten years and three hypocholesterolemic drug trials. In none did he find a positive effect of high polyunsaturated fat, low saturated fat or low cholesterol diets on mortality. Levy[89] discussed 18 trials between 1955 and 1980 designed to determine the effect of lowering serum cholesterol. In most it was possible to reduce the cholesterol by 10-15% with diet alone but analyzed individually, none demonstrated significant difference in heart deaths or heart attacks. The individual benefit of a group reduction in serum cholesterol level of 10 to 15% must be questioned and covariance of serum cholesterol and the clinical or preferably pathological benefit must be demonstrated for the study to be meaningful.

Levy[89] considered a decrease of only 10-15% in serum cholesterol in a human trial makes it difficult to demonstrate a treatment benefit in man but this may reflect poor correlation between diet and serum cholesterol as previously indicated. Levy was critical of other trials believing some results were suggestive but inconclusive. Pooling dyslipidemic subjects with other CHD patients causes bias in the experimental design of clinical trials if the aim is to determine the cause and management of atherosclerosis. The exclusion of females from many trials rouses suspicion and the expensive Lipid Research Clinics Coronary Primary Prevention Trial (LRCC PPT)[87,88] was to provide the crucial answer. In all, 3806 asymptomatic middle-aged men 35 to 59 years of age) with primary hypercholesterolemia (type II hyperlipoproteinemia) and serum cholesterol levels 265 mg/dL or greater (95th percentile) were subjected to a moderate cholesterol-lowering diet. The mean serum cholesterol level was 292 mg/dL. The randomly chosen treatment group received cholestyramine and controls received a placebo for seven to ten years. In view of the unpalatability of and digestive upsets associated with cholestyramine medication, whether or not the study was truly blind is doubtful. The total cholesterol level of the cholestyramine group fell to 239 mg/dL at the end of the first year but was 257 mg/dL at year seven, whilst the placebo group was 275 mg/dL at year one and 277 mg/dL at year seven. Most of the fall was in the LDL fraction. As well as suggestive evidence of adaptation in the cholestyramine group, the mean total cholesterol level was only 7.2% lower than the control group at the end of the study despite the fact that this difference is within the possible range of technological, individual, diurnal and seasonal variability.

The alleged reduction in "definite" CHD mortality after seven years was small, there being 30 in the cholestyramine group (1.6%) and 38 in the placebo group (2.0%). There were 158 "definite" nonfatal infarcts in the placebo group (8.3%) and 130 in the cholestyramine group (6.8%). The results were interpreted as demonstrating a percentage reduction in risk of 19%, but such a calculation is misleading being widely misunderstood in the literature. The results were considered significant statistically (using a one-tailed test) but the application of statistics does not indicate that this very expensive investigation produced supportive evidence that a reduction in blood cholesterol significantly reduces the incidence of CHD and by their extrapolation, the severity of atherosclerosis. Using the two-tailed test, considered essential in such a trial,[93-95] the results were not statistically significant.[84] Even so, the lack of reliability of the clinical diagnosis of CHD in the absence of difference in overall mortality between the two groups, the high frequency of asymptomatic CHD, the variation in diagnostic accuracy in the 12 centers participating in the trial and misuse of clinical CHD as a surrogate monitor placed the results beyond the limits of scientific acceptability. Even without considering diagnostic error, Kronmal[94] was critical of the statistical analysis and regarded any relationship of serum cholesterol to CHD in the study to be weak. This study did not apply to women in whom the incidence of CHD is less than for males and he considered that the long-term benefits in women may well have been different. Moreover the subjects were suffering from primary hypercholesterolemia and FH and FDB which are probably the commonest human genetic disorders responsible and thus the trial result cannot be said to have bearing on atherosclerosis. Yet dietary recommendations for the entire population (male and female) were based on the results of this trial which Simons[96] regarded as the nearest proof likely to be obtained for the lipid hypothesis which he considered proven!

The incidence of noncoronary deaths was higher in the experimental group, the possible significance of this statistic being discussed later. What is certain however is that the trial did not prove that those below the 95th percentile of serum cholesterol, or those not suffering from primary hypercholesterolemia, are likely to derive benefit from a cholesterol lowering regime[97] and there was no reduction in overall mortality in the cholestyramine-treated group. In a six year follow-up of the trial there was no conclusive evidence of benefit,[98] the overall mortality was not significantly different in the two groups although there was a nonsignificant increase in malignancies in the cholestyramine treated group.

The Helsinki Heart Study[99] was a double blind trial involving 4081 asymptomatic dyslipidemic men (40 to 55 years of age). The total number of cardiac endpoints was 27.3 per 1000 (gemfibrozil-treated) and 41.4 per 1000 for the placebo group, the differences being regarded as significant though no allowance was made for the maldiagnostic error. There was no statistically significant difference in total mortality or specific cause of death. The results are inapplicable to the general population because the men were dyslipidemic and in a restricted age group and no women were included.

More recently Strandberg et al[100] reported that five years after the end of the Multifactorial Primary Prevention Trial, there were 67 deaths in the intervention group since the commencement of the trial and only 46 in the control group. These deaths consisted of 34 and 14 cardiac deaths, 2 and 4 due to other cardiovascular diseases (not significant), 13 and 21 deaths due to cancer and 13 and 1 deaths due to violence respectively. The authors concluded that the results could not necessarily jeopardize the prevention strategy by lowering blood cholesterol levels but considered more careful selection of subjects was required. We must concur with this view. The authors indicated that the trial must be considered in the light of all the available data and that it is difficult to match two groups of human subjects in every respect. This of course applies to every clinical trial but rationalization is incongruous when the bias for inclusion of FH subjects is recognized.

Miettinen et al[101] reported on a five-year multifactorial prevention trial and despite markedly improved risk-factor status, CHD incidence was higher in the treated group, though stroke incidence was decreased.

Wilson et al[102] allege that if the total fat intake was lowered to 35% and the saturated fat lowered to 15% of the energy intake, and dietary cholesterol maintained below 300 mg/day, mean cholesterol levels could fall by about 6% to 10% and CHD mortality diminish by up to 31%. Although opinions differ, it is apparent that the benefits of such therapy even with more powerful hypolipidemic drugs have not yet been realized. Cobbe and Shepherd[103] reviewed 22 randomized clinical trials of dietary and hypolipidemic drug therapy and concluded that there was a reduction in risk of myocardial infarction and coronary death but that there was also a parallel increase in noncoronary mortality that offset the beneficial effects on coronary mortality. However the important issue is that no change in mortality has yet been demonstrated as the result of the hypocholesterolemic regimen. In view of the substantial diagnostic error for CHD and its syndromes,[104] the absence of autopsy verification of the causes of death, the inclusion of FH in the series and other methodological faults, the trials have been in vain. Since many lipid protagonists allege that CHD is preventable, it is important to know whether this also applies to subjects with FH, FDB, type III hyperlipoproteinemia and nonlipid metabolic disorders associated with CHD. By pooling all cases of CHD the effect of therapy on these dyslipidemic subjects is masked.

Holme[105] concluded from a meta-analysis of trials that there was a beneficial effect of cholesterol lowering programs on nonfatal and fatal CHD events combined although the reductions in plasma cholesterol were alleged to be too low to have an effect on mortality. The most prominent and extensive meta-analysis was reported by Jacobs et al[106] and incorporated clinical trials from several nations because of the concern for the effect of low blood cholesterol levels. These trials consisted of vastly different populations, races, customs and geography while adjustments were made for age, blood pressure, smoking, body mass index and alcohol intake "as available". Precisely how these adjustments were made was not explained. A significantly increased risk of noncardiovascular death in both men and women with total cholesterol levels below 160 mg/dL was reported from a variety of causes (cancers, respiratory disease, digestive diseases, trauma and other causes). A positive relationship was found between the serum cholesterol levels and CHD mortality but since FH was not excluded from the trials and some cohort studies consisted almost entirely of such hypercholesterolemic subjects, this result is not unexpected. The high mortality at low blood cholesterol levels was

not attributed to preexisting illness since the conclusion was the same even after excluding deaths within the first five years. In primary prevention trials of cholesterol intervention the increase in noncoronary death rate was similar to the decrease in CHD death rate. However an alleged reduction in CHD mortality in clinical trials cannot be said to be significant without a corresponding reduction in total mortality unless verified by an autopsy study in every death. Otherwise it is as Becker said "analogous to the stewards rearranging the deck chairs on the Titanic".[107]

Interestingly no association was found between high blood cholesterol and cardiovascular deaths in women.[108] This may be due to the greater use of men than women in clinical trials and/or to the later onset of CHD in females with heterozygous FH. The relationship of high rates of cerebral hemorrhage with low blood cholesterol levels is relevant to Japanese mortality rates but these vital statistics have been demonstrated to be invalid.[109,110]

This meta-analysis was praised for its performance by O'Brien[111] but curiously he and Jacobs[106] considered the relationship between low blood cholesterol levels and excess mortality, though unproven, merely in need of further research to explain possible epidemiological confounding. Yet no suggestion of confounding or reconsideration of CHD epidemiological methodology has been suggested despite criticisms and the inclusion of subjects with FH. O'Brien[111] declared that if efforts to increase blood cholesterol levels among persons with very low levels should ever be found beneficial, "there would be no inconsistency in undertaking such effort in this subgroup". Yet the current recommendations are for all subjects to reduce their blood cholesterol levels for the public good and specific recommendations have been made to reduce levels below 180mg/dL and even 150 mg/dL.[112]

Hulley et al[108] concluded their commentary by saying "We need to pull back on national policies directed at identifying and treating high blood cholesterol in the primary prevention setting and put on hold well-meant desires to intervene while we await convincing evidence that the net effects will be beneficial". Whilst these conclusions may stimulate caution, they are not likely in the near future to revoke the worldwide dietary recommendations that have resulted from past policies.

The trials reviewed in the National Heart, Lung and Blood Institute (NHLBI) meta-analysis[106] were extremely different one from another and to consider that there were sufficient similarities to incorporate 19 such trials to obtain more meaningful results than from the individual trials with all their methodological faults defies credibility. It is difficult to imagine how modern day scientists can believe that pooling inconsistent and inconclusive results of multiple trials can provide a more reliable response by statistical manipulation of such mixed data of variable quality, the purpose seems to be to provide the positive answer originally sought whilst ignoring the fundamental flaws in the methodology.

The failure to provide positive support for these clinical trials was recently virtually acknowledged by Castelli[113] from the Framingham Study who speculates that if the cholesterol campaigns are successful, an increase in longevity of three to five years could be expected but few would suffer angina or heart failure. In other words life would be easier and Davies[114] interpreted this as meaning that a happy life was as valuable as the total life span. It is difficult to know how Castelli can justify such a statement as no mention was made of aneurysms, strokes or peripheral vascular disease nor of the fact that atherosclerosis is not the only cause of heart failure. No mention was made of regression of atherosclerosis or of the many thousands of lives that were to be saved because CHD was supposed to be preventable. Oliver[115] too considered that the most significant result of the trials is reduction in nonfatal coronary events leading to an improvement in the quality of life but only for drug trials. This view ignores the diagnostic error for CHD. However Castelli's statement[113] is the first indication of some degree of retraction by lipid protagonists.

RADIOLOGICAL ASSESSMENT OF ATHEROSCLEROSIS

Radiological calcification of the prelumbar aorta has been considered to predict CHD mortality and in men aged 45 years was associated with a six-fold increase in the likelihood of the development of CHD, independent of major "risk factors".[116] Little is known of the factors leading to calcification in atherosclerosis and disturbances of calcium metabolism may enhance mineralization without affecting the severity of the disease. Calcification is a late event and as such is an unsatisfactory method of assessing the severity of atherosclerosis. The technique has not been pursued. The radiological technique predominantly used is angiography, a particularly crude form of assessment with serious limitations for it relies merely on the silhouette of the lumen. It can provide information on deformities of the lumen as indicators of severity and on the time course of their development but does not reveal the nature of the lesion. Changes in silhouettes may indicate gross alterations in caliber and in short-term studies are most likely to be caused by spasm, thromboembolism, thrombolysis, ulceration or repair. It has been estimated that 68% of regression lesions were due to recanalization[117] and likewise Stary[118] concluded that angiographic reduction in lesion size was mostly due to lysis of occlusive mural thrombi. Regression of lesions in FH was attributed to lipid resorption and dissolution of foam cells and held to be analogous to regression of dietary-induced fat lesions in rabbits. Hennerici et al[119] found no evidence of regression in conventional atherosclerosis consisting predominantly of collagen. This was confirmed for carotid atherosclerosis by a specially designed high-resolution ultrasound duplex system.

There are many limitations in the use of angiography, e.g., angiographers' skills, inter- and intraobserver variations,[120] the quality of the angiographic techniques, factors associated with the patient and difficulties in accurately measuring the stenosis. Two directional angiography is better than unidirectional angiograms but minor or major variations in lumen caliber can still be missed depending on the site, whether the stenosis is concentric or eccentric, vascular tone, the phase of the cardiac cycle and vasospasm. With the most accurate mensuration, errors in determining the degree of stenosis are considerable and even worse with subjective naked eye analysis. The cross-sectional area varies with the square of the radius and reduction of a fraction of a millimeter in diameter can mean a reduction in the lumen of from 10-25%. A reduction of 10% is equivalent to a reduction of 19% in the cross-sectional area and 25% reduction in diameter is equivalent to a reduction of 56% in lumen area. Halving the diameter leads to a reduction of 75% in lumen area.[121] In large vessels such as the aorta, a change in dimension of 1mm is much less significant than in arteries of the caliber of coronary or cerebral arteries.

Angiographically the lumen may appear quite cylindrical, whereas considerable eccentric atherosclerotic thickening of the wall may not be appreciated. Angiographers seek irregularities in the silhouette of the lumen either longitudinally or in the diameter and compare "stenosis" with the adjacent lumen which may be ectatic or concentrically narrowed. Qualitative and quantitative changes in the wall cannot be appreciated and even the pathologist at autopsy cannot assess mural fragility and the likelihood of intimal tears or ulceration. Subtle changes in the wall cannot be assessed by any modern technique.

At best modern ultrasound technology has serious limitations in measurements of the lumen, the wall and its constituent parts. Angiographically misclassification of arteries with at least 70% stenosis is about 31% and the greatest error in visual assessments is said to occur with 30-60% narrowing.[86,122] Over and underestimation are frequent with stenoses greater than 60%. Subtle changes in diameter of a fuzzy silhouette can be missed and vasospasm can alter the diameter by at least 15%.

Sensitivity[123] in detecting ulceration is only 59% with ulcers often missed in carotid arteriograms[124] as has been confirmed by angioscopic observations.[125] Even at autopsy superficial erosions are overlooked by macroscopic inspections. Mural thrombi and intimal tears filled with thrombus may not be sufficiently irregular in contour to give a suspicion of their presence. Such assessments cannot compare with careful histological evaluation postmortem, and even this technique has its deficiencies.

Qualitative changes in the wall can occur and little is known of the vagaries and rapidity of progression of atherosclerosis and regression of some complicating ulcers and thrombi in different vascular beds. Angiography cannot provide such data. It remains a crude and unsatisfactory method of assessment of the severity, extent and progression of atherosclerosis. Advanced plaques are not angiographically visible and therefore assessment of the severity of atherosclerosis as distinct from the degree of stenosis is not possible.[126]

Comparison of angiography with postmortem study of arteries reveals that (i) angiography underestimates the degree of stenosis,[127,128] (ii) the lumen shape is difficult to assess angiographically and (iii) changes in the wall and ectasia cannot be determined. Moreover as a colleague said, "Who judges a doughnut by the hole in the middle?"

Angiography has revealed that lesions appear stationary with intermittent periods of progression,[129-132] the most important determinant being the time interval between angiograms, a factor that could affect the results of clinical trials. Alleged regression may be due to resolution of a mural thrombus by lysis or organization, assuming that vasospasm has been excluded and some changes could be secondary to catheter trauma.

Venous bypass grafts are not architecturally designed to withstand arterial hemodynamics and can rapidly undergo mural changes consistent with phlebosclerosis and atherosclerosis. Stenosis at the anastomotic site due to surgical technique, a disadvantageous anastomotic angle and the disparity in caliber can affect the end result. The rapidity of mural changes may be affected by those hemodynamic factors and also by individual variability of mural connective tissues. Experimentally hemodynamic stress has been shown to govern lipid deposition in hypercholesterolemic rabbits[133,134] and the same may apply in the case of venous bypass grafts and coronary arteries of subjects with FH, FDB or type III hyperlipoproteinemia. Cholesterol-lowering drugs may reduce the lipid deposition in such subjects as Stary[118] suggests with secondary enlargement of the lumen. This could be interpreted erroneously as regression of atherosclerosis whereas in reality it is regression of lipid storage. Whether lipid depletion can occur to any significant degree in normolipidemic individuals is unknown and remains to be proven. Gensini and Kelly[135] investigated

1263 subjects by coronary angiography without confirming significant coronary disease in 32% of males and 63% of females. Clinically silent but significant disease was detected in 6% of males and 3% of females investigated for other reasons. Serial cineangiography revealed progression in 78% of patients affected at the initial investigation and 95% of patients with normal coronaries remained free during the period of observation (average of 3 years). Bemis et al[136] found progression in 52% of subjects re-examined 2 to 75 months after initial angiography (average 23.8 months), the progression being independent of the initial state of the vessels.

Kramer et al[137] reported that in 262 patients with 50% or greater narrowing of at least one coronary artery, progression had occurred in 128 when recatheterized 2 to 182 months later, there being no correlation with the usual risk factors including serum cholesterol. The incidence of progression increased with increase in the time interval between studies. In a series of 256 patients progression was reported in 53.6% of patients with coronary atherosclerosis recatheterized within one year, 92% when recatheterized after five years or longer[130] and only 12 (4.7%) revealed evidence of so-called regression. Unstable angina has been found associated more frequently with progression angiographically than has stable angina.[138]

Those investigations by sequential catheterization analyze survivors only thereby underestimating both incidence and degree of progression. Patients with changing symptoms are more likely to be recatheterized and there is a tendency to overestimate the progression.[137] However in most studies significant change in lumen diameter (20 to 25%) is required angiographically before it is considered a change has occurred,[136,137,139] thus excluding from the tally the more subtle changes in lumen diameter. It is often not stated whether the incremental steps (20 to 25%) refer to diameter or cross-sectional area but even so each step indicates a very significant change in the lumen.[121] Only the very optimistic would accept that lesser changes in diameter could be reliably measured. Angiographic stenosis cannot be equated with atheroma.[140] Variation in time between studies drastically alters the incidence of progression and consequently this must be taken into account to avoid bias which can also occur with inappropriate bypass surgery in multicenter trials.[141]

Perhaps the most serious defect in this type of study stems from the need to ensure that the study groups are initially of equal severity since the rate of progression and the likelihood of detection are prone to change with increasing severity of disease. It is important to acknowledge that progression and regression are used in a restricted angiographic sense indicating changes in the silhouettes and also that regression does not necessarily indicate regression of atherosclerosis in the absence of information concerning the nature of the mural changes. It cannot be assumed that changes in the silhouette indicate variations in atherosclerosis itself.

ANGIOGRAPHIC STUDIES AND TRIALS

The NHLBI Type II Coronary Intervention Study[142,143] was double-blind, placebo-controlled and randomized involving 115 male type II hyperlipoproteinemic subjects on a low-fat, low-cholesterol diet. Half were given cholestyramine and others a placebo. After five years 25.4% of the cholestyramine-treated group were said to have definite progression of lesions compared with 35.4% in the placebo-treated group but the differences were not significant. Definite regression was observed in only one of the placebo group and two in the cholestyramine group. No definite conclusion was drawn due to the sample size but when probable changes were included, it was suggested that the results indicated that cholestyramine treatment prevents or retards the rate of progression of atherosclerosis in type II hyperlipoproteinemic males. Since most subjects were probably suffering from heterozygous FH, no such conclusion can legitimately be made regarding atherosclerosis. Even so it is unlikely that subjects can be categorized as showing progression, regression or no change in atherosclerosis, since individual segments of arteries behave differently. The study was extended to examine the relationship of the lipid response and angiographic changes irrespective of the treatment group.[143] The analyses were said to demonstrate an inverse relationship between progression at five years and a combination of an increase in HDL cholesterol and a decrease in LDL cholesterol. No significant relationship with definite or probable progression and LDL cholesterol reduction was found. In view of the crude assessment provided by angiography, no cause and effect relationship between the lipid and the angiographic changes can be claimed. Considering the difficulties inherent in angiographic assessment at two time periods, the small number of subjects in these trials does not substantiate the benefit of plasma lipid reduction in FH and certainly not in atherosclerosis.

In 10 retrospective studies[144] in which coronary angiography was repeated presumably because of increasing symptoms and the severity of the disease, progression was observed in 53% of subjects and regression in 2%. In 8 prospective studies,[144] progression occurred in 50% of patients and regression in approximately 20%. In six prospective angiographic studies of lower limbs,[144] progression was observed in 30% of cases and regression in 20%. It is likely that progression and repair of lesions and resolution of thrombi occur concomitantly in various parts of the arterial tree in the same individual. However in seven of the studies reporting regression, in about 50% of the subjects there was a change from occlusion to subtotal obstruction, suggesting that the change was due to lysis and resolution of occlusive thrombus.

Glueck[145] reviewed angiographic studies of lipid-lowering therapy on coronary atherosclerosis in patients with dyslipoproteinemia. No angiographic change in luminal diameter predominated and regression was either absent or rare. The remaining subjects showed progression of lesions (12-45% of subjects). The lack of adequate design in the trials does not detract from the significance of the results since most studies were aimed at demonstrating regression.

Hombach et al[146] claimed regression of coronary atherosclerosis in 10 patients with FH following specific LDL immunabsorption but extrapolation from FH to atherosclerosis is invalid. The Montreal Heart Institute Study[147] involved 82 subjects 10 years after coronary vein bypass grafting. It was concluded that plasma lipoprotein levels may have influenced the angiographic deterioration of the grafts postoperatively and 92% of those subjects with new lesions had hyperlipoproteinemia. However the study design precludes this investigation from

consideration in atherogenesis. In another study by Lamas et al[148] involving coronary bypass grafting the subjects had an unspecified mixture of internal mammary artery and saphenous vein grafts. This basic design fault precludes this study from consideration but even so subjects who underwent regrafting "tended to be younger, to have higher serum cholesterol levels, fewer previous myocardial infarctions, fewer diseased vessels and less distal disease" than those who underwent one graft operation only. This suggests a bias by inclusion of FH subjects and is also inconsistent with the role of elevated plasma cholesterol in atherogenesis.

In the Cholesterol-Lowering Atherosclerosis Study[149] 162 men (40 to 59 years of age) who had previously undergone coronary venous bypass grafting were randomized into a control group given methocel as a placebo and a group was treated with cholestipol and niacin. Serum cholesterol levels ranged from 185 to 350 mg/dL. After two years each subject was assessed by a crude global appraisal to indicate overall improvement, no change or angiographic worsening of the circulation. Greater subjective improvement was reported in the treated group though there was no difference in cardiovascular events in the two groups and no suggestion that those initially with cholesterol levels in excess of 300 mg/dL derived the greatest benefit from the therapeutic regimen. The incidence of dyslipidemia was not indicated and caution is needed in the use of methocel which parenterally in rabbits induced arterial tears and tissue storage.[150] The value of such short-term experiments on small numbers of patients including subjects with FH, a mixture of variables and the inability to assess accurately the effect on coronary and graft atherosclerosis must be discounted. Such trials mislead the undiscerning practitioner into believing that this sort of therapy is beneficial and as a consequence patients are subjected to long-term drug therapy, the ill-effects of which are unknown.

In the St.Thomas' Atherosclerosis Regression Study (STARS) 74 men under the age of 66 years with previous angina or myocardial infarction were divided into three groups.[151] One group was given their usual diet, and the other two were given special diets either fortified with omega fatty acids and pectin or cholestyramine.

Following repeat angiography at the end of the trial, the mean differences in overall change in diameter of the coronary segments studied were compared one with another, the mean differences being compared in millimeters to the third decimal point. The control group allegedly showed an increase of 0.003 mm and 0.103 mm respectively. In view of the inclusion of FH subjects in the study, the small caliber of the arteries, the fuzzy margin of angiographic silhouettes and the small number of subjects, no conclusion could be reached, and demonstrating alleged mean differences in millimeters to the third decimal point is farcical.

In the Familial Atherosclerosis Treatment Study[152] the results in those subjected to drug-induced reduction of blood cholesterol levels and the controls were almost identical. Kane et al[153] studied the effect of lowering blood cholesterol levels in FH heterozygotes. The control group received dietary advice whilst the experimental group also received various combinations of drugs. The subjects were examined again by angiography after two years and the degree of area stenosis as a mean was estimated to have been reduced in the experimental and treated group and there was a slight increase in stenosis in the controls. Amongst the controls 13 had progression and 4 had regression and in the treated group 13 had regression and 8 had progression. Statistically however the differences between progression and regression in the treated group were not significant. They concluded that reduction could be induced, their estimate being 2% reduction in total cross-sectional area of stenosis of several lesions in two years. Such differences are insignificant and well within the range of error for the overall differences in the width of the silhouettes which would be measured in mμ.

In a randomized controlled clinical trial of lipid-lowering therapy involving 24 dyslipoproteinemic subjects,[154] regression was said to be indicated by a decrease in edge irregularity of demonstrable lesions. The change was found in 33% of segments in subjects on lipid-lowering therapy and in 15% in the control group. The therapy was considered beneficial but the number of subjects benefited was not indicated and the criteria for regression is questionable as change in the edge of lesions could be due to

repair, further intimal proliferation or a change in mural thrombus. Furthermore computerized analysis of the digitized arteriogram demonstrated progression of disease in most segments examined. This finding was at variance with the conclusions reached by the authors.

Whilst benefit from hypocholesterolemic therapy was alleged in these studies, other studies have reported no correlation between the severity of the angiographic changes in coronary arteries or bypass grafts and serum lipid values.[129,130,137,155-158] Bemis et al[136] found that changes in serum cholesterol had no effect on coronary arterial disease on repeat angiography. In a trial of 39 subjects with stable angina exhibiting 50% stenosis of at least one artery,[159] dietary intervention was associated with progression of coronary artery lesions in 53.8% and the remainder were stationary, a result similar to that of untreated subjects (56.3%) reported by Bruschke et al.[130]

Angiography (i) does not depict the atherosclerotic lesions and seriously underestimates the severity and extent of the disease, (ii) often fails to reveal superficial erosions with mural thrombus, (iii) is not sensitive to functional and subtle changes in the vessel wall and (iv) does not reveal old complicated lesions[125] nor identify plaques likely to rupture. Moreover angiographically demonstrable progression and development of new coronary lesions are variable and unpredictable. Therefore the validity of alleged regression is questionable and must be considered with great caution. In view of the serious methodological limitations of these short-term trials on such small numbers of patients, valid assessment of the severity of atherosclerosis in vivo demands considerably improved technology. Newer ultrasonographic techniques are being introduced and used but the mensuration errors are of significance and measurements involving hazy margins of angiograms or ultrasonograms will always be associated with imprecision and error. Thrombosis has similar acoustic properties to flowing blood and so even a total thrombotic occlusion may be missed.[160] Measurements of the lumen diameter, mural thickness or intima-media thickness of restricted segments of arteries, irrespective of accuracy of mensuration, provide data of limited value. No pathologist would make a diagnosis of the changes in the vessel wall, assess the severity of the presumed atherosclerosis or prognosticate on the likely outcome of such pathology. It is doubtful that comparative study of the natural history of angiographic changes with the coronary arteries at autopsy in a very large number of subjects would overcome the weaknesses of the methodology. Even histological study of a restricted segment of artery does not necessarily reflect the pathological changes or the severity of atherosclerosis in other arteries and vascular beds. The results of the present clinical trials involving a mixture of normolipidemic and hyperlipidemic subjects are of no relevance to atherosclerosis or to the lipid dystrophies. The trials on hypercholesterolemic subjects alone have relevance only to those subjects with this affliction but even then they could be improved by assessment of the effects specifically on the vascular pathology of each genotype.

The basic concept of hypocholesterolemic therapy is still based on false and contradictory premises, the concept that reduction of blood cholesterol levels will prevent progression of atherosclerosis or even induce regression of its pathology being but a forlorn and seemingly vain hope. New and powerful drugs can lower the serum cholesterol level profoundly by reducing its synthesis or increasing its excretion but until we are sure of the ideal or optimal plasma cholesterol level for health, interfering with its metabolic pathway is unwise and fraught with considerable potential hazard without sound justification. Reduction in plasma cholesterol may well deplete lipid from vascular storage deposits in FH and other lipid dystrophies as evidence indicates[161] but pure cohorts of these disorders are required and therapy should probably be instituted early in life. However to suggest that it retards, impedes or causes regression of atherosclerosis is unproven conjecture. Efficacy and long-term safety of such lipid depletion from atherosclerotic lesions of normolipidemic subjects are undetermined, and we can be assured that lowering blood cholesterol levels does not reduce mortality as is so often alleged.

LOW SERUM CHOLESTEROL LEVELS

In the Gaussian distribution of plasma cholesterol levels those above or below "statistically normal" values are regarded as possibly indicative of some unusual or unhealthy state requiring investigation. Those with levels above the upper discrimination value often have some lipid dystrophy as indicated earlier but in a few the higher values could be at an individualistic high level without denoting demonstrable disease or a shortened life span. It may also be an indicator of some as yet unknown benefit or even an undetermined disease state. On the other hand low values are known to be associated with several disease states including infections, acquired immune deficiency disease and neoplasia. The plasma cholesterol level is lowest early in life when atherosclerosis commences, but in recent years increasing concern has been expressed about the secondary effects of hypocholesterolemic regimens whether dietary, drug-induced or a combination of the two. In the Los Angeles Veterans Administration Study[162] there were more deaths from cancer in the test group than amongst controls.[163] The possibility is that low cholesterol levels may be due to occult or preclinical cancer but this should be manifested in the control group also. Since that time there has been increasing interest in the subject and several studies have indicated a similar trend.[164] Kagan et al[165] reported that in the Honolulu Heart Program the mortality from cancer was invariably related to blood cholesterol levels. The highest death rate occurred with the highest serum cholesterol levels, the latter no doubt reflecting biased inclusion of FH subjects. Kozarevic et al[166] reported the highest mortality amongst Yugoslav men 35 to 62 years of age, mostly from respiratory disease and cancer was associated with low blood cholesterol levels but the relationship between cancer and low cholesterol levels was not statistically significant. Salmond et al[167] found an inverse relationship between total serum cholesterol levels and total mortality in Maori women and also cancer for both males and females over a 17-year period. Some early deaths may conceivably have been associated with preexisting tumors but the authors considered it unlikely that this accounted for all cases and the association was maintained in women after exclusion of cases dying within the first five years.

The literature on this relationship is inconsistent and Kritchevsky[168] reported an inverse relationship between serum cholesterol and cancer in the National Health and Nutrition Survey Epidemiological Follow-up Study conducted between 1971 and 1984. This supposed relationship is at variance with allegations that diets high in saturated animal fat increase the risk of certain cancers particularly those of the colon and breast and possibly lung. The evidence for such a causative role for animal fat is controversial and by no means proven. The association between cholesterol lowering programs and an increase in the risk of cancer is sufficiently common to warrant close monitoring and restriction of such therapy to those with lipid storage disorders.

The possibility of an excess of deaths from accidental suicides and violence in those on hypocholesterolemic therapy was noted in the LRCCPPT and the Helsinki Heart Study. Review of these trials has shown that many of the suicides and accidental deaths were associated with previous histories of alcoholism and psychiatric disorders after withdrawal of active therapy.[169] In a recent epidemiological study there was also an association between low cholesterol and short-term excess risk of suicide in men.[170] Muldoon et al[171] reviewed six primary prevention trials of serum cholesterol reduction and collated the results. The total mortality from all causes was unaffected although it was alleged that CHD mortality was reduced by cholesterol lowering therapy, but in view of the diagnostic error for CHD this cannot be accepted as valid. No consistent relationship was found with cancer and there was a significant relationship in the deaths from accidents, suicides and violence. The authors suggested that low cholesterol regimens may be associated with changes in cell membrane function effecting neurochemical and behavioral consequences as seen in rats with altered maze learning, thermoregulation and physical activity and increased aggression in monkeys on a diet of low cholesterol and saturated fat content. Their review of epidemiological studies also suggested that low cholesterol levels in humans correlated with criminals, violence and similar behavioral problems.

Hulley et al[108] were quite adamant that the results of the NHLBI meta-analysis[106] clearly indicate an association between low blood cholesterol levels and noncardiovascular deaths from various causes in men and women. The results certainly suggest the need for caution given these facts alone since some subjects may be susceptible to low cholesterol diets. It again reinforces the necessity to restrict such therapy to those with lipid dystrophies.

A recent report of 12 cases of acute rhabdomyolysis during combined treatment with lovastatin and gemfibrozil[172] may be a harbinger of what is yet to come. In four cases there was myoglobinuria and five had acute renal failure. This complication may have been specifically due to the combination of the two drugs concerned or else it may be the consequence of interference with the metabolic activities of cholesterol and LDL. In this respect it could indicate that interference with cholesterol metabolism, its synthesis and utilization may be nonspecific and far-reaching in its general ill-effects. The associated increase of *trans* fatty acids in margarines and shortening due to cholesterol phobia may be deleterious and if membrane fragility is increased, the result may be a substantial increase in matrix vesicle production with augmented lipid accumulation in the intima. A further recent report has indicated that *trans* fatty acids increase the LDL/HDL cholesterol.[173] The increase of fatty acids was estimated from dietary questionnaires in 85,095 women not suffering from CHD, stroke, diabetes or hypercholesterolemia in 1980. In an eight-year follow-up, there were 431 new cases of CHD, and after adjustment for age, and total energy uptake, the intake of *trans* isomers was directly related to the risk of CHD, the risk appearing greatest in those women whose margarine intake had been stable over the past 20 years. Since the study is based on CHD as a surrogate for atherosclerosis and dietary questionnaires are not likely to provide reliable information on the diet over eight years, the findings are not valid even though *trans* fatty acids may be detrimental.

CONCLUSIONS

Randomized blind trials have been regarded as the best evidence contributing to a causal inference because the role of confounders, whether measured or not, is thought to be limited to chance maldistributions that are taken into account in the tests for statistical significance.[108] This however presupposes that (i) the trials are well conducted, (ii) the subjects are a good representation of the population as a whole, (iii) the numbers are sufficiently large, (iv) confounders are not influenced by the program of intervention, (v) the intervention program has a similar affect on the confounders as on the remaining subjects and (vi) the endpoint or parameter measured is the desired endpoint. In the case of atherosclerosis these criteria are not met.

If the benefit of a cholesterol lowering regimen requires elaborate statistical analysis to indicate that a statistically significant difference exists between a treated and a control group and is not due to chance with p values less than 0.05, the value of the therapy cannot be regarded as biologically significant and does not warrant the dietary and lifestyle regulations that lipid protagonists seek to impose on the public at large.

There is no scientific evidence that atherosclerosis can regress nor that intervention can prevent progression of the disease. Nor is there evidence that the various clinical trials increase longevity or reduce the mortality. If the intervention programs do not reduce the overall mortality of a large group of individuals when subjected to a cholesterol reducing program, it cannot be said to have an effect on CHD mortality in the absence of autopsy confirmation of deaths in each group. Autopsy confirmation of diagnostic accuracy is essential in view of the magnitude of the maldiagnostic rate which is consistently ignored in all clinical trials.

The claim that the causal role of blood cholesterol in the production of CHD occurs over the entire range of blood cholesterol levels is inconsistent with the concept of regression of atherosclerosis by cholesterol lowering programs. The recent indication from the NHLBI meta-analysis[106,108] that high blood cholesterol levels have no positive association with CHD in women is a further contradiction of the lipid hypothesis since it follows that lowering blood cholesterol levels in women is futile and cannot therefore cause regression or reduced progression of atherosclerosis. Moreover it provides yet another reason why dietary fat is not a cause of CHD or atherosclerosis because in western cultures men and women eat the same food.

The long-term effects of a low cholesterol and polyunsaturated diet, the effects of pharmacological interference with cholesterol metabolism and the effect of *trans* fatty acid incorporation in cell membranes and other metabolic pathways have yet to be realized. The risk may be considered acceptable by those affected by FH and FDB but on the available pathological and epidemiological evidence for the lipid hypothesis, to recommend that normolipemic subjects should be subjected to a cholesterol-lowering regimen is unwarranted, unscientific and potentially hazardous. Progress in medical science can only result from the pursuit of truth and therefore there is need for exactitude and reliability of data in clinical trials. There has been too much faith in CHD mortality and morbidity rates and angiography and the low quality data provided by CHD epidemiologists in the belief that these can be used to monitor the severity of atherosclerosis. The epidemiological data and the methodology do not bear close scrutiny or critical analysis and this is confounded by the inclusion of subjects with FH. It will not be possible to assess therapy or prevention of atherosclerosis until it is technologically possible to grade the severity of the disease during life. In view of the variable severity of atherosclerosis from vascular bed to vascular bed and since the severity in one vessel is independent of that in other vessels, the task will indeed be difficult. Moreover to conclude from these trials that lowering blood cholesterol levels reduces the morbidity of CHD is false, and misleads the public, the medical fraternity and governments and does a great disservice to medicine and science.

In no way do the clinical trials, flawed from their inception by virtue of their fallacious methodology, confirm the lipid hypothesis of atherogenesis. It is of concern that so many "knowledgeable experts" can continue to allege that these trials support the lipid hypothesis and that lowering blood cholesterol can prevent CHD in the community or actually cause regression of atherosclerosis.

References

1. Hopkins PN, Williams RR. Identification and relative weight of cardiovascular risk factors. Cardiovasc Clin 1986; 4:3-31.
2. Kannel WB. Recent highlights from the Framingham Study. Aust NZ J Med 1976;

6:373-86.

3. Medalie JH, Goldbourt U. Unrecognized myocardial infarction: Five-year incidence, mortality, and risk factors. Ann Int Med 1976; 84:526-31.

4. Rose GA. Ischemic heart disease. Chest pain questionnaire. Milbank Mem Fund Quart 1965; 43:32-9

5. De Backer IG, Kornitzer M, Sobolski J et al. Intermittent claudication—epidemiology and natural history. Acta Cardiol 1979; 34:115-24.

6. Rose G. Standardisation of observers in blood-pressure measurements. Lancet 1965; 1:673-4.

7. Meade TW, Gardner MJ, Cannon P et al. Observer variability in recording the peripheral pulses. Br Heart J 1968; 30:661-5.

8. Ludbrook J. Clarke AM, McKenzie JK. Significance of absent ankle pulse. Br Med J 1962; 1:1724-6.

9. Roberts WC. Fat versus fatigue: Comments on causes of atherosclerosis. Cardiovasc Med 1977: 2:593-5.

10. McGill HC, Stern MP. Sex and atherosclerosis. Atherosclerosis Reviews 1979; 4:157-242.

11. Report of the Inter-Society Commission for Heart Disease Resources. Primary Prevention of the Atherosclerotic Diseases. Circulation 1970; 42:1-44. Revised 1972.

12. Page IH, Stamler J. Diet and coronary heart disease. Mod Concepts Cardiovasc Dis 1968; 37:119-23.

13. Oliver MF. Diet and coronary heart disease. Br Med Bull 1981; 37:49-58.

14. Kannel WB, Castelli WP, Gordon T. Cholesterol in the prediction of atherosclerotic disease. New perspectives based on the Framingham Study. Ann Int Med 1979; 90:85-91.

15. Oliver MF, Boyd GS. The plasma lipids in coronary heart disease. Br Heart J 1953; 15:387-92.

16. The Pooling Research Group. Relationship of blood pressure, serum cholesterol, smoking habit, relative weight and ECG abnormalities to incidence of major coronary events: Final report of the Pooling Project. J Chr Dis 1978; 31:201-306.

17. Levy RI, Feinlab M. Risk factors for coronary artery disease and their management. In: Braunwald E, ed. Heart Disease. Philadelphia: W B Saunders, 1984: 1205-34.

18. Keys A, Fidanze F. Serum cholesterol and relative body weight of coronary patients in different populations. Circulation 1960; 22:1091-106.

19. Mathur KS, Patney NL, Kumar V et al. Serum cholesterol and atherosclerosis in man. Circulation 1961; 23:847-52.

20. Paterson JC, Cornish BR, Armstrong EC. The serum lipids in human atherosclerosis. An interim report. Circulation 1956; 13:224-34.

21. Reed DM, Strong JP, Resch J et al. Serum lipids and lipoproteins as predictors of atherosclerosis. An autopsy study. Arteriosclerosis 1989; 9:560-4.

22. Ravnskov U. An elevated serum cholesterol level is secondary, not causal in coronary heart disease. Med Hypothesis 1991; 6:238-41.

23. Smith RL. Diet, Blood Cholesterol and Coronary Heart Disease: A Critical Review of the Literature. Vol 2. Santa Monica: Vector Enterprises Inc, 1991.

24. Pickering GW. High Blood Pressure. London: J & A Churchill Ltd, 1955.

25. Stamler J. Population studies. In: Levy RI, Rifkind BM, Dennis et al, eds. Nutrition, Lipids, and Coronary Heart Disease. New York: Raven Press, 1979: 25-88.

26. Epstein FH. The epidemiology of coronary heart disease. J Chr Dis 1965; 18:735-74.

27. Dawber TR. The Framingham Study. The Epidemiology of Atherosclerotic Disease. Cambridge: Harvard Univ Press, 1980.

28. Deming QB, Mosbach EH, Bevans M et al. Blood pressure, cholesterol content of serum and tissues, and atherogenesis in the rat. J Exp Med 1958; 107:581.

29. Mann GV, Muñoz JA, Scrimshaw NS. The serum lipoprotein and cholesterol concentration of central and north Americans with different dietary habits. Am J Med 1955; 19:25-32.

30. Hubert HB, Feinlab M, McNamara PM et al. Obesity as an independent risk factor for cardiovascular disease: A 26-year follow-up of participants in the Framingham Heart Study. Circulation 1983; 67:968-77.

31. Schmeider RE, Messerli FH. Obesity hypertension. Med Clin Nth Amer 1987; 71:991-1001.

32. Brunzell JD. Obesity and coronary heart disease. A targeted approach. Arteriosclerosis 1984; 4:180-3.

33. Roberts JC. Epidemiology for Clinicians. Bath: Pitman Medical, 1977. 170-2.

34. Havlik RJ, Feinlab M. Epidemiology and genetics of hypertension. Hypertension 1982; 4 Suppl III:III.121-7.

35. Reaven GM, Hoffman BB. A role for insulin in the etiology and course of hypertension . Lancet 1987; 2:435-7.

36. Lundman T. Smoking in relation to coronary heart disease and lung function in twins. A co-twin control study. Acta Med Scand 1966; Suppl 455:

37. Laurent P, Janoff A, Kagan HM. Cigarette smoke blocks cross-linking of elastin in vitro. Am Review Resp Dis 1983; 127:189-92.

38. Crofton E, Crofton J. Influence of smoking on mortality from various diseases in Scotland and in England and Wales. Br Med J 1963; 2: 1161-4.

39. Jenkins CD. Recent evidence supporting psychological and social risk factors for coronary disease. N Engl J Med 1976; 294:987-94, 1033-8.

40. Friedman M, Rosenman RH. Association of specific overt behavior pattern with blood and cardiovascular findings. JAMA 1959; 169:1286-96.

41. Glass DC. Stress, behavior pattern, and coronary disease. Am Scient 1977; 65:177-87.

42 Stehbens WE. The epidemiological relationship of hypercholesterolemia, hypertension, diabetes mellitus and obesity to coronary heart disease and atherogenesis. J Clin Epidemiol 1990; 43:733-41.

43. Cochran WG. Methodological problems in the study of human populations., Ann NY Acad Sc 1963; 107:476-89.

44. Kannel WB. Status of coronary heart disease risk factors. J Nutr Res 1978; 10:10-4.

45 Stehbens WE. Basic precepts and the lipid hypothesis of atherogenesis. Med Hypotheses 1990; 31:105-13.

46. Meade TW, Chakrabarti R. Arterial-disease research: Observation or intervention. Lancet 1972; 2:913-6.

47 Haines AP. Catching up the Europeans in preventing heart disease. Br Med J 1985; 291:1667-8.

48. Rose G. Sick individuals and sick populations. Int J Epidemiol 1985; 14:32-8.

49. Whyte HM. Potential effect on coronary heart disease morbidity of lowering the blood cholesterol. Lancet 1975; 1:906-10.

50. Walker ARP. Studies bearing on coronary heart disease in South African populations. S A Med J 1973; 47:85-90.

51. Oliver MF. Prevention of coronary heart disease—

propaganda, promises, problems and prospects. Circulation 1986; 73:1-9.

52. Stehbens WE. The controversial role of dietary cholesterol and hypercholesterolemia in coronary heart disease and atherogenesis. Pathology 1989; 21:213-21.

53. Shaper AG, Pocock SJ. British blood cholesterol values and the American consensus. Br Heart J 1985; 291:480-1.

54. Oliver M. Dietary cholesterol, plasma cholesterol and coronary heart disease. Br Heart J 1976; 38:214-8.

55. Editorial. Very early recognition of coronary heart disease, Br Med J 1977; 1:1302.

56. Jenkins CD. Psychologic and social precursors of coronary disease. N Engl J Med 1971; 284:244-55, 307-17.

57. Heller RF, Chinn S, Tunstall Pedoe HD et al. How well can we predict coronary heart disease? Findings in the United Kingdom Heart Disease Prevention Project. Br Med J 1984; 288:1409-11.

58. Oliver MF. Mass or selective control of lipids in the primary prevention of coronary heart disease. In: Carlson LA, Olson AG, eds. Treatment of Hyperlipoproteinemia. New York: Raven Press, 1984: 197-209.

59 Taylor WC, Pass TM, Shepherd DS et al. Cholesterol reduction and life expectancy. Ann Int Med 1987; 166:605-14.

60. Holme I, Enger SC, Helgeland A et al. Risk factors and raised atherosclerotic lesions in coronary and cerebral arteries. Arteriosclerosis 1981; 1:250-6.

61. Kannel WB. The role of cholesterol in coronary atherogenesis. Med Clin Nth Amer 1974; 58:363-79.

62. Marmot MG. Epidemiology and the art of the soluble. Lancet 1986; 1:897-900.

63. Blackburn H. Population strategies of cardiovascular disease prevention: Scientific base, rationale and public health implications. Ann Med 1985; 21:157-62.

64. Jackson R, Beaglehole R. What should be done about hypercholesterolemia. N Z Med J 1988; 101:506-7.

65. Tunstall-Pedoe H. Paunches and the prediction of coronary heart disease. Br Med J 1984; 288:1629-30.

66. Bruhn JG, Wolf S. Studies reporting "low rates" of ischemic heart disease: A critical review. Am

J Publ Health 1970; 60:1477-95.

67. St Clair RW. Atherosclerosis regression in animal models: Current concepts of cellular and biochemical mechanisms. Progr Cardiovasc Dis. 1983; 26:109-32.

68 Daoud AS, Jarmolych J, Angustyn JM et al. Sequential morphologic studies of regression of advanced atherosclerosis. Arch Pathol Lab Med 1981; 105:233-9.

69 Armstrong ML, Warner ED, Connor WE. Regression of coronary atheromatosis in rhesus monkeys. Circ Res 1970; 27:59-67.

70. Ahrens EH, Hirsch J. Insull W et al. The influence of dietary fats on serum-lipid levels in man. Lancet 1957; i:943-53.

71. Nakamura T, Veyama Y, Funahashi T et al. Nonmacrophage-related accumulation of cholesterol during probucol treatment in familial hypercholesterolemia: Report of two cases. Atherosclerosis 1992; 92:193-202.

72. Fishman JA, Ryan GB, Karnovsky MJ. Endothelial regression in the rat carotid artery and the significance of endothelial denudation in the pathogenesis of myointimal thickening. Lab Invest 1975; 32:339.

73. Norman RM, Urich H. Dissecting aneurysm of the middle cerebral artery as a cause of acute infantile hemiplegia. J Pathol Bacteriol 1957; 73:580-2.

74. Haudenschild CC, Chobanian AV. Blood pressure lowering diminishes age-related changes in the rat aortic intima. Hypertension 1984; 6 Suppl 1:I.62-8.

75. Stehbens WE. Cerebral atherosclerosis. Arch Pathol 1975: 99:582-91.

76. Scott RS, Lintott J, Bremer J et al. Hyperlipidemia and the prevention of coronary heart disease. NZ Med J 1987; 100:717-9.

77. Stamler J. Wentworth D, Neaton JD. Is relationship between serum cholesterol and risk of premature death from coronary heart disease continuous and graded? Findings in 356,222 primary screens of the Multiple Risk Factor Intervention Trial (MRFIT). JAMA 1986; 256:2823-8.

78. Kannel WB, Garcia MJ, McNamara PM et al. Serum lipid precursors of coronary heart disease. Human Pathol 1971; 2:129-51.

79. Smith RL. The abuse of logic. Am Clin Lab 1993; March: 28-9.

80. Roussouw JE, Lewis B Rifkind BM. The value of lowering cholesterol after myocardial infarction, N Engl J Med 1990; 323:1112-9.

81. Criqui MH. Cholesterol, primary and secondary prevention, and all-cause mortality. Ann Int Med 1991; 115:973-7.

82. Blackburn H, Gillum RF. Heart disease In: Last JE, ed. Maxcy-Rosenau Public Health ahd Preventive Medicine. 11th Ed. New York: Appleton-Century-Crofts, 1980:1168-201.

83. Werkö L. Risk factors and coronary heart disease-facts of fancy? Am Heart J 1976; 91:87-98.

84. Olson RE. Mass intervention vs screening and selective intervention for the prevention of coronary heart disease. JAMA 1986; 255:2204-7.

85. Ahrens EH. Dietary fats and coronary heart disease: Unfinished business. Lancet 1979; 2:1345-48.

86. Corday E, Corday SR. Arteriosclerosis remains a dilemma. Int J Cardiol 1983; 4:216-20.

87. Lipid Research Clinics Program. The Lipid Research Clinics Coronary Primary Prevention Trial Results. I. Reduction in incidence of coronary heart disease. JAMA 1984; 251:351-64.

88. Lipid Research Clinics Program. The Lipid Research Clinics Coronary Primary Prevention Trial Results. II The relationship of reduction in incidence of coronary heart disease to cholesterol lowering. JAMA 1984; 251:365-74.

89. Levy RI. Changing perspectives in the prevention of coronary artery disease. Am J Cardiol 1986; 57:17G-26G.

90. Editorial. Cholesterol metabolism. Lancet 1972; 1:524-5.

91. Kannel WB. Prevention of coronary heart disease by control of risk factors. JAMA 1974; 227:338.

92. Olson RE. Is there an optimum diet for the prevention of coronary heart disease? In: Levy I, Rifkind BM, Dennis BH et al, eds. Nutrition, Lipids. and Coronary Heart Disease. New York: Raven Press, 1979: 349-64.

93. Editorial. Is reduction of blood cholesterol effective? Lancet 1984; 1:317-8.

94. Kronmal RA. Commentary on the published results of the Lipid Research Clinics Coronary Primary Prevention Trial. JAMA 1985; 253: 2091-3.

95. Pinckney ER, Smith RL. Statistical analysis of Lipid Research Clinics Program. Lancet 1987; 1:503-4.

96. Simons L. The lipid hypothesis is proven. Med J

Aust 1984; 140:316-7.

97. Kolata G. Heart Panel's conclusions questioned. Science 1985; 227:40-41.

98. The Lipid Research Clinics Coronary Primary Prevention Trial. Results of 6 years of post-trial follow-up. Arch Int Med 1992; 152:1399-410.

99. Frick MH, Elo O, Haapa K et al. Helsinki Heart Study: Primary-Prevention Trial with gemfibrozil in middle-aged men with dyslipidemia. N Engl J Med 1987; 317:1237-45.

100. Strandberg TE, Salomaa VV, Naukkarinen VA et al. Long-term mortality after 5-year multifactorial primary prevention of cardiovascular diseases in middle-aged men. JAMA 1991; 266:1225-9.

101. Miettenen TA, Huttunen JK, Naukkarinen VA et al. Multifactorial primary prevention of cardiovascular diseases in middle-aged men. JAMA 1985; 254:2097-102.

102. Wilson A, Leeder S, Isacsson S-O. Health education, health promotion or drugs? Cholesterol and coronary heart disease. Med J Aust 1990; 152:561-3.

103. Cobbe SM, Shepherd J. Cholesterol reduction in the prevention of coronary heart disease: Therapeutic rationale and guidelines. Br Heart J 1993: 69 Suppl:S63-9.

104. Stehbens WE. An Appraisal of the epidemic rise of coronary heart disease and its decline. Lancet 1987; 1:606-11.

105. Holme I. Relation of coronary heart disease incidence and total mortality to plasma cholesterol reduction in randomized trials: Use of meta-analysis. Br Heart J 1993; 69 Suppl:S42-7.

106. Jacobs D, Blackburn H, Higgins M et al. Report of the conference on low blood cholesterol: mortality associations. Circulation 1992; 28:1046-60.

107. Becker MH. The cholesterol saga: Whither health promotion? Ann Int Med 1987; 106:623-6.

108. Hulley SB, Walsh J, Newman TB. Health policy on blood cholesterol. Time to change directions. Circulation 1992; 86:1026-9.

109. Stehbens WE. Pathology of the Cerebral Blood Vessels. St Louis: C V Mosby, 1972.

110. Stehbens WE. Validity of cerebrovascular mortality rates. Angiology 1991; 42:261-7.

111. O'Brien PC. Meta-analysis: Its role in medical research and in assessment of the association between low levels of cholesterol and excess mortality. Mayo Clin Proc 1993; 68:91-3.

112. Roberts WC. Factors linking cholesterol to atherosclerotic plaques. Am J Cardiol 1988; 62:495-9.

113. Castelli WP. The facts and fiction of lowering cholesterol concentrations in the primary prevention of coronary heart disease. Br Heart J 1993; 69 Suppl:S70-3.

114. Davies MJ. Atherosclerosis. Br Heart J 1993; 69 Suppl:S1.

115. Oliver MF. Reducing cholesterol does not reduce mortality. J Am Coll Cardiol 1988; 12:814-7.

116. Witteman JCM, Kok FJ, van Saase JLCM et al. Aortic calcification as a predictor of cardiovascular mortality. Lancet 1986; 2:1120-1.

117. Bruschke AVG, Kramer JR, Bal ET et al. The diagnosis of progression of coronary atherosclerosis studied in 168 medically treated patients who underwent coronary arteriography three times. Am Heart J 1989; 117:296-305.

118. Stary HC. What is the nature of the coronary atherosclerotic lesions that have been shown to regress in experiments with nonhuman primates and by angiography in man? Vasa 1984; 13:298-304.

119. Hennerici M, Rautenberg W, Trockel U et al. Spontaneous regression and regression of small carotid atheroma. Lancet 1985. 1:1415-9.

120. Zir LM, Miller SW, Dinsmore RE et al. Interobserver variability in coronary angiography. Circulation 1976; 53:627-32.

121. Stehbens WE. Reduction of serum cholesterol levels and regression of atherosclerosis. Pathology 1991; 23:45-53.

122. De Rouen TA, Murray JA, Owen W. Variability in the analysis of coronary arteriograms. Circulation 1977; 55:324-328.

123. O'Donnell TF, Erdoes L, Mackey WC et al. Correlation of B-mode ultrasound imaging and arteriography with pathological findings at carotid endarterectomy. Arch Surg 1985; 120:443-9.

124. Mohr JP. Asymptomatic carotid artery disease. Stroke 1982; 13:431-2.

125. Uchida Y, Hasegawa K, Kawamura K et al. Angiographic observations of the coronary luminal changes induced by percutaneous transluminal coronary angioplasty. Am Heart J 1989; 117:769-76.

126. Davies MJ, Woolf N. Atherosclerosis: What is it and why does it occur? Br Heart J 1993; 69

Suppl:S3-11.

127. Blankenhorn DH, Curry PJ. The accuracy of arteriography and ultrasound imaging for atherosclerosis measurement. Arch Pathol Lab Med 1982; 106:483-9.

128. Vlodaver Z, Frech R, van Tassel RA et al. Correlation of the antemortem coronary arteriogram and post mortem specimen. Circulation 1973; 47:162-9.

129. Bruschke AVG, Proudfit WL, Sones FM. Clinical course of patients with normal, and slightly or moderately abnormal coronary arteriograms. A follow-up study on 500 patients. Circulation 1973; 47:936-45.

130. Bruschke AVG, Wijers TS, Koliters W et al. The anatomic evolution of coronary artery disease demonstrated by coronary arteriography in 256 nonoperated patients. Circulation 1981; 63:527-36.

131. Frick MH, Valle M, Harjola P-T. Progression of coronary artery disease in randomized medical and surgical patients over a 5-year angiographic follow-up. Am J Cardiol 1983; 52:681-5.

132. Ambrose JA, Winters SL, Arora RR et al. Angiographic evolution of coronary morphology in unstable angina. Am J Cardiol 1986; 7:472-8.

133. Stehbens WE. Experimental arteriovenous fistulae in normal and cholesterol-fed rabbits. Pathology 1973; 5:311-4.

134. Stehbens WE. Predilection of experimental arterial aneurysms for dietary-induced lipid deposition. Pathology 1981; 13:735-47.

135. Gensini G, Kelly AE. Incidence and progression of coronary artery disease. Arch Int Med 1972; 129:814-27.

136. Bemis CE, Gorlin R, Kemp HG et al. Progression of coronary artery disease. A clinical arteriographic study. Circulation 1973;3; 7:455-64.

137. Kramer JR, Matsuda Y, Mulligan JC et al. Progression of coronary atherosclerosis. Circulation 1981; 63:519-26.

138. Moise A, Théroux P, Taeymans Y et al. Unstable angina and progression of coronary atherosclerosis. N Engl J Med 1983; 309:685-9.

139. Schwartz JN, Kong Y, Hackel DB et al. Comparison of angiographic and postmortem findings in patients with coronary artery disease. Am J Cardiol 1975; 36:174-8.

140. Norris JW, Bornstein NM. Progression and regression of cardiac stenosis. Stroke 1986; 17:755-7.

141. Winslow CM, Kosecoff JB, Chassin M et al. The appropriateness of performing coronary artery pass surgery. JAMA 1988; 260:505-9.

142. Brensike JF, Levy RI, Kelsey SF et al. Effects of therapy with cholestyramine on progression of coronary arteriosclerosis: Results of the NHLBI Type II Coronary Intervention Study. Circulation 1984; 69:313-24.

143. Levy RI, Brensike JF, Epstein SE et al. The influence of changes in lipid values induced by cholestyramine and diet on progression of coronary artery disease: Results of the NHLBI Type II Coronary Intervention Study. Circulation 1984; 69:325-7.

144. Malinow MR. Regression and resolution in atherosclerosis. In: Tulenko TN, Cox RH, eds. Recent Advances in Arterial Diseases: Atherosclerosis, Hypertension, and Vasospasm. New York: Alan Liss, 1986: 31-6.

145. Glueck CJ. Role of risk factor management in progression and regression of coronary and femoral artery atherosclerosis. Am J Cardiol 1986; 57:35G-41G.

146. Hombach V, Borbeng A, Gadzkowski A et al. Regression der Koronarsklerose bei familiärer Hypercholesterinämie IIa durch spezifische LDL-Apherese. Deutsch Med Wochenschr 1986; 111: 1709-15.

147. Campeau L, Enjalbert M, Lesperance J et al. The relation of risk factors to the development of atherosclerosis in saphenous-vein bypass grafts and the progression of disease in the native circulation. A study 10 years after aortocoronary bypass surgery. N Engl J Med 1984; 21:1329-32.

148. Lamas GA, Mudge GH, Collins JJ et al. Clinical response to coronary artery reoperations. Am J Coll Cardiol 1986; 8:274-9.

149. Blankenhorn DH, Nessim SA, Johnson RL et al. Beneficial effects of combined colestipol-niacin therapy on coronary atherosclerosis and coronary venous bypass grafts. JAMA 1987; 257:3233-40.

150. Stehbens WE, Silver MD. Arterial lesions induced by methyl cellulose. Am J Pathol 1965; 48:483-501.

151. Watts GF, Lewis B, Brunt JNH et al. Effects on coronary artery disease of lipid-lowering diet, or diet plus cholestyramine, in the St.Thomas' Atherosclerosis Regression Study (STARS). Lancet 1992; 339:563-9.

152. Gibson CM, Rosner B, Hillger L et al. A comparison of outcomes and sample sizes using lesion and patient-based analysis of coronary regression data: Results of the Familial Atherosclerosis Treatment Study (FATS). J Am Coll Cardiol 1993; 21:71A.

153. Kane JP, Malloy MJ, Ports TA et al. Regression of coronary atherosclerosis during treatment of familial hypercholesterolemia with combined drug regimes. JAMA 1990; 264:3007-12.

154. Duffield RGM, Lewis B, Miller NE et al. Treatment of hyperlipidaemia retards progression of symptomatic femoral atherosclerosis. A randomized controlled study. Lancet 1983; 2:639-42.

155. Fuster V, Frye RL, Connolly DC et al. Arteriographic patterns early in the onset of the coronary syndromes. Br Heart J 1975; 37:1250-5.

156. Kuo PT. Diet-drug treatment of hyperlipidemia in coronary artery disease. A rational and beneficial approach. Chest 1983; 83:165-6.

157. Petch MC. The progression of coronary artery disease. Br Med J 1981; 283:1073-4.

158. Editorial. The progression of atherosclerosis. Lancet 1985; 1:791-3.

159. Arntzenius AC, Kromhout D, Barth JD et al. Diet, lipoproteins, and the progression of atherosclerosis. The Leiden Intervention Trial. N Engl J Med 1985; 312:805-11.

160. Strandness DE. Noninvasive evaluation of arteriosclerosis. Comparison of methods. Arteriosclerosis 1983; 3:103-16.

161. Buchwald H, Moore RB, Rucker RD et al. Clinical angiographic regression of atherosclerosis after ileal bypass. Atherosclerosis 1983; 46:117-28.

162. Dayton S, Pearce ML, Hashimoto MC et al. A controlled clinical trial of diet high in unsaturated fat in preventing complications of atherosclerosis. Circulation 1969; 39 & 40 Suppl II:II-1; II-63.

163. Mann GV. Diet-heart: End of an era. N Engl J Med 1977; 297:644-50.

164. Oliver MF. Might treatment of hypercholesterolemia increase non-cardiac mortality? Lancet 1991; 337:1529-31.

165. Kagan A, McGee DL, Yano K et al. Serum cholesterol and mortality in a Japanese-American population. Am J Epidemiol 1981; 114: 11-20.

166. Kozarevic D, McGee D, Vojvodic N et al. Serum cholesterol and mortality. The Yugoslavia cardiovascular disease study. Am J Epidemiol 1981; 144:21-28.

167. Salmond CE, Beaglehole R, Prior IAM. Are low cholesterol values associated with excess mortality. Br Med J 1985; 290:422-4.

168. Kritchevsky SB. Dietary lipids and the low blood cholesterol-cancer association. Am J Epidemiol 1992; 135:509-20.

169. Wysowski DK, Gross TP. Deaths due to accidents and violence in two recent trials of cholesterol-lowering drugs. Arch Int Med 1990; 150:2169-72.

170. Lindberg G, Råstam L, Gullberg B et al. Low serum cholesterol concentration and short-term mortality from injuries in mane and women. Lancet 1992; 305:277-9.

171. Muldoon MF, Manuck SB, Mathews KA. Lowering cholesterol concentrations and mortality: A quantitative review of primary prevention trials. Br Med J 1990; 301:309-14.

172. Pierce LR, Wysowski DK, Gross TP. Myopathy and rhabdomyolysis associated with Lovastatin-Gemfibrozil combination therapy. JAMA 1990; 264:71-5.

173. Willett WC, Stampfer MJ, Manson JE et al. Intake of *trans* fatty acids and risk of coronary heart disease among women. Lancet 1993; 341:581-5.

CHAPTER 7

EPIDEMIOLOGY, ATHEROGENESIS AND THE FUTURE

The lipid hypothesis currently dominates the field of atherogenesis. Dissidents have been classified as biased or extremists not cognizant of the "strong epidemiological evidence" for links between dietary fat and coronary heart disease (CHD).[1] The truth of this statement, based on the philosophical approach of those who favor a middle of the road course, is not inviolate and depends on logic and the weight of evidence for and against the dietary lipid hypothesis. The voices of dissidents are drowned by the majority and their research grants[2] and publications run the gauntlet of appraisal by lipid protagonists. There is increasing public awareness of the scientific confusion that prevails and genuine worldwide concern the public is being subjected to changes in lifestyle, the chronic effects of which, as yet unknown, are potentially hazardous.[1-8]

Epidemiology, of particular value in acute infectious and occupational diseases, has less applicability to ubiquitous chronic degenerative diseases such as atherosclerosis. The first step in the investigation of atherogenesis should be to become acquainted with the pathology and to appreciate that atherosclerosis is ubiquitous and not species-specific. Unfortunately most investigators are not well acquainted with the modern pathology of the disease. Rather than appraising the basic scientific evidence many have assumed the lipid hypothesis is valid because of the weight of opinion. Pathologists too have had preconceived ideas which led to misappraisal and misrepresentation of the pathology of the cholesterol-fed animal[9,10] and familial hypercholesterolemia (FH)[11,12] on which all the prolipid epidemiological studies rely in vain for biological plausibility. Warnings that the pathology of these conditions differs substantially from spontaneous atherosclerosis were either not heeded or simply ignored.

With the best of intentions many clinical attempts have been made over the years to search for epidemiological factors which might be used to interrupt the chain of events from the initiation of atherosclerosis to the development of clinical and possibly fatal complications of the end-stage disease. Unfortunately no such factor has yet been identified in atherosclerosis analogous to the role of swamps or mosquitoes in malaria or the contamination of the water supply in typhoid epidemics. Some lipid protagonists have mistakenly believed that cholesterol and latterly low density lipoproteins (LDL) fulfill such a role but that is not the case. The empirical approach was unlikely to be successful since atherosclerosis is ubiquitous with a prolonged developmental phase prior to the onset of complications (Fig. 2.2) and because correlations of indirect observations were sought with an unsatisfactory surrogate. It is also unlikely that a universal disease in man which is also widespread in lower animals would be due to an essential circulating metabolite or to environmental factors as postulated by the growing school of CHD epidemiology. The difficulties do not excuse the basic errors in methodology that pervade CHD epidemiology.

When Robert Koch discovered the tubercle bacillus, the general epidemiological view was that tuberculosis was a disease of malnutrition and when Joseph Goldberger began to investigate pellagra in southern USA, the prevailing view, based on epidemiology, was that pellagra was an infectious disease.[13] The discovery of the tubercle bacillus as the cause of tuberculosis was a major scientific advance. The solution was the result of the rigid application of scientific criteria (the Henle-Koch postulates) to exclude secondary or noncausative factors from consideration in causality. Progress in the identification of causes of other important chronic diseases also depends on logic and exactitude in the appraisal of evidence and the use and availability of accurate and reliable data. High scientific standards increase the likelihood of correct interpretations and minimize the effect of time wasting extraneous factors inherent in uncontrolled observations.

FLAWS IN THE EPIDEMIOLOGICAL APPROACH TO CORONARY HEART DISEASE AND ATHEROGENESIS

1. MISUSE OF CAUSE (SEE CHAPTER 3)

At the very crux of the controversy of the lipid hypothesis and the "cholesterol myth" is the misuse of "cause". If statistical methods do not prove causality in acute infectious diseases, they are less likely to indicate it in chronic degenerative diseases. To seek one specific cause may seem unreal in the current climate of multicausal etiologies, as indeed it must have seemed to many before Robert Koch opened

the door to the monocausal concept of infectious diseases which brought in its train such profound benefit to medicine and humanity. The elucidation of atherosclerosis is faced with similar obstacles. Imperfect and inadequate knowledge of atherosclerosis can only be overcome by diligent and accurate observations and the maintenance of high scientific standards and not by the lack of formal logic acknowledged by some epidemiologists or by the "make do" philosophy of the contemporary school of CHD epidemiology.

According to Aristotle[14] language is the instrument of thinking and knowing. In science clear specific meanings must be given to words, otherwise neither critical judgment nor critical thinking is possible. All philosophical con games rely on using words as vague approximations.[15] The misuse of cause personifies the lack of precision of the CHD school of epidemiology whereby an approximation of the definition and lack of specificity are sufficient for its purpose. The meaning of cause has become deliberately altered to falsely inflate the capabilities and potential of the role of epidemiology in medical science. In science "epidemiology" can only indicate possible contenders for the causal role, and following further investigation, each of these must be discarded or classified according to its participation in the pathogenesis of the specific disease. The cause may not be amongst them. Cause and effect must be proven by nonepidemiological means. The use of risk factors interchangeably and synonymously with cause, the denigration of the concept of cause, the assumption of causation[16] and the unconscionable declaration that cause is merely a matter of judgement[17] typify the unscientific epidemiological concept of causality. To leap from statistical association to risk factor to cause on the basis of assumption and personal "judgment" is not worthy of 20th century medicine. Such views are not designed to exclude spurious causes and have actively impeded the determination of the cause of atherosclerosis. This misuse and manipulation of cause besmirches the very fabric of scientific logic and threatens to lead medicine back into the dark ages.[18] The cause must be the sole prerequisite without which the disease cannot occur.

2. INAPPROPRIATE SURROGACY

Atherosclerosis is responsible for the highest mortality in western countries. It is not possible to assess the severity of the disease during life and it is unlikely that agreement could be reached regarding the parameter that should be measured even if it were possible. Reference to Chapter 3 will indicate that the incidence of CHD is quite an inappropriate surrogate for the severity of atherosclerosis. Using CHD incidence in a population study instead of the severity of atherosclerosis contravenes a basic precept in science that the desired parameter and no other should be measured. To suggest that the incidence of CHD, irrespective of the diagnostic error entailed, is a satisfactory monitor of the severity of atherosclerosis is unscientific. It is an abuse of the basic epidemiological model of comparing and contrasting diseased subjects with nondiseased subjects when all have atherosclerosis, the difference between individuals being variation in severity that is never assessed. This makes the identification of possible causal characteristics from population samples impossible.

This fundamental and incontrovertible fallacy cannot be overcome nor allowance made for in epidemiological attempts to find possible causes and is in itself sufficient to invalidate CHD epidemiology. All that can be said is that those with CHD in general have a more severe but undefinable and unpredictable degree of atherosclerosis than the others. The degree of overlap is indeterminate but the difference between the two is in degree not of kind.

The second basic error underlying the use of CHD as a surrogate of atherosclerosis is that CHD is not a specific disease and does not represent CHD due to atherosclerosis alone. It is an imprecise clinical diagnosis signifying myocardial ischemia of whatever cause and is no more specific than terms like dermatitis, peritonitis or subarachnoid hemorrhage. Use of such a general pathological state as CHD is totally at variance with modern day medicine. Clinicians endeavor to determine the cause of subarachnoid hemorrhage or peritonitis and provide therapy directed at the specific cause. To practice medicine contrary to this principle would be regarded as malpractice, yet in CHD epidemiology all cases of CHD are treated as if they are one disease, when they are not.

No metabolic disorder affecting blood vessels should be included in this category whether cases of lipid storage disorders, mucopolysaccharidoses, connective tissue disorders, Menke's kinky hair disease, homocystinuria, progeria or Werner's syndrome. Most of these are rare disorders but the dyslipidemias have led to selection bias.

This inappropriate surrogacy has been perpetuated by special reports from (i) The National Heart, Lung and Blood Institute[19] stating that coronary atherosclerosis "is also termed arteriosclerotic or atherosclerotic heart disease, coronary heart disease, or coronary artery disease" and that "most men and many women over 50 years of age in the United States have moderately advanced coronary atherosclerosis even though they are presymptomatic", and (ii) the Royal Society of New Zealand[20] defining CHD as "a specific disease in which the essential lesion is the deposition of cholesterol and other lipids in the arterial walls associated with abnormalities of lipid metabolism and/or transport". Such erroneous and misleading statements, based on ignorance of the pathology of atherosclerosis and myocardial ischemia, are more in keeping with medicine of a century ago.

Stroke or cerebrovascular disease (CVD) and peripheral vascular disease (PVD) are also nonspecific surrogates of atherosclerosis and more inappropriate than CHD. Each could include secondary lesions not primarily atherosclerotic in nature. CVD, used more frequently than PVD, is a heterogeneous mix of pathological lesions that vary with age and the type of atherosclerotic lesion. Scientific medicine demands that treatment and management of CVD, CHD and PVD depend on the underlying disease responsible for each of these disorders. This is not current practice in CHD epidemiology. Their inclusion provides fallacious, unscientific data. The absence of a satisfactory alternative parameter to the "severity of atherosclerosis" for epidemiological use does not condone use of false surrogates that have no place in scientific medicine. Many clinicians, including cardiologists swept along by the fervor and zealotry of CHD epidemiologists, have relied on consensus opinion and unthinkingly misuse CHD and CVD in like manner.

3. THE CONCEPT OF RISK FACTORS

The concept of risk factor in medicine should be abandoned. Risk implies exposure to some noxious factor but with no certainty of sustained injury of any sort. Yet risk factor is in essence a factor that has a statistical association with CHD and whilst epidemiologists and others acknowledge that statistical associations and parallel graphs do not prove cause and effect, in practice causality is assumed[16] because proof is difficult.

Most of the more than 270 risk factors for CHD can have no biological significance. Their relationship to end-stage disease and possibly to secondary or tertiary complications (Fig. 2.2) rather than the primary complication of an intimal tear, indicates that they may not even be related to atherosclerosis at all and reveals the pseudoscientific approach of CHD epidemiology and the lack of validity in the extrapolations to the etiology of atherosclerosis.

PVD is rarely used as a monitor and stroke and CVD are coming into more frequent use with the diagnostic error even greater although FH is not a confounding factor. In addition to the inappropriate use of the incidence of CHD and CVD as surrogates of the severity of atherosclerosis, the current practice of using the incidence of a risk factor or characteristic being studied rather than the grade and duration of exposure to the risk serves to further reduce the validity and precision of the data sought. It is therefore not surprising that the predictive value of risk factors is of little value even for CHD.

It has been calculated from Framingham data that adults with blood cholesterol levels between 180 to 300 mg/dL could expect to lengthen their lives by a few days to several months at most by adhering to a bland, life long, low cholesterol diet.[21] Jackson and Beaglehole[22] consider that New Zealand could not afford to treat individually the one-third of the population with blood cholesterol levels above 240 mg/dL (the critical level requiring intensive treatment according to US recommendations) and admit "the benefit to most of those treated would be minimal". On these grounds they recommend the entire adult population should change to a low cholesterol/saturated fat diet! Such is the predictive value of the risk, yet it is also acknowledged that the risk of CHD

is present at all blood levels since there is no discrimination level below which it cannot occur. Underlying this "logic" is the school's concept that CHD is a mass disease of western populations all of whom Rose[23] considers to be sick because the average blood cholesterol levels exceed the average of third world countries.

The gross misuse of risk implying an effect on the person and the assumption that CHD risk factors are causes of atherosclerosis are gross misrepresentations of fact. Even worse is the concept of relative risk whereby the ratio of the numerators of two rates provides the relative risk without any reference to the absolute difference. Without reference to the event incidence in the control group, the true clinical significance cannot be appreciated. In the Lipid Research Clinics Trial [24,25] a difference of 1.6 events per 100 between control and treatment groups was reported as a 19% reduction in events and in the gemfibrozil study,[26] a difference of 1.41 events per 100 was reported as 34% reduction in incidence of coronary heart disease[11] but no difference in mortality. This mathematical ploy was used by lipid protagonists because of the appeal of the high percentage value to exaggerate the value of their epidemiological findings.[27,28] It serves to mislead the reader regarding the value of their therapeutic program, to alarm the public, persuade the government health agencies to invest more money in such research and also promulgates the pontifications of this school of CHD epidemiologists. The use of risk factor and risk reduction by the lipid protagonists, unscientific as it is, is evidence that they must fully appreciate that the relationship of blood cholesterol levels to CHD mortality is extremely weak or they would not resort to such creative computations. One questions whether their purpose is first and foremost the promulgation of scientific truth. Given the underlying fallacies and invalid interpretations in the risk factor concept (Fig. 2.2) and its misuse, their concept of risk should be erased from the scientific literature.

4. THE USE OF FALLACIOUS MORTALITY AND MORBIDITY RATES

It is not widely recognized that clinical diagnoses are based on probabilities and the maldiagnostic error for CHD is substantial and unquantifiable in the community. It varies from center to center and even with time in the one institution. There is little doubt that it will also vary with the individual clinician and comparison of death certificates with autopsies from literature surveys reveals that the false positive rate for CHD ranged from 14-76.9% (average 34.2%) and the false negative rate from 20-85.7%.[29] Many countries and institutions have not attempted to monitor the diagnostic accuracy which is even greater for CVD.[30]

Up to 70% of attacks of myocardial ischemia are silent[31] and as many as 20 or 30% of subjects with angina pectoris have normal or near normal coronary angiograms.[32,33] The incidence of silent myocardial infarctions is unknown but it has been suggested that there is a subject with a silent myocardial infarct in the community for every case diagnosed.[34] It is also a fact that epidemiologists who review clinical histories and case notes often do not have the clinical experience or expertise of practicing clinicians. There are many sources of error in clinical diagnosis of CHD[35] and mortality rates or vital statistics are associated with additional sources of error other than in diagnosis[36] and indeed monocausal vital statistics provide additional substantial errors, their extent leading Feinstein[37] to declare that "no knowledgeable clinician or pathologist in the second half of the 20th century believes that single choices of death certificate diagnoses can indicate disease specific causes of death and that those choices can represent the actual occurrence of the specified disease". Then again the incidence of CHD is not the desired parameter and such vital statistics, even when available, provide fallacious data unsuitable for scientific purposes. Clinical studies also entail substantial error and considerable overlap, the correlation of the severity of atherosclerosis with the clinical severity of CHD being poor.[38] Such errors permit substantial but unquantifiable overlap. Adhering to a protocol allegedly to validate diagnoses cannot be accepted as providing other than fallacious data. Neither can it be assumed that positive and negative errors cancel each other out. Proof of this is required rather than an unsubstantiated assumption. CHD epidemiologists rely heavily on national mortality rates and have never taken into account the substantial but variable diagnostic error in any clinical study or clinical trial. It is routinely ignored.

The lack of reliable mortality rates for specific diseases and the inability to assess the severity of atherosclerosis does not condone continued use of fallacious data. A cardinal rule in epidemiology and in science generally should be that if a particular parameter cannot be measured satisfactorily, it is better to refrain from embarking on the project than to use some other unsatisfactory parameter as being the alleged nearest or the only one available. To continue to use vital statistics for analysis of rates in specific diseases and demographic groups, "to speculate uninhibitedly about generic or environmental causes of change in those rates, and to initiate elaborate new epidemiological projects based on the unproved causal speculations are activities that seem as strange in modern medical science as would the methods of alchemy applied to molecular biology".[39] It is worse when the endpoint or parameter is ill-defined and the calibration system inappropriate.

5. DIETARY DATA

In many respects human nutrition is a relatively neglected field, understandably so in view of the difficulty in experimenting with free living persons especially in the long-term, the accurate assessment of dietary intake, heterogeneity of response and the many variables involved in the investigation of individuals and populations.

Diet is largely a socio-culturally determined characteristic and is said to be a central influence on the population distribution of elevated lipids.[40] Many investigators believe the composition of the diet to be the essential factor in the prevalence of hypercholesterolemia, CHD and severe atherosclerosis and consequently make recommendations for change in diet particularly with respect to the intake of cholesterol and saturated fats. Opinions have varied concerning the relative importance of cholesterol, saturated fats, polyunsaturated fats and total fat but the current consensus is that all four dietary factors are involved in atherogenesis, though the mechanisms have not been clearly explained.

Anyone wishing to explore the dietary aspect of the lipid hypothesis of atherogenesis must become cognizant of the methodology used and the quality of data. The evidence ultimately is dependent on the following:

(i) Vital Statistics

These are provided by the World Health Organization (WHO) and are crude inaccurate estimates of the number of deaths in which CHD was given as the primary cause of death in monocausal death certificates. They do not provide scientifically acceptable data on the national incidence of any specific disease at death as explained earlier (Chapter 4). They are not available for many of the undeveloped countries with which comparisons are so often made and the causes of death determined by autopsy are from a nonrepresentative minority of the population. If mortality rates for geographic regions within countries or for cohorts in clinical studies are used, the death certificate and clinical diagnoses are grossly inaccurate and the errors are never taken into account. Comparison with undeveloped countries also provides fallacious statistics because of further differences in the populations other than nutrition and serum cholesterol levels, differences which include genetic, racial, cultural and socioeconomic factors of the people, the mean age and longevity, indigenous diseases, body build, physical activity, and socio-cultural stresses.

(ii) Food Intake

National food production does not equate with the national food intake. These are crude estimates that do not account for spoilage and wastage. Individual intake varies widely and there is no accurate or feasible means of determining the intake of a sizable number of subjects over a protracted period of time. Chemical analysis of equal servings cannot be performed for large numbers of free-living individuals. Compositional dietary data are inaccurate, inadequate and unsuitable for scientific use and even so such diets are not representative of the food intake during the 50 years or more of the quiescent phase of atherogenesis. Neither is the consumption of occasional items that may be beneficial or detrimental allowed for.

The biased focus on fat intake has been emphasized and correlations with the fallacious CHD mortality rates and mean cholesterol values demonstrated with the per capita income,

animal fat intake and also with protein, refined carbohydrates, the use of telephones, motor vehicles, radios and telephones, educational standards and energy consumption all indicate nonspecificity and therefore noncausality.[41] They are merely characteristics of affluent societies and all that is entailed by such categorization, and yet in affluent societies it is alleged paradoxically that CHD is most frequent in the lowest socioeconomic group.[42] To focus merely on the dietary intake of fat, an essential dietary commodity, and to assume causality is scientifically untenable when populations differ in so many more ways. Moreover they respond in different ways. The lack of correspondence in CHD mortality amongst men 45 to 65 years of age in 26 countries over time[43] is only one of many observations that contradicts or casts serious doubt on the importance of lifestyle, risk factors and diet on CHD mortality.

Extremes of fat intake have been accompanied by the same blood cholesterol levels and conversely no difference in nutrient or caloric intake was found when subjects were grouped according to blood cholesterol levels except for carbohydrate intake.[44] Currently we do not know what is the ideal blood cholesterol level. In controlled experiments blood cholesterol levels may be reduced or elevated in the short-term but suggesting that this affects the rate of development of atherosclerosis is speculation and fails to take into account long-term adaptability to the dietary intake of any commodity. In free living subjects it is not possible to specify how the blood cholesterol level will respond. Some individuals may be responders and others nonresponders. It is inappropriate to assume that all humans react in a manner similar to the rabbit or rhesus monkey. Currently it would seem that genetics is the most important determinant of our individual blood cholesterol levels and the effects of consuming eggs, milk and yogurt are inconsistent with the current lipid hypothesis and the dietary recommendations of the lipid protagonists. The higher blood cholesterol levels in developed countries may be the effect of better nutrition, immunity and body growth together with the absence of indigenous diseases rather than being indicative of a sick population as Rose alleged.[23] It is possible that the higher blood cholesterol levels in affluent countries are a biological necessity because of the diverse stresses associated with our active, competitive life styles. Quite apart from the contrary pathological and experimental evidence, the effect of diet on most individuals cannot be of paramount importance since (i) men and women tend to eat the same foods yet the time trends of CHD mortality rates are different for each sex,[43] (ii) it is now admitted that CHD occurs over the full range of cholesterol levels and (iii) atherosclerosis is initiated prior to birth with the development of intimal proliferation at forks, junctions and curvatures and when cholesterol levels are at their lowest. There are many other inconsistencies in the dietary hypothesis.[41,45-47] The manner in which such dietary data have been misrepresented is dealt with in detail by Smith.[28,47]

Lipid protagonists and those who accept their edicts and postulations remain impressed by the differences in vital statistics of populations with which epidemiologists are primarily concerned rather than with individuals within the population. Yet the working group of the National Institutes of Health in 1981 concluded that in epidemiological studies of large national or regional population groups, there was generally (but not invariably) a correlation between dietary cholesterol and both the concentration of serum cholesterol and the morbidity and mortality rates for CHD.[48] However they also added that it had "not been possible to show an unequivocal association between the ingestion of dietary cholesterol and either the concentration of serum cholesterol or the incidence and prevalence of atherosclerotic disease through surveys of individuals within population groups".

A similar statement was expressed by McGill.[49] Few appear to appreciate that continuing to invoke population statistics and ignoring the absence of relationships in individuals is an ecological fallacy, an elementary error in epidemiology. This lack of association in the individual and the current emphasis on population changes in diet, lifestyle and blood cholesterol is a perpetuation of the ecological fallacy.

The corollary of the alleged relationship between dietary saturated fat and cholesterol is the concept that a cholesterol lowering diet should reduce the mortality from CHD. It is apparent (Chapter 6) that there is no scientific evidence of a reduction in mortality or any direct effect on atherogenesis but there has been increased mortality in the intervention groups in some trials. Whilst some allege that there is a reduction in CHD mortality and morbidity this cannot be accepted in view of the methodology, the bias resulting from inclusion of FH, the absence of consideration of the diagnostic error and the lack of autopsies.

In 1976 Oliver[1] said, "Many who study cardiovascular epidemiology, nutrition, or cardiology have neither the will, the wish, nor the time to examine the fabric of the case for and against causal relationships". He added that many advocates of "a significant relation between, for example, dietary fat and coronary heart disease .....endanger their own good case by appearing to be uncritical and to overlook inconvenient facts. Exactly the same is true of those who chose to disregard the links between dietary fat and coronary heart disease." Yet he added "The evidence incriminating dietary cholesterol as a cause of coronary heart disease in developed countries is virtually nonexistent" and there is certainly no evidence of a causal relationship in less well developed countries. Oliver estimated that from the ordinary mixed diet in the U.K. only about 250 mg of cholesterol per day (chiefly from eggs, milk, liver, shellfish and meat) was absorbed into the body pool. In this quantity dietary cholesterol had no measurable effect on plasma cholesterol levels and even in the extremes of cholesterol intake the effect on blood cholesterol is usually transient before a new homeostatic balance is achieved. A high intake is counterbalanced by reduced absorption and variation in blood cholesterol or LDL levels is modulated by changes in neutral cholesterol, excretion, conversion to bile acids and intracellular uptake mediated by regulation of LDL receptors. Overall dietary cholesterol is a minor contributor to blood cholesterol levels.[1] In 1981 Oliver[50] wrote, "raised serum cholesterol is undoubtedly the knave of hearts in many developed and affluent communities, where it interacts with endothelial injury to produce atherosclerosis" and recommended that the public should "eat less saturated fat". In the same year he declared,[51] "There are no sound correlations between diet and CHD within the same community or for individuals". In 1983 in reference to the results of the LRC Trial published the following year he said, "If they are negative or inconclusive, the era of dietary fat modification will pass into history".[52] Although the authors[24] misrepresented the results[27,28] they were not statistically significant. Yet the dietary fat hypothesis continues to linger on with its perpetuation dependent not on logic and scientific evidence but on human credulity.

6. SELECTION OF SUBJECTS ON THE BASIS OF AGE

The valid selection of subjects in "case-control" studies is a problem in epidemiology.[53] Attention has been drawn to the nonrepresentative sampling of subjects in CHD studies including the Framingham Study and the National Pooling Project.[53] The tendency in CHD epidemiology is to restrict studies to middle-aged subjects (usually under 55 years) and therefore most clinical studies and trials have been concerned with a nonrepresentative young age group. Curiously enough women have generally been excluded although this too has not deterred lipid protagonists from extrapolating from their spurious results to the entire population. By virtue of this biased selection of a young age group in which four risk factors (blood cholesterol levels, hypertension, diabetes mellitus, obesity) are on the increase as is the severity of atherosclerosis and the incidence of CHD, their results are skewed towards a desired outcome.[55] Moreover the risk factors also have an unexplained interrelationship one with another and are each genetically dependent. Sophisticated statistics cannot therefore isolate the specific relationship between blood cholesterol levels and the incidence of CHD and certainly cannot suggest a causal relationship with atherosclerosis. The absence of a demonstrable causal relationship in the individual was acknowledged by the Working Group on Arteriosclerosis of the NIH.[48] It is also supported by (i) the lack of correlation between declining blood cholesterol levels in men over the age of 55 years when the CHD mortality is increasing exponentially (Chapter 5), (ii) the absence of predictive power of blood cholesterol levels after the age of 50 years[56,57] when most CHD deaths occur after the age of 60 years and (iii) the absence of a relationship of CHD and

hypercholesterolemia in women reported in a meta-analysis of clinical trials.[7]

The fact that both blood cholesterol levels and CHD mortality in men 32 to 57 years increase with age does not indicate a causal relationship any more than does Yudkin's demonstration of parallel graphs between the sale of radios and televisions and CHD mortality.[58] Assuming there is no causal relationship and providing sufficient subjects are used, it is inevitable that serum cholesterol and CHD mortality would show a graded relationship even if the subjects are divided into quintiles on the basis of age. Yet this is precisely what Stamler et al[59] reported inferring this was a causal relationship rather than each factor being independently both age and genetically dependent. The value of and relevance of their study and conclusions to atherogenesis are thrown further into doubt by (i) the failure to exclude FH and other metabolic disorders and (ii) the failure to include women who, it is stated, exhibit no relationship between CHD and hypercholesterolemia.[7]

This type of fallacious statistics has led to the concept that the relationship between serum cholesterol and CHD is not a threshold one with increased risk confined to the highest quintile, but a continuously graded relationship over virtually the whole range of cholesterol levels. Rather than facing reality and acknowledging the absence of a causal relationship, compensatory rationalization resulted in the abandonment of the conventional discrimination values based on statistical analysis of the normal distribution of biochemical parameters in the community even though originally CHD was linked with subjects with unduly elevated blood cholesterol levels.

It is scientifically untenable that cholesterol, at least 80% of which is synthesized endogenously and more if required and being an essential metabolite of every cell in the body, a precursor of hormones, vitamin D and bile salts, and constituting 17% of the dry weight of the brain can be regarded as noxious at all blood levels. All the available evidence here reviewed confirms the basic physiological importance of cholesterol and denies it is the cause of atherosclerosis.

7. THE BIAS OF FAMILIAL HYPERCHOLESTEROLEMIA (FH)

Berkson[60] demonstrated that the results of clinical studies can be fallacious when (i) the occurrence of the two diseases or disorders in the same person provides an increased probability of admission to a hospital or clinic and (ii) the persons with the disorders under investigation are not represented in the hospital or clinic population in the same proportions as in the general population.[60,61] This further flaw is applicable to CHD studies particularly with lipid dystrophies but the possibility of taking Berkson's bias into account is not usually considered in regard to FH.[61]

It is well recognized that FH is a genetic disorder and that both the homozygous and the heterozygous forms are associated with premature death from CHD but not from other fatal complications of atherosclerosis. There is no doubt that FH constitutes a very distinct clinical entity although until recently it included a small percentage of subjects now classified as familial apolipoprotein B-100 (FDB). The etiology, pathology, pathogenesis and associated manifestations of FH are so vastly different from those of atherosclerosis[11,12] that it is bad medical practice and certainly bad science not to exclude these subjects from clinical studies and clinical trials from which results are applied to the population at large. The bulk of the population does not suffer from a lipid metabolic disorder.

Therapy and management of subjects with FH are directed at lowering serum cholesterol and LDL levels not at the prevention of coronary thrombosis. FH should be excluded from any study of atherosclerosis which is the disease that CHD epidemiologists are primarily concerned with. Even if the vascular lesions of FH were truly atherosclerotic, the premature and rapid development of CHD and the other clinical features are sufficiently distinctive as to warrant their separation for independent study.

Clinical trials of FH subjects alone are warranted but prevention of CHD due to FH can be directed at reducing the serum LDL levels and fat storage or at the genetic defect responsible for the defective or absent LDL receptors. This is certainly not the approach to prevention of atherosclerosis for most of the population

without such a defined genetic disorder of lipid metabolism and treating them under the same cholesterol lowering regimens is bad medicine being potentially hazardous.

The selection of a young nonrepresentative age group for clinical studies and clinical trials has led to an unduly large representation of FH subjects with CHD. Thus inclusion of FH in clinical studies[41] ensures a correlation between serum cholesterol levels and CHD. Furthermore in young and middle aged subjects the unduly high proportion of subjects with FH will suggest that rapidly formed lesions develop in subjects with high or increasing blood serum cholesterol levels. Angiographically progression of lesions has been reported to be more pronounced and widespread in young subjects with lipid dystrophies than in older patients.[62] Moreover in almost all studies alleging a relationship between serum cholesterol levels and atherosclerosis, it is impossible to evaluate the influence of this selection bias for inclusion of FH because nothing but correlation coefficients and p-values were presented.[63] This gives a false impression of the frequency of hypercholesterolemia in subjects with CHD.

CHD epidemiologists extrapolate from clinical trials on male subjects consisting wholly or predominantly of FH sufferers to the whole population but it would be considered malpractice to apply the genetic therapy for FH to all other subjects with CHD. Moreover hyperhomocystinemia has recently been reported[64] in 14% of CHD men under 60 years of age leading to the conclusion that this partly genetically determined disorder may be an important contributor to CHD. By analogy the wise scientist would investigate subjects with hyperhomocystinemia and FH as separate categories and would not incorporate them in studies of CHD subjects without such metabolic disorders. To do other wise is contrary to acknowledged medical practice.

It is difficult to accept that so many trained physicians and scientific personnel have unwittingly overlooked this serious defect in CHD epidemiology and are continuing to ignore the error and to use the data so derived to promulgate their views on the lipid hypothesis and hypercholesterolemia.

The application of molecular genetics to produce lipid storage disorders in blood vessels of transgenic mice may be of value for subjects with lipid metabolic disorders and a propensity for CHD and may assist in elucidating aspects of lipid metabolism. However it offers little promise of assistance for the other 99.8% or 99.5% of the population with atherosclerotic CHD or in elucidating the pathogenesis of vascular fragility and aneurysms in atherosclerosis. Gene therapy may assist in reducing the rapidity of development of true atherosclerosis but first it will be necessary to understand the initial development and underlying mechanisms of atherosclerosis and then to elucidate the means of genetic transmission. In view of the universal susceptibility of blood vessels to atherosclerosis it is most likely that no one genetic defect underlies the etiology of the disease but rather that multiple genetic factors may indirectly aggravate its severity.

8. INTERPRETATION OF STATISTICS AND EPIDEMIOLOGICAL RESULTS

There are two conditions under which statistics are of value. The first requirement is that the data must be accurate. CHD epidemiologists have shown scant concern for the quality and specificity of their data. There must be some limit to the magnitude of error in scientific measurements but in CHD epidemiology the fallacious methodology has ensured the data are lacking in precision and are of such low quality as to endanger the future of epidemiology as a scientific discipline.

Not all are aware of the difficulties in any epidemiological study of such a chronic ubiquitous disease as atherosclerosis but the difficulties should be recognized and taken into account before embarking on over-ambitious projects. If desired parameters are unavailable and unmeasurable, reality must be faced and it would be wiser to investigate the disease by other means. This has not been the attitude taken by CHD epidemiologists. Their zealous desire to measure what is currently unmeasurable (severity of atherosclerosis) has triumphed over logic and scientific exactitude—hence the many methodological errors that have swamped their results.

Avoidance of bias in study groups of atherosclerosis is more difficult than in acute infectious diseases where numerical difference between those that are and those not afflicted hardly requires statistical evaluation. Epidemiological studies are constantly faced with the problem of comparability in all respects of two population samples under investigation. This is seen in studies of bus drivers and postal workers in the UK where confounding factors (constitutional differences) were uncovered[65,66] revealing that men entering sedentary occupations were constitutionally different from those choosing more active occupations. In the Framingham study the subjects willing to participate differed from the general American population in blood pressure, blood cholesterol levels and mortality from cardiovascular disorders[53] suggesting that nonrespondents and those lost to follow-up make the study population nonrepresentative and the results inapplicable to the general population.

Bruhn and Wolf[67] asserted that (i) the design of CHD studies was often poor, (ii) methods of diagnosis of CHD and of dietary assessments often varied and (iii) the criteria for elevated blood pressure or cholesterol levels were not constant. Methods of study varied and basic data regarding prevalence rates, diet, and behavioral characteristics, sometimes of the same population group changed with the author. Being very much indirect, Feinstein[37,39] considers it impossible to control all factors in human populations with their remarkable heterogeneity. When the "outcome event" occurs unequally in both groups there is the possibility of detection bias particularly since the diagnosis of CHD is inexact.[37,39] Moreover epidemiologists have paid inadequate attention to the quality of data in their studies. Qualitative and quantitative errors are often excused in the belief that errors, being in both directions, will compensate one for another. To assume that all errors in mortality rates or other epidemiological data will be uniform time-wise, nationally and geographically is untenable. Sophisticated statistical analyses cannot overcome indeterminate and fluctuating errors or convert bad data into good data.

Riegelman[68] also drew attention to the fallacy of comparing one population with another and drawing conclusions about specific factors (such as CHD mortality and diets) whilst ignoring the multitude of other overriding differences in the populations.

Detection bias in clinical trials can result (i) from variation in the standard of surveillance, diagnostic testing or diagnostic interpretation especially in multicenter trials since it is already known diagnostic fashions can affect national death certification[69] and (ii) when the trial is not truly blind, because the patient often inadvertently provides clues to the investigator.

It is not surprising that such errors in addition to the more significant methodological errors when taken together have provided fallacious, unreliable data, the shortcomings being of such magnitude as to discredit most of the widely accepted evidence for the lipid hypothesis on these grounds alone.

The second and equally important prerequisite is that the interpretation of the results must be valid. Naturally they must be based on knowledge of the source and nature of the data, sound knowledge of the disease and an understanding of the limitations of statistical analysis in respect of biological significance and of the disease itself.

Causality is basic to science and determination of the cause of atherosclerosis has been the highest priority ever since its recognition as a disease. Indirect observational studies used by epidemiologists are of very limited value in chronic diseases such as atherosclerosis. Observational investigations of this sort rarely establish with reasonable certainty that the observed differences are due to predicated variables under investigation and not to extraneous variables.[70] Such studies may provide useful leads but not definitive answers[71] for they never prove cause and effect which requires confirmation by other means. Examples of these were provided by Cochrane et al[72] who studied the relationship of age-specific mortality rates up to the age of 64 years with various health, environmental and dietary factors in 18 developed countries. Positive correlations were found (i) between the prevalence of doctors and pediatricians and mortality up to the age of 44 years, (ii) cigarette smoking and all death rates and (iii) dietary factors other than sugar consumption had consistently positive associations especially protein and total caloric intake. A nega-

tive correlation was found with the gross national product per head except between 5 and 24 years of age. The authors indicated that such studies contained methodological weaknesses, e.g., (i) only Western-type countries were included because of the lack of reliable information from underdeveloped countries, (ii) mortality rates and input variables were averaged across each country without allowance for the heterogeneity within each country, (iii) the validity and causal role of these factors cannot be assumed. The application of statistics indicates the relative probability of an association being due to chance alone and does not indicate biological significance. A statistically significant result will often be given weight disproportionate to its scientific import. Biologically it may be of no consequence. The association may be due to unrecognized mutually related factors, thus stressing the need for verification by substituting evidence of diverse nature. Some associations may appear attractive and be eagerly accepted without corroborative evidence whilst others are dismissed out of hand. This is particularly pertinent to CHD because causality of statistical associations (risk factors) is usually assumed[16] whilst others have acknowledged that determination of cause and effect was a matter of judgement.[17] It is understandable how in such antiscientific environments overzealous operators would accept what was consistent with preconceived ideas and discard unwelcome results. It is not surprising that over 270 risk factors have now been recognized.[73]

Wood[74] indicated that a widespread disease could have positive and negative correlative associations with such factors as rainfall, water, calcium, sugar and fat even if no real relationship exists. He then recorded apparent high positive relationships between per capita consumption of vegetable fat (percentage of all fat, 1961 to 1973) and the number of spells in hospital in England and Wales for several major disease categories for males, including rheumatic fever, hypertension and cardiac disease. Some had a strong negative association and others a zero correlation, thus emphasizing the need for proof of causality.

It is appreciated that epidemiologists are concerned with populations rather than individuals but such ecological studies (as they are so often called) have to be valid for the individuals within that population or the results are worthless. To allege otherwise is an ecological fallacy for it must be remembered that mean values provide limited information and do not necessarily even represent the features of the majority. An ecological fallacy involving the national dietary intake of fat, blood cholesterol levels and the incidence of CHD and severity of atherosclerosis has been perpetuated. A similar error is a common feature of CHD epidemiology. For example differences between group averages may be statistically significant but unless the participants are examined individually the differences may well not be of biological significance nor representative of the majority. There may be no evidence that those allegedly exposed to a causal maneuver were exposed nor evidence that the effect was not present at the commencement of the study. The biased inclusion of FH by virtue of the age group selected can radically modify average cholesterol levels and those with the highest blood cholesterol levels may not have developed CHD or vice versa. More emphasis should be given to individual responses than to group responses. Only when the correlation is true at the individual level are group or national responses valid. Robinson[75] categorically denied any validity in substituting ecological correlations for individual correlations and went so far as to make the ruling that ecological correlations almost invariably produce meaningless results.

There is also danger in extrapolating from the study of a population group directly to the general population without taking into account the frequency of a condition, e.g., FH, in the general population. Likewise it is inappropriate to extrapolate from a study of males only or males with a variable mixture of FH to the entire population when at least half of the population is female and subjects with FH have a genetic defect which in general is not true for 99.8% of the population.

"Heterogeneity of responsiveness to diet and/or drug interventions will be glossed over if data are presented as averages".[76] Making broad recommendations for the general population about reducing cholesterol intake is inappropriate when responders and nonresponders are mixed and a mean result is taken, especially

given the prevailing diagnostic error in determining endpoints.[69] Moreover when statistics are required to demonstrate statistical significance between the results in an intervention group and a control group, the intervention maneuver is more likely to be concerned only as a modifying factor rather than a causal factor. Even quite trivial differences in response can be made statistically significant if sufficiently large numbers are used and automatically regarded as of therapeutic value and used to substantiate the lipid hypothesis and the validity of methods of prevention of CHD or atherosclerosis.

It has become common practice to relate measured parameters to an intermediary variable such as serum cholesterol levels instead of to CHD or to the severity of atherosclerosis. A possible correlation is said to indicate the possibility of the measured parameter being a risk factor, a practice referred to as the substitution game[77] without actually demonstrating a direct cause and effect relationship to CHD or atherosclerosis. Such parameters are then regarded as atherogenic. A further extension of this occurs where an inverse relationship to the blood cholesterol level is considered to be protective or of benefit for CHD or atherosclerosis, e.g, HDL. Such extrapolations, like that of risk factors of CHD to the cause of atherosclerosis are invalid and require direct experimental evidence of the effect assumed.

9. Inconsistencies and Contradictory Evidence

It is a basic rule of logic that the presence of one unexplained inconsistency negates a hypothesis and it is therefore mandatory that investigators review the premise on which the hypothesis is based. It is always advisable to undertake periodic review particularly when there is a lack of progress. Some reliance must be placed on the many inconsistencies in the lipid hypothesis of atherosclerosis that have been acknowledged but lipid protagonists rationalize by invoking a multifactorial etiology, attributing discrepancies to methodological differences and calling for further research.

The most glaring inconsistency is the iatrogenic induction of severe accelerated atherosclerosis in venous bypass grafts and arteriovenous shunts for renal dialysis when the veins if left intact and in situ like other veins elsewhere would show minimal change for the remaining years of life. Their atherosclerosis cannot be caused by an ever present circulating humoral agent be it cholesterol, LDL or any noxious agent. This incontrovertible inconsistency is ignored although by itself it is sufficient to refute the lipid hypothesis. The atherosclerosis so induced must be due to the hemodynamic stresses which the veins are not architecturally designed to withstand. The evidence is further substantiated by the experimental production of atherosclerosis by hemodynamic means [18,46,78] in herbivores on a stock diet.

The search for truth is a professional and moral requirement in scientific investigations and of late scientists have been exhorted to expose bad science.[79] However dissenting criticisms of the deeply ingrained dogma are regarded by the consensus majority as heretical activity[80] and are silenced by rejection of publications and denial of research grants and even exclusion from meetings—academic equivalents of being burnt at the stake.[80] Contradictory evidence is difficult to publish and when accepted can be ignored by the prevailing consensus opinion determined by consensus conferences of selected "authorities".[80] This manipulation of a research field by the "consensus syndrome" has been regarded as inhibiting the normal progress of research activity.[80] There is always security in numbers and as Pickard[81] said, "there will be but few who dare to stir the waters of consensus. Indeed there are few who remain free to do so." This is not a new phenomenon as it is characteristic of human nature that resentment rather than scientific interest is roused when new evidence dictates that long-held beliefs, concepts or dogma are false.

Free, open and detailed debate in a scientific forum of criticisms, contradictory evidence and inconsistencies is essential for progress. Inconsistencies of evidence usually receive only passing attention and negative results are less acceptable to editorial review than those providing positive correlations. How studies with equivocal results fare in editorial processing has not been assessed. Inconsistencies in the pathological and experimental evidence have been discussed in detail but thenceforth ignored. In view of the many methodological flaws it is inevitable that inconsistencies are abundant and associations weak. The most extensive documentation of the epidemiological inconsistencies, statistical manipulations, biased reportings, illogical and contradictory statements and flagrant misrepresentations made by the lipid protagonists have been presented by Smith[28,47] in his extensively referenced writings and in this sense his valuable analyses constitute in themselves a damning indictment of the CHD school of epidemiology.

10. Atherogenesis

It has always been unlikely that the cause of atherosclerosis would be determined by epidemiological or clinical studies because of the slow, insidious and protracted course of this ubiquitous disease and the limitations of the epidemiological approach for such research. To date the epidemiological research effort has been a most expensive venture but its amassed evidence cannot prove cause and affect. Epidemiology always requires pathological and experimental corroborative evidence. Progressively much new pathological data has been acquired over the last 20 years.

11. Corroborative Evidence

Corroborative evidence invoked by epidemiologists consists of three aspects.

(a) Cholesterol and Lipid in the Advanced Atherosclerotic Plaque

The presence of lipid and cholesterol crystals is a common feature in old, degenerate, necrotic lesions, tumors, fibromyomata and old cerebral infarcts. Their presence is no more indicative of cause than calcification, fibrosis or the presence of smooth muscle cells. However it must be emphasized that the lipid hypothesis is basically an explanation for the influx of lipid into the vessel wall in the mistaken belief that the presence of lipid and cholesterol is the hallmark of atherosclerosis. The assumption has always been that once lipid is present the full gamut of changes of atherogenesis and the complications follow in its wake. Yet LDL and cholesterol are needed by the cells of the blood vessel wall and are therefore continuously percolating through the walls. No explanation based on the lipid hypothesis has ever been provided for the intimal tears, ulceration, tortuosity, ectasia and aneurysms nor for the lipid accumulation that occurs in the vesiculogranular debris (matrix vesicles).[46,82] Nor has an adequate explanation been provided for (i) the absence of a minimal change in some veins and arteries, (ii) the disparate severity in various vascular beds or adjacent segments even in the same vessel,[46] (iii) the surgical induction of accelerated atherosclerosis in venous bypass grafts and veins of arteriovenous shunts for renal dialysis or (iv) the experimental production of atherosclerosis in herbivores with low blood cholesterol levels under conditions analogous to those in man.[18,46] No continuously circulating humoral agent can be responsible for such changes and spontaneous development of atherosclerosis in herbivores, omnivores and carnivorous lower animal species argues against the lipid hypothesis.

It is also widely accepted now that the initial lesion of atherosclerosis is fibromusculoelastic intimal thickening, the lipid being a later secondary manifestation. This early lesion seen in the fetus and neonate is more likely to provide clues to the etiology than the end-stage disease which originally inspired the lipid hypothesis. Yet atherosclerosis is initiated and progresses at a stage of life when serum cholesterol levels are lower than levels which have been alleged to cause regression of disease and are said to be capable of preventing CHD.

(b) Familial Hypercholesterolemia

Adequate reasons have been provided for not accepting the vascular lesions of FH as atherosclerotic (Chapter 2). Homozygotes like all other humans suffer from atherosclerosis. Consequently the vascular changes must be mixed lesions and the diagnosis has to be dependent on the overall picture, the pathogenesis of the early lesions, the topography, complications and associated changes, not merely on the advanced lesion with fibrosis. Scars and the end-stages of very destructive diseases can look similar although there are usually accompanying and persistent features or a specific topography that could provide clues as to origins. FH must be regarded as a metabolic storage disease and has characteristic features of metabolic vascular storage disorders (aortic valvular disease and

polyarthritis). Extravascular fat storage and the general absence of complications of atherosclerosis substantiate this view. The pathogenesis of myocardial ischemia in FH differs from that of atherosclerotic CHD. Under the circumstances this disease cannot be used as evidence of the validity of the lipid hypothesis. Any epidemiological study or clinical trial incorporating these subjects in unspecified numbers is invalidated for this reason quite apart from the other methodological flaws.

(c) Cholesterol Overfed Animals

It is unfortunate that so many pathologists went along with the dogma that cholesterol overfeeding of susceptible animals results in atherosclerosis. Many prominent pathologists in the field of atherogenesis have at one time or another acknowledged differences but continued to refer to dietary induced lipid deposition in blood vessels as atherosclerosis, possibly assuming that the differences were due to a species difference and an accelerated rate of development. Such facile assumption can no longer be accepted as explanation for irreconcilable differences between cholesterol-induced lesions and spontaneous atherosclerosis of man. To ignore the differences is to deny the need for scientific exactitude. The vascular lesions closely resemble the early lesions of homozygous FH in humans. Vascular storage disorders in rabbits can be induced by the use of high molecular weight polysaccharides and genetically determined lipid storage disorders similar to FH occur in several lower animal species.

The very fact that some animals require thyroid gland ablation to induce susceptibility to cholesterol overfeeding supports the concept that there are animals, e.g., rabbits, that are naturally susceptible to cholesterol overdosage. Humans do not manifest this high degree of susceptibility. It is important to note however that many vessels, e.g., veins, even in the presence of extreme hypercholesterolemia exhibit limited or no susceptibility at all to lipid accumulation but can be made highly susceptible by subjecting the vessel to hemodynamic stresses.[83,84]

Cholesterol overfeeding of rabbits and other susceptible animals does not reproduce the pathogenesis or complications of atherosclerosis. Ingenious attempts have been made to reproduce its complications but they do not meet the requirements of modified Koch's postulates and therefore cannot be accepted.

12. LACK OF CORROBORATIVE PATHOLOGICAL AND EXPERIMENTAL EVIDENCE

It has to be stressed that epidemiology cannot prove cause and effect. It always requires pathological and experimental substantiation of epidemiological hypotheses and without such corroboration, epidemiological evidence lacks validity. Epidemiologists placed unwarranted faith in the validity of the pathological and especially experimental evidence. Over the years they have totally ignored the frequent warnings in the literature of the pathological differences between the vascular lesions in FH and cholesterol induced hypercholesterolemia. This cannot continue for on these grounds alone the epidemiological evidence remains unsubstantiated.

To invoke clinical trials as evidence in support of the lipid hypothesis is unjustified. Consideration of the methodological flaws, the selection bias for FH, the use of young nonrepresentative minority age groups, the diagnostic error for CHD, the fallacious and inexact nature of angiographic and ultrasonic estimations, and the failure to reduce the overall mortality denies support for any significant effect on CHD and there is no evidence of a beneficial effect on atherosclerosis.

Schwartz et al[85] declared "that human atherosclerotic plaques can regress is no longer in doubt." Others disagree with this assessment. Some day in the future it may be possible to retard progression of atherosclerosis but we have no good evidence for this to date. The space-occupying capacity of lipid accumulation in the wall in atherosclerosis may be reduced but we have no evidence currently that lowering the blood cholesterol level enlarges the lumen or has any beneficial effect on the blood vessel wall. Some amelioration and reduction of lipid storage in the intima of subjects with FH may be possible but again the dangers of reducing blood cholesterol levels in normolipidemic subjects and even in FH subjects are not known. Effects of major reduction of cholesterol levels and side effects of the new powerful cholesterol lowering drugs are still uncertain.

That there are dangers in lowering blood cholesterol levels was becoming appreciated even in early clinical trials and more recently [7,86] was sufficient to suggest a possible moratorium or change in direction until there is more convincing evidence of benefit from the cholesterol-lowering program.[86] There are serious side effects particularly in children in whom failure to thrive and nutritional dwarfism have been reported.[87] The risks of iron and calcium deficiency particularly in women, the increase in orthopedic problems and other possible sequelae from jogging and marathon running, the alleged benefits of which are also based on the same fallacious methodology, have yet to be assessed.

THE ULTIMATE PROOF OF CAUSALITY

In Chapter 2 the basic features of atherosclerosis were presented and it should have become apparent to the reader that hemodynamics or hydraulic factors play an important role.

Important clues to the etiology should always be sought in the earliest demonstrable lesions. From study of serial histological sections of several hundred arterial forks (cerebral and extracranial), the early intimal proliferation with its preceding elastic tissue changes was considered the early lesion of atherosclerosis. The localization is highly suggestive of hydraulic forces being responsible and both the progressive development and extension are consistent with this view. There is progression to overt atherosclerosis in adulthood with no sharp line of lesion demarcation. Similar thickenings occur at vessel junctions and curvatures which are regions of particular hydraulic stress and it is at such sites that atherosclerosis occurs in later life. Ultrastructurally degenerative changes present in the intimal proliferation at forks are but the early stages of those characterizing more advanced atherosclerosis.

Since atherosclerosis is ubiquitous and the intimal proliferations at arterial forks have been found in every lower animal so far examined by serial section technique, special criteria had to be formulated to exclude spurious causes from consideration.[18] In compliance with these criteria it is possible to reproduce atherosclerosis in herbivorous animals under conditions analogous to those occurring in man.

In 1958 I[88] postulated that atherosclerosis constituted the degenerative and reparative processes consequent upon hemodynamically induced engineering fatigue of the blood vessel wall. I contended that the vibrations consisting of the pulsations associated with cardiac contractions and the vortex shedding generated in the blood vessels at branchings, unions, curvatures and fusiform dilatations (carotid sinus) over a lifetime were responsible for the fatigue failure after a certain but individually variable number of vibrations. Shear stresses being pulsatile are vibrations and increased mural tension associated with a large diameter or hypertension accelerates the onset of fatigue. Under these circumstances age is merely a time factor and the vibrational stress is cumulative throughout life although unlike inanimate objects such as metals, airplane wings, timber and rubber etc. living biological tissues undergo repair.

Pursuant to this hypothesis, the experimental production of atherosclerosis follows surgical production of arteriovenous fistulas in sheep and rabbits under conditions analogous to those occurring in humans and the iatrogenic production of atherosclerosis in veins of arteriovenous shunts for renal dialysis.[46] Likewise experimental aneurysms and curvatures were followed by a similar phenomenon, commencing with intimal proliferation analogous to that occurring in humans. As well as proliferative lesions atrophic lesions of atherosclerosis can be reproduced in several hemodynamic models in herbivores on stock diets.[46,78] Complications such as ectasia, aneurysmal dilatation and complete mural atrophy can occur together with intimal tears and mural thrombosis. Moreover intimal proliferation can be induced at experimental arterial forks[89] and curvatures[90] where no intimal proliferation had been present preoperatively as occurs spontaneously in humans. Recently it has been demonstrated in the rabbit that the intimal proliferation of arterial branching sites proximal to an experimental femoral arteriovenous fistula enlarges and progresses to overt atherosclerosis and this extends also up the posterior wall of the abdominal aorta as in man.[78] Such progression has been attributed predominantly to the grossly augmented flow (by a factor exceeding 10 times). The atrophic lesions were attributed primarily to the water hammer ef-

fect of the pulse. Whilst this hemodynamic explanation for the two lesions may require modification, the fact remains that atherosclerosis histologically, ultrastructurally and pathologically similar to human atherosclerosis can be produced without dietary manipulations or the administration of pharmacological or toxic agents in herbivores and the conditions are analogous to those prevailing in man. Such experimental models constitute ultimate proof and (i) provide strong evidence refuting the lipid or cholesterol hypothesis of atherosclerosis, (ii) should replace the cholesterol overfed animal as the preferred experimental model of atherosclerosis and (iii) constitute the ultimate proof of causality for the "wear and tear" or more correctly the hemodynamically induced fatigue hypothesis of atherogenesis.[88]

DOGMA AND THE LIPID HYPOTHESIS

Dogma derives from and thrives on broad and often vague generalizations, misuse of words and imprecise and ambiguous terminology[91] not from scientific facts and reliable data. The massive edifice of epidemiological data is illustrative of this definition of dogma.

The epidemiological approach has been concerned with CHD rather than atherogenesis and as atherosclerotic arteries are never assessed in pathological terms, opinions on their pathology rely on preconceived assumption rather than scientific appraisal. The epidemiological data dominates research in atherogenesis and the lipid hypothesis encompasses the concept that in any one person atherosclerosis is due to a variable mix of risk factors, none of which is necessary. As a consequence the role of any one factor whether dietary fat or serum cholesterol levels can never be proven or disproven. This objection, not in itself reason for discrediting the concept, has been used to discredit criticisms or demonstrated inconsistencies and added to the other faults in the epidemiology of CHD ensures the current lipid hypothesis is unequivocally dogma.

Loose and ambiguous writings of the lipid protagonists are typified by such statements as for example, the evidence is overwhelming that elevation of serum cholesterol levels is strongly associated with or a major cause of CHD.[92] Though this ambiguous statement is true for

FH, it does not follow that all subjects with CHD have elevated blood levels yet this is precisely the basis for the current regression programs. The contention is either an instance of the ambiguity of intelligent dogmatists or merely bad scientific writing which is the outward manifestation of an inward confusion of thought.[93]

Scientific truth is established on the basis of irrefutable evidence and not by faith, fantasy or majority opinion. Medicine must be a precise science. The CHD epidemiological approach by providing fallacious results and conclusions that are unacceptable, has retarded scientific progress. Its rebuttal has not been a matter of refuting or disproving the lipid hypothesis but rather one of demonstrating that the evidence, methodology and logic on which the hypothesis is founded are false.

The current school of CHD epidemiology has not only misrepresented and subverted science but misled and seduced into its ranks many followers who, unwittingly led by the epidemiological halter, unthinkingly and assiduously spread the dogma. A high grade psychologist might one day shed light on the reasons why so many blindly followed along like a fanatical sect.

Undoubted financial, funding, career, publication and political advantages have accrued for the adherents and the lipid school has been aided and abetted by commercial interests and the false representation of atherosclerosis to the public. Uncritical faith in such unscientific work culminated in recommendations to governments and the public for changes in lifestyle and legislation to facilitate and promote such change.[94] Despite admonitions from skeptics and even fence sitters the committed were unprepared to wait for conclusive proof before calling for changes in diet and life styles as life saving measures for western populations.

In 1976 Werkö[53] expressed concern that some physicians and official organizations wished to implement "preventive" measures at that time without awaiting more scientific results even though in 1984 it was considered that no clinical trial up till that time had a satisfactory protocol.[24,25] After reviewing the cholesterol program Corday and Rydén[4] said, "to propose dietary interventions in the entire population is misleading at best and intellectually dishonest at worst". Cholesterol-lowering programs have still not been shown to reduce mortality. Consistently the lipid protagonists have refused to listen or debate. They invoke the consensus views of their own organizations. With a basis of bad science and bad data they have embarked on their anticholesterol campaign inflicting probably the largest and completely uncontrolled and unmonitored experiment ever on the populations of the world.

It is understandable that in an inherited metabolic storage disease such as FH, therapeutic measures should be taken to reduce excessive blood cholesterol levels, but when these same therapeutic measures are used on normolipidemic subjects in the mistaken expectation of relief from atherosclerosis, iatrogenic disorders must be anticipated. Interference with nature often brings unforeseen malign consequences.

Lipid protagonists, convinced of the validity of the lipid hypothesis and under the guise of promoting health, set about their task of indoctrinating the public, to promote establishment of their concept of heart-healthy foods, to influence their availability or to manipulate prices.[95] It was recommended that governments should legislate accordingly and prevent dissidents from interfering in any way with their plans to alter national diets.[94] Despite criticisms of these policies and their data, requests to wait for more conclusive evidence[5] were again ignored. The promotion of the cholesterol campaign has been unrelenting.

"Throughout the centuries the greatest single obstacle to progress has been the uncritical acceptance of dogma"[42] and the "agreement of experts has been a traditional source of all the errors that have been established throughout medical history".[80] Unfortunately erroneous beliefs based on unscientific evidence are habitually perpetuated in the literature. Once established in the literature they acquire what Bean[96] regarded as "the mystical potency of the written word in an age when mere literacy exposes the reader to the hazard of believing whatsoever they read". Nevertheless it would appear that the tide is turning and in due course the lipid hypothesis could be dismantled as swiftly as the Berlin wall.

THE HUMAN DIET

Homo sapiens is essentially omnivorous and individual diets have largely been dependent on geographic, socioeconomic and cultural characteristics. Animal food products have been a basic ingredient in the human diet for millennia and humans in the absence of metabolic diseases generally cope with the ingestion of animal fats far better than rabbits. With more pervasive affluence the consumption of animal food products increased but milk, eggs and meat remain the major source of high quality protein. These commodities in association with fruit and vegetables have been considered the basis of good nutrition, greater body size, immunity and brain development. Poor nutrition on the other hand, seen for the most part in communities with poor access to animal protein, is associated with poor physical and mental development, apathy, susceptibility to infectious diseases and a shortened life span. Fat, consumed in many varieties of food, provides a good source of energy. In general it satiates the appetite better than carbohydrate which traditionally has often been used as a filling agent but few can eat much fat at any one sitting and its consumption tends to be self limiting. Much fat is lost in cooking and often meat and sausages cook in their own fat which adds flavor and moistness. There are anecdotal tales about the need for a high fat diet by the Inuit and Arctic fisherman who, sustaining very adverse climatic conditions, need a high fat intake to cope with hard labor and to maintain health. This observation could provoke an interesting scientific investigation.

The consumption of eggs, milk, cream, butter and cheese has been actively discouraged for some time. Because there has been emphasis on cholesterol and fat in meat, this too has suffered a bad press although some softening of this attitude is becoming apparent and portions of lean meat are now permissible. The acknowledged absence of demonstrable effect of these cholesterol containing foods in the diet on serum cholesterol levels in individuals and the evidence that some have a hypocholesterolemic effect indicate that the current dietary recommendations are based on superstition and an ecological fallacy rather than science. With the implementation of current dietary recommen-

dations of the lipid protagonists across the spectrum of the human population concern must be expressed regarding the adequacy of the diet. Common sense is not proving to be as common as is necessary, e.g., (a) It is usually not possible to reduce the intake of a major dietary constituent such as fat (more specifically animal fat) without provoking secondary effects on the adequacy of intake of animal protein, vitamins, calcium and iron in readily assimilable forms. Low fat milk is a case in point.

(b) The emphasis on carbohydrate in particular may contribute indirectly to an increased incidence of obesity in the community.

(c) The greatest concern must be for the adequacy of protein intake and animal products remain the best and most convenient source. There is already evidence of nutritional deprivation and dwarfism. Children deprived in early life of adequate protein-caloric intake develop hypogammaglobulinemia and even agammaglobulinemia. Immunological deficiency can persist after the institution of adequate nutrition.

(d) The adequacy of iron and calcium intake particularly in women must be a cause for concern and reduction in animal fat and protein could be accompanied by vitamin deficiencies.

(e) The adverse effects of *trans* fatty acids, other commercial modifications and substitute foods and preserving agents are unknown but the evidence is that some may be distinctly "unhealthy".

Food is to be enjoyed and tasty: nutritious food can be a source of immense pleasure. This observation does not condone gluttony and as with all things prudence will avoid a lot of problems. Currently the advice that should be given to the population is to eat a varied diet in moderation, preferably fresh natural foods with a minimum of food additives or preservatives. Animal foods are highly nutritious and can provide considerable variation in gustatory pleasures in contrast with the unpalatable monotony of some currently recommended diets.

Milk, eggs and meat remain the major source of high quality protein and these commodities in association with fruit and vegetables should constitute the basis of what we call good nutrition. Emphasis should be on the ingestion of animal protein, fresh natural foods, an adequate source of vitamins and minerals and variety. These recommendations rely to a large extent on common sense and are made with the realization that additional rations of salt and iodine are needed according to geographical and environmental conditions in the same way that fluid intake should be adequate.

THE CONSEQUENCES AND THE FUTURE

The epidemiology of atherosclerosis has been expressed in terms of the imprecise clinical diagnosis of CHD and there is currently no scientific evidence to indicate that a high fat and cholesterol diet or hyperlipoproteinemia plays a causative role in atherogenesis. There is need for a new epidemiological school to review the existing epidemiological data in the hope that worthwhile data pertaining to the lipid dystrophies can be extracted by review of such data on as many individuals as possible taking into account the inherent errors in mensuration and the limitations of such data and conclusions derived therefrom. This appears to be the only hope of resurrecting something from what has shown itself to be the cholesterol epidemiological debacle.

The lipid hypothesis was a strong stimulus to lipid research and resulted in much new knowledge on lipid, cholesterol metabolism and FH. Additional information is needed on the lipid dystrophies. It would be very unfortunate if this tragic episode in medical research interfered in any way with funding of research in the field of atherogenesis. New directions of research in atherosclerosis are needed rather than an intensification of the study of traditional risk factors. The major emphasis should be directed at the physico-chemistry and metabolism of the constituents of the blood vessel wall and the role of hemodynamics in atherogenesis and the pathogenesis of the complications.

Eagerness to identify causes of diseases that might be readily controlled is understandable. However the hunger for results in atherogenesis has led to lapses in scientific logic, lack of precision in terminology and data, nonstringent criteria of proof and validity, poor pathology, invalid extrapolations, spurious arguments, rationalization, premature conclusions and the sacrifice of truth. Any error or lapse in scientific logic can mislead and result in fallacious

data and the wrong questions being asked and the errors multiplied. As a consequence of bad science, the suggestive association between dietary fat, serum cholesterol and atherosclerosis created the impression that the relationship was truly valid and it ultimately acquired the status as a supporting link in a chain of presumed proof.[77] Epidemiologists were less concerned with the quality of data than devising new statistical techniques[37] which can neither overcome methodological weaknesses nor launder bad data. When the cumulative effect of the methodological errors is taken into account, we have the lipid hypothesis and it is as if the aim was to obfuscate rather than elucidate the etiology of atherosclerosis.

Rather than review long-established and deeply ingrained beliefs and the evidence on which their theory was based, the CHD epidemiologists consistently ignored criticisms, contrary experimental evidence and serious inconsistencies. They adopted the characteristics of the three unwise monkeys that see, hear and expound no doubts, inconsistencies or contrary evidence. Smith's documentation[28,47] of the many inconsistencies, contradictions, and flagrant misrepresentations of their evidential material reveals the lipid protagonists to have rationalized, altered the standard discrimination values for blood cholesterol to suit their data and continued to assiduously disseminate their dogma at the expense of science and now it appears of the general health of many of the public.

Not all are endowed with the same analytical acuity nor infected by that rare trait scepticemia.[97] Most of us are not independent thinkers nor intellectual initiators. But it appears many can readily become inculcated with the antirational thinking that pervades the milieu in which we live and work instead of maintaining a critical, logical and rational approach to our way of life. Many are gratefully reassured by the consensus majority which attracts supporters and deters dissidents. Others believe only what they want to believe, and no doubt abhor evidence particularly if it is contrary to the beliefs on which their research program is based. The consensus opinion is vigorously encouraged and actively enforced.[80]

Other lessons to be learned that can affect the future have been the subject of limited discussion in medical journals and relate to bias and peer review in journals and research funding. These require reconsideration because historically the dissident individuals or minority with heterodox views are vulnerable, the opposition coming not from the so-called ignorant but from educated contemporaries that are professional and chronological but not intellectual peers.

The credibility of the medical profession may be damaged irreparably in the eyes of the trusting public although if it means that medical graduates will be in future more open to and amenable to listen to new ideas and contrary evidence, this sad episode in medicine will not have been in vain though it is claimed history always repeats itself.

CONCLUSION

The basis and evidence for the lipid hypothesis has been reviewed from a broad perspective revealing the poor pathology that so obviously misled early investigators. However misplaced faith in the validity of the pathological and experimental evidence cannot excuse the unscientific methodology on which the epidemiological case has been based. The methodological flaws are mostly indicated as basic errors listed in text books of epidemiology. Errors due to incompetence, lack of logic or ignorance, even though unintentional, are nevertheless scientific misrepresentation. It should be of concern to all that so many have willingly and unquestioningly accepted the fallacious epidemiological methodology and data for so many years and still do so. In the face of the current evidence, lipid protagonists continue to allege success for the cholesterol lowering program and are unwilling to face reality and the possibility that they are wrong.

Some CHD epidemiologists may be unable to critically appraise scientific literature but their continued activity cannot be condoned. Criticisms of the nature and quality of the data used in CHD epidemiology and contrary pathological and experimental evidence have been ignored. This is reprehensible behavior for any professional person especially when they regard themselves as experts in the field representing august scientific bodies allegedly interested in the advancement of science and the public good, a view further substantiated by Smith's evidence.[47] Such persons have demonstrated their unsuitability for membership on any scientific committee. It is to be hoped that the lessons that deserve to be learnt from this sorry state of affairs will be duly acquired.

Progress in atherogenesis depends on compliance with the fundamental requirements of science in maintaining high standards in communication, quality of data, logical and dispassionate analysis, rational scientific debate and valid extrapolations.

As Le Fanu[98] said of the lipid protagonists, "In all their self-righteous admonitions to the public they appear blind to the various consequences of their propaganda, that it misinforms the public about the complexity of disease, trivializes tragedy, blames patients for their illnesses, stigmatizes the dairy industry and degrades medicine as a science-based profession."

This book has related the rise of the lipid hypothesis and its insidious, sedulous propagation. I have attempted to draw together and explain the methodological flaws that have led to this episode in medical science. In truth it must constitute the perpetration of the greatest scientific blunder in medicine of the century and the iatrogenic, nutritional and economic consequences may be more far reaching than can currently be imagined. My hope is that this account will play its part in leading to the deservedly ignominious demise of the lipid hypothesis of atherogenesis and in providing a more profitable direction for future research. In all the years of its preeminence the lipid hypothesis of atherogenesis had a facade of science but no substance.

REFERENCES

1. Oliver M. Dietary cholesterol, plasma cholesterol and coronary heart disease. Br Heart J 1976; 38:214-8.
2. Mann GV. Diet-heart: end of an era. N Engl J Med 1977; 297:644-50.
3. Becker MH. The cholesterol saga: whither health promotion? Ann Int Med 1987; 106:623-6.
4. Corday E, Rydén L. Why some physicians have concerns about the cholesterol awareness program. J Am Coll Cardiol 1989; 13:497-502.
5. Werkö L. The enigma of coronary heart disease and its prevention. Acta Med Scand 1987; 221:323-33.

6. Berger M. The cholesterol nonconsensus. Bibl Nutr Diet (Basel) 1992; 49:125-30.

7. Hulley SB, Walsh JMR, Newman TB. Health policy on blood cholesterol. Time to change directions. Circulation 1992; 86:1026-9.

8. McCormick J, Skrabanek P. Coronary heart disease is not preventable by population interventions. Lancet 1988; 2:839-41.

9. Stehbens WE. An appraisal of cholesterol-feeding in experimental atherogenesis. Progr Cardiovasc Dis 1986; 29:107-28.

10. Stehbens WE. Vascular complications in experimental atherosclerosis. Progr Cardiovasc Dis 1986; 29:221-37.

11. Stehbens WE, Wierzbicki E. The relationship of hypercholesterolemia to atherosclerosis with particular emphasis on familial hypercholesterolemia, diabetes mellitus, obstructive jaundice, myxedema and the nephrotic syndrome. Progr Cardiovasc Dis 1988; 30:289-306.

12. Stehbens WE, Martin M. The vascular pathology of familial hypercholesterolemia. Pathology 1991; 23:54-61.

13. Olson RE. Is there an optimum diet for the prevention of coronary heart disease? In: Levy RI, Rifkind BM, Dennis BH et al, eds. Nutrition, Lipids, and Coronary Heart Disease. New York: Raven Press, 1979: 349-64.

14. Randall JH. Aristotle. New York: Columbia Univ Press, 1960.

15. Rand A. Philosophy: Who Needs It? Indianapolis: Bobbs-Merrill Co, 1982.

16. Epstein FH. The epidemiology of coronary heart disease. A review. J Chr Dis 1965; 118:735-74.

17. Beaglehole R. Does passive smoking cause heart disease? Br Med J 1990: 301:1343-4.

18. Stehbens WE. Causality in medical science with particular reference to coronary heart disease and atherosclerosis. Perspect Biol Med 1992;36:97-119.

19. National Heart, Lung and Blood Institute. Arteriosclerosis. The Report of the 1977 Working Group to Review the 1971 Report by the National Heart and Lung Institute Task Force on Arteriosclerosis. Washington: DHEW Publication No (NIH) 78-1526, 1977.

20. Report of the Committee of the Royal Society of New Zealand. Coronary Heart Disease. Wellington: David Jones Ltd, 1971.

21. Taylor WC, Pass PM, Shepherd DS et al. Cholesterol reduction and life expectancy. Ann Int Med 1987; 106:605-14.

22. Jackson R, Beaglehole R. What should be done about hypercholesterolaemia. NZ Med J 1988; 101:506-7.

23. Rose G. Sick individuals and sick populations. Int J Epidemiol 1985; 14:32-8.

24. Lipid Research Clinics Program. Lipid Research Clinics Coronary Primary Prevention Trial Results. I. Reduction in incidence of coronary heart disease. JAMA 1984; 251:351-64.

25. Lipid Research Clinics Program. The Lipid Research Clinics Coronary Primary Prevention Trial Results. II. The relationships of reduction in incidence of coronary heart disease to cholesterol lowering. JAMA 1984; 251:365-74.

26. Frick MH, Elo O, Haapoa K et al. Helsinki Heart Study: Primary-prevention trial with gemfibrozil in middle-aged men with dyslipidemia. N Engl J Med 1987; 317:1237-45.

27. Weissler AM, Miller BI, Boudoulas H. The need for clarification of percent risk reduction data in clinical cardiovascular trial reports. J Am Coll Cardiol 1989; 13:764-

28. Smith RL, Pinckney ER. The Cholesterol Conspiracy. St Louis: Warren H Green Inc, 1991.

29. Stehbens WE. The cholesterol-heart controversy. Asean Food J 1990; 5:131-42.

30. Stehbens WE. Validity of cerebrovascular mortality rates. Angiology 1991; 42:261-7.

31. Maseri A, Chierchia S, Davies G et al. Mechanisms of ischemic cardiac pain and silent myocardial ischemia. Am J Med 1985; 79 Suppl 3A:7-11.

32. Gazes PC. Angina pectoris: Classification and diagnosis. Part 2. Mod Concepts of Cardiovasc Dis 1988; 57:25-7.

33. Mukerji V, Alpert MA, Newett JE et al. Can patients with chest pain and normal coronary arteries be discriminated from those with coronary artery disease prior to coronary angiography? Angiology 1989; 40:276-82.

34. Editorial. Unrecognized myocardial infarction. Lancet 1976; 2:449-50.

35. Stehbens WE. Imprecision of the clinical diagnosis of coronary heart disease in epidemiological studies and atherogenesis. J Clin Epidemiol 1991; 44:999-1006.

36. Stehbens WE. Review of the validity of national coronary heart disease mortality rates. Angiology 1990; 41:85-94.

37. Feinstein AR. Clinical Epidemiology. The Ar-

chitecture of Clinical Research. Philadelphia: WB Saunders, 1985.

38. Buja LM, Willerson JT. The role of coronary artery lesions in ischemic heart disease: Insights from recent clinicopathologic, coronary arteriographic and experimental studies. Human Pathol 1987; 18:451-61.

39. Feinstein AR. Clinical epidemiology. II. The identification rates of disease. Ann Int Med 1968; 69:1037-61.

40. Blackburn H, Gillum RF. Heart disease. In: Last JM, ed. Maxcy-Rosenau Public Health and Preventive Medicine. 11th Ed. New York: Appleton-Century-Crofts, 1980: 1168-201.

41. Stehbens WE. The controversial role of dietary cholesterol and hypercholesterolemia in coronary heart disease and atherogenesis. Pathology 1989; 21:213-21.

42. Gorringe JAL. A fresh look at what everybody knows about ischaemic heart disease: Discussion paper. J Roy Soc Med 1984; 77:390-8.

43. Thom TJ, Epstein FH, Feldman JJ et al. Trends in total mortality and morbidity from heart disease in 26 countries from 1950 to 1978. Int J Epidemiol 1985; 14:510-20.

44. Browe JH, Morlley DM, Logrillo VM et al. Diet and heart disease in the cardiovascular health center. J Am Diet Assoc 1967; 50:376-84.

45. Stehbens WE. Diet and atherogenesis. Nutr Rev 1989; 47:1-12.

46. Stehbens WE. The lipid hypothesis and the role of hemodynamics in atherogenesis. Progr Cardiovasc Dis 1990; 33:119-36.

47. Smith RL. Diet, Blood Cholesterol and Coronary Heart Disease: A Critical Review of the Literature. Vol 2. Santa Monica: Vector Enterprises Inc, 1991.

48. Report of the Working Group on Arteriosclerosis of the National Heart, Lung and Blood Institute. Arteriosclerosis. Vol 2. U.S. Dept Health & Human Service, NIH, 1981.

49. McGill H. The relationship of dietary cholesterol to serum cholesterol concentration and to atherosclerosis in man. Am J Clin Nutr 1979; 32:2664-702.

50. Oliver MF. Serum cholesterol—the knave of hearts and the joker. Lancet 1981; 2:1090-5.

51. Oliver MF. Diet and coronary heart disease. Br Med Bull 1981; 37:49-58.

52. Oliver MF. Should we not forget about mass control of coronary risk factors. Lancet 1983; 2:37-8.

53. Werkö L. Risk factors and coronary heart disease—facts or fancy? Am Heart J 1976; 91:87-97.

54. Miettinen OS. The "case-control" study: Valid selection of subjects. J Chr Dis 1985; 38: 543-48.

55. Stehbens WE. The epidemiological relationship of hypercholesterolemia, hypertension, diabetes mellitus and obesity to coronary heart disease and atherogenesis. J Clin Epidemiol 1990; 43:733-41.

56. Gordon T, Castelli WP, Hjortland MC et al. Predicting coronary heart disease in middle-aged and older persons. The Framingham Study. JAMA 1977; 238:497-9.

57. Anderson KM, Castelli WP, Levy D. Cholesterol and mortality. 30 years of follow-up from the Framingham Study. JAMA 1987; 257:2176-80.

58. Yudkin J. Diet and coronary thrombosis. Hypothesis and fact. Lancet 1957; 2:155-62.

59. Stamler J, Wentworth D, Neaton JD. Is relationship between serum cholesterol and risk of premature death from coronary heart disease continuous and graded? Findings in 356,222 primary screens of the Multiple Risk Factor Intervention Trial (MRFIT). JAMA 1986; 256:2823-8.

60. Berkson J. Limitations of the application of four-fold table analysis to hospital data. Biometrics Bull 1946; 2:47-53.

61. Mainland D. The risk of fallacious conclusions from autopsy data on the incidence of diseases with applications to heart disease. Am Heart J 1953; 45:644-54.

62. Bemis CE, Gorlin R, Kemp HG et al. Progression of coronary artery disease. A clinical arteriographic study. Circulation 1973; 47: 455-64.

63. Ravnskov U. An elevated serum cholesterol level is secondary, not causal in coronary heart disease. Med Hypotheses 1991; 36:238-41.

64. Genest JJ, McNamara JR, Upson B et al. Prevalence of familial hyperhomocyst(e)inemia in men with premature coronary artery disease. Arteriosclerosis Thromb 1991; 11:1129-36.

65. Oliver RM. Constitutional differences between men recruited for driving and non-driving occupations. Br J Indust Med 1969; 26:289-93.

66. Morris JN, Heady JM, Raffle PAB. Physique of London busmen. Epidemiology of uniforms. Lancet 1956; 2:569-70.

67. Bruhn JG, Wolf S. Studies reporting "low rates"

of ischemic heart disease: A critical review. Am J Publ Health 1970; 60:1477-95.

68. Riegelman R. Contributory cause: Unnecessary and insufficient. Postgrad Med 1979; 66: 177-79.

69. Stehbens WE. An appraisal of the epidemic rise of coronary heart disease and its decline. Lancet 1987; 1:606-11.

70. Lew EA. Biostatistical pitfalls in studies of atherosclerotic heart disease. Fed Proc 1962; 21 Suppl 11:62-70.

71. Yerushalmy J, Hilleboe HE. Fat in the diet and mortality from heart disease. New York State Med J 1957; 57:2343-53.

72. Cochrane AL, St Leger AS, Moore F. Health service "input" and mortality "output" in developed countries. J Epidemiol Comm Health 1978; 32:200-5.

73. Hopkins PN, Williams RR. Identification and relative weight of cardiovascular risk factors. Cardiol Clinics 1986;4:3-31.

74. Wood PDP. A statistical look at the main evidence considered in the diet/heart controversy. In: Fats on Trial. Tunbridge Wells: Butter Information Council, 1980:38-43.

75. Robinson WS. Ecological correlations and the behavior of individuals. Amer Sociol Rev 1950; 15:351-7.

76. Ahrens EH. The diet-heart question in 1985: Has it really been settled? Lancet 1985; 1: 1085-7.

77. Yerushalmy J, Palmer CE. On the methodology of investigations of etiologic factors in chronic diseases. J Chr Dis 1959; 10:27-40.

78. Stehbens WE. Experimental induction of atherosclerosis associated with femoral arteriovenous fistulae in rabbits on a cholesterol-free diet. Atherosclerosis 1992; 95:127-35.

79. Comar C. Bad science and social penalties. Science 1978; 200:1225.

80. Feinstein AR. Fraud, distortion, delusion and consensus: The problems of human and natural deception in epidemiologic science. Am J Med 1988; 84:475-8.

81. Pickard B. Dairy products and red meat—villains or victims? In: Anderson D, ed. A Diet of Reason. London: Esmonde Pub Ltd, 1986: 21-39.

82. Stehbens WE. The role of lipid in the pathogenesis of atherosclerosis. Lancet 1975; 1:724-7.

83. Stehbens WE. Experimental arteriovenous fistulae in normal and cholesterol-fed rabbits. Pathology 1973; 5:311-24.

84. Stehbens WE. Predilection of experimental arterial aneurysms for dietary-induced lipid deposition. Pathology 1981; 13:735-47.

85. Schwartz CJ, Valente AJ, Sprague EA et al. Atherosclerosis. Potential targets for stabilization and regression. Circulation 1992; 86 Suppl III:III-117-23.

86. Strandberg TE, Salomaa VV, Naukkarinen VA et al. Long-term mortality after 5-year multifactorial primary prevention of cardiovascular diseases in middle-aged men. JAMA 1991; 266:1225-9.

87. Lifshitz F, Moses N. Growth failure. A complication of dietary treatment of hypercholesterolemia. Am J Dis Child 1989; 143:537-42.

88. Stehbens WE. Intracranial Arterial Aneurysms and Atherosclerosis, Univ Sydney: Thesis, 1958.

89. Stehbens WE, Martin BJ, Delahunt B. Light and scanning electron microscopic changes observed in experimental arterial forks in rabbits. Int J Exp Pathol 1991; 72:183-93.

90. Stehbens WE. Experimental arterial loops and arterial atrophy. Exp Mol Path 1986; 44:177-89.

91. Altschule MD. Dogmas in medicine. Med Science (Phil) 1963; 13:837-44.

92. Gotto AM, La Rosa JC, Hunninghake D et al. The Cholesterol Facts. A Joint statement by the American Heart Association and The National Heart, Lung, and Blood Institute. Circulation 1990; 81:1721-33.

93. Woodford FP. Sounder thinking through clearer writing. Science 1967; 156:743-5.

94. Report of a WHO Expert Committee. Prevention of coronary heart disease. Technical Report Series 678. Geneva: World Health Organization, 1982.

95. Peto R. Screening in adults. Discussion. The Value of Preventive Medicine. Ciba Foundation Symposium 110. London: Pitman, 1985: 82-3.

96. Bean WB. Vascular Spiders and Related Lesions of the Skin. Springfield: CC Thomas, 1958.

97. Skrabanek P, McCormick J. Follies and Fallacies in Medicine. Buffalo: Prometheus Books, 1989.

98. Le Fanu J. Diet and disease: Nonsense and nonscience. In: Anderson D, ed. A Diet of Reason. Sense and Nonsense in the Healthy Eating Debate. Exeter: Esmonde Publishing Ltd, 1986: 109-24.

INDEX

Items in italics denote figures (f) and tables (t).

A

Abramson JH, 66, 80

Accidental deaths, of patients receiving hypocholesterolemic therapy, 155

Acheson RM, 72

Affluence
age and, serum cholesterol levels and, *110f*, 110-111
better nutrition and, 101
cholesterol and, 116
coronary heart disease incidence and, 107

African tribes, serum cholesterol levels in, 100, 101

Age
as risk factor for coronary heart disease, 137, 139-140
serum cholesterol levels and, *110f*, 110-111

Age dependence
coronary heart disease and, 139-140
in epidemiological approach, 170

Ahrens EH, 106

Analogy, as criteria of causality, 57

Anderson JT, 106

Angina pectoris
in coronary heart disease, 69-70
lipid profile in, 112
myxedema associated with, 35

Angiography
atherosclerosis assessment by, 151-154
limitations of, 149-150, 153-154
versus post mortem studies, 150
retrospective studies, 152

Animal fats, role in atherogenesis, 107

Animals, experimental. See Experimental animals

Anitschkow N, 97

Anitschkow NN, 4, 26, 27

Aortic valve stenosis, incidence in familial hypercholesterolemia, 33

Apolipoprotein E, 120

Apolipoproteins
apo E, 120
characteristics of, 102, *103t*
synthesis of, 102

Arachidonic acid, 123

Aristotle, 53, 164

Armstrong ML, 143

Armstrong VW, 119

Aro A, 111

Arterial calcification, 92

Arterial forks
effect of high fat diet on, 116
intimal proliferation at, 20-21
pseudoaneurysmal changes, 23

Arterial wall, matrix vesicle population in, 104-105

Asnaes S, 67

Assman G, 40

Association, statistical. See Statistical association

Atheroma, 2

Atherosclerosis
angiographic studies and trials, 151-154
aortic morphology in, 12-15, *13f-16f*, 17, *17f*
complications arising from, 17-20, *18f-20f*
deaths from, 1
described, 1
in diabetics, 34-35
versus dietary-induced lipid deposition in animals, 42
experimental studies, 34
and familial hypercholesterolemia lesions, 41
genetics of, 125
investigative steps into, 164
lipid accumulation in, 104
lipid hypothesis of, 2, 41-42
multicausal approach to, 55-56
nature of, 10, *11f*
pathology of, 10-11, *11f*
radiological assessment of, 149-151
regression of
in clinical trials, 144-149
lowering of blood cholesterol and, 145
serum cholesterol levels and, 114-116
topographical distribution of, 11-12
ultrastructure of, *21f*, 21-23, *22f*

Atherosclerotic plaques
advanced, cholesterol and lipid in, 175-176
lipoprotein (a) in, 118

Atrophic lesion, at arterial forks, 23

Autopsies
death certificates and, 75-76
diagnostic errors at, 64
circulatory disease, 80